Freestanding Birth Centers

Linda J. Cole, DNP, CNM, received her bachelor of science in nursing at the University of Colorado in 1985, her master of science in nursing at the Medical University of South Carolina in 1994, and her doctorate in nursing practice at Frontier Nursing University, Hyden, Kentucky, in 2012. Dr. Cole has spent most of her professional life in full-scope practice at a freestanding birth center, Lisa Ross Birth and Women's Center in Knoxville, Tennessee. Dr. Cole joined Frontier Nursing University in 2012 as an assistant professor in the Department of Midwifery and Women's Health. She served as president of the American Association of Birth Centers (AABC) from 2009 to 2013. She continues to volunteer at the national level with the AABC Foundation. Her professional interests are focused on the birth center model of care and the triple aim of cost, quality, and patient satisfaction.

Melissa D. Avery, PhD, CNM, FACNM, FAAN, received her bachelor of science in nursing at Northern Illinois University, her master of science in nursing at the University of Kentucky, and her PhD at the University of Minnesota. She is a professor in the School of Nursing, University of Minnesota, Minneapolis, Minnesota, and directs the nurse-midwifery education program there. Dr. Avery has 25 years full-scope midwifery practice experience. Her current research involves examining prenatal care practices to enhance maternal confidence for physiologic labor and birth. Dr. Avery has been a pioneer in distance education and is currently partnering with colleagues to develop interprofessional learning opportunities for midwifery students and OB/GYN residents. She is a member of the Academy of Distinguished Teachers at the University of Minnesota and is a past president of the American College of Nurse-Midwives (ACNM).

Freestanding Birth Centers

Innovation, Evidence, Optimal Outcomes

LINDA J. COLE, DNP, CNM
MELISSA D. AVERY, PHD, CNM, FACNM, FAAN

Editors

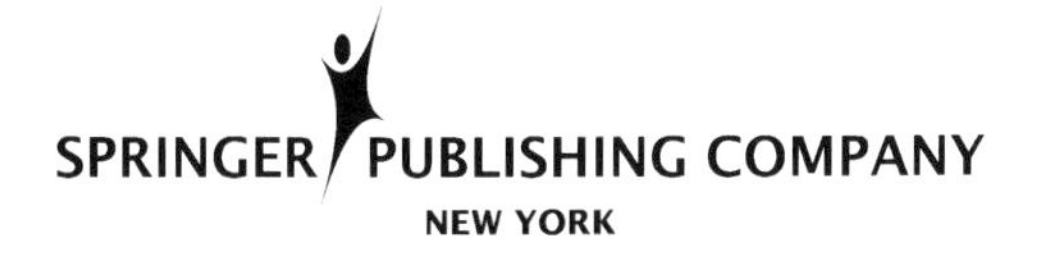

Springer Publishing Company, LLC
11 West 42nd Street
New York, NY 10036
www.springerpub.com

Acquisitions Editor: Elizabeth Nieginski
Senior Production Editor: Kris Parrish
Compositor: Westchester Publishing Services

ISBN: 978-0-8261-2589-7
e-book ISBN: 978-0-8261-2592-7

18 19 20 21 22 / 6 5 4 3 2

Library of Congress Cataloging-in-Publication Data

Names: Cole, Linda J., editor. | Avery, Melissa D., editor.
Title: Freestanding birth centers : innovation, evidence, optimal outcomes / [edited by] Linda J. Cole, Melissa D. Avery.
Description: New York, NY : Springer Publishing Company, LLC, [2017] | Includes index.
Identifiers: LCCN 2017000292 (print) | LCCN 2017001038 (ebook) | ISBN 9780826125897 (hard copy : alk. paper) | ISBN 9780826125927 (ebook)
Subjects: | MESH: Birthing Centers | United States
Classification: LCC RG960 (print) | LCC RG960 (ebook) | NLM WQ 27 AA1 | DDC 362.198200973—dc23
LC record available at https://lccn.loc.gov/2017000292

Printed in the United States of America by McNaughton & Gunn.

Contents

Contributors

Jill Alliman, DNP, CNM
Chair, Government Affairs Committee
American Association of Birth Centers
Course Faculty, Frontier Nursing University
Hyden, Kentucky

Barbara A. Anderson, DrPH, CNM, FACNM, FAAN
Professor Emeritus
Frontier Nursing University
Hyden, Kentucky

Melissa D. Avery, PhD, CNM, FACNM, FAAN
Professor
Director, Nurse-Midwifery Program
School of Nursing, University of Minnesota
Minneapolis, Minnesota

Kate E. Bauer, MBA
Executive Director
American Association of Birth Centers
Perkiomenville, Pennsylvania

Brianna Honea Bennett, MBA
Business Director
Women's Birth and Wellness Center
Chapel Hill, North Carolina

Jesse S. Bushman, MA, MALA
Former Director of Federal Government Affairs
American College of Nurse-Midwives
Silver Spring, Maryland

Erika R. Cheng, PhD, MPA
Assistant Professor
Department of Pediatrics, Section of Children's Health Services Research
Indiana University School of Medicine
Bloomington, Indiana

Linda J. Cole, DNP, CNM
Assistant Professor
Frontier Nursing University
Hyden, Kentucky

Kathleen Danhausen, MPH, CNM
Instructor of Clinical Nursing
Vanderbilt University School of Nursing
Nashville, Tennessee

Eugene R. Declercq, PhD
Professor
Community Health Science Department
Boston University School of Public Health
Boston, Massachusetts

Cynthia Flynn, PhD, CNM, FACNM
Principal
FlynnCNM Birth Center Consulting
Kennewick, Washington

Diana R. Jolles, PhD, CNM
Instructor
Frontier Nursing University
Hyden, Kentucky

Kaye Kanne, CDM, CPM
Founder (retired)
Juneau Family Health and Birth Center
Juneau, Alaska

Paula Pelletier-Butler, MSM, LM, CPM
Founder and Co-Owner
Flagstaff Birth and Women's Center
Flagstaff, Arizona
Faculty
Bastyr University
Kenmore, Washington

Julia C. Phillippi, PhD, CNM, FACNM
Assistant Professor
Vanderbilt University
School of Nursing
Nashville, Tennessee

Kathryn M. Schrag, MSN, CNM, FNP
Senior Instructor
Frontier Nursing University
Hyden, Kentucky
Workshop Chairperson
American Association of Birth Centers
Perkiomenville, Pennsylvania

Rosemary Senjem, BA
Former Executive Director of the Commission for the Accreditation of Birth Centers
White Bear Lake, Minnesota

Neel T. Shah, MD, MPP
Assistant Professor of Obstetrics
Gynecology and Reproductive Biology
Harvard Medical School
Boston, Massachusetts

Susan Rutledge Stapleton, DNP, CNM, FACNM
Data Coordinator
American Association of Birth Centers
Perkiomenville, Pennsylvania

Autumn Versace Vergo, MSN, CNM, CPM
Certified Nurse-Midwife
Dartmouth-Hitchcock
Keene, New Hampshire

Alisha H. Wilkes, DNP, CNM, ARNP
Owner, Three Moons Midwifery
Issaquah, Washington

Victoria G. Woo, MD
Fellow, Clinical Excellence Research Center
Stanford University
Stanford, California
Obstetrician and Gynecologist
Kaiser Permanente Oakland Medical Center
Oakland, California

Foreword

The birth center idea is not new. It is an answer to the cries of the childbearing public heard in large measure by women and caring professionals. As shown in Washington, DC, since the year 2000, it can be the "glue" that binds together a spectrum of health, social, and educational care that begins with conception and follows brain development through early childhood.

The editors of this book have brought together experts in the fields of midwifery, obstetrics, and public health to craft the first textbook in the United States dedicated to the birth center model. It is imperative that students, professionals, lawmakers, and anyone involved in maternity care—not the least, expectant parents—are introduced to this innovative model. Topics such as health care innovation, cost, clinical outcomes, education, policy, and quality are all integrally tied to the success of the birth center model and are explored in this book.

The timing of this book could not be better. As birth centers grow in number across our nation, more families are choosing this option. All clinicians providing care to childbearing families should read this book to broaden their understanding of the possibilities for delivery of care in a manner that addresses the triple aim of optimal outcomes, cost, and satisfaction.

As you read about the development of the birth center innovation and evidence provided by research on birth centers in this text, think about the potential return of such an investment at the beginning of life in the United States for childbearing families, the health care delivery system, and even the future development of a nonviolent society. Think about what Mary Breckinridge, founder of the Frontier Nursing Service, said almost a century ago—that "All health care begins with the care of the mother."

Ruth Watson Lubic, CNM, EdD, FACNM, FAAN
Founder, Developing Families Center
Washington, DC
Kitty Ernst, CNM, MPH, FACNM
Mary Breckinridge Chair of Midwifery
Frontier Nursing University,
Hyden, Kentucky

Preface

Maternity care in the United States has been in an unsteady state for many years. The fine tuning of the national health care lens has resulted in the implementation of evidence-based care and the Triple Aim of the Institute for Healthcare Improvement. This process of improving the care experience, health outcomes, and costs of care has made apparent to providers, policy makers, insurers, educators, businesses, and, most importantly, consumers the need for change in care at the beginning of life. The free-standing birth center model is well positioned as an important part of the necessary change. Health care professionals and students have the opportunity to learn about the community-based birth center, its history, and opportunities for expansion of this model in this timely book about birth centers.

The first chapter introduces the rich history accompanying the formation of birth centers in the United States and internationally. As you read the stories told by the midwives who founded this movement, sit back, take some time, and imagine the passion and vision of the early proponents of this model. Most of these women are still alive, a few into their 80s and 90s, and they continue to actively promote and expose newcomers to the model they created with the support of many others. To them, we owe much for their vision, persistence, stamina, and faith. They had a belief that there was a healthier and more humane way to care for women and babies beyond unnecessary and costly hospital routines designed for the few but applied to most.

Many important health care issues are addressed in this book. Health system structure and function, innovation, the triple aim, policy, quality, and education all impact the expansion of the community-based birth center model. Birth centers are making a difference locally in the communities in which they are built, as well as nationally as the spotlight shines on models of care demonstrating improved outcomes.

There are many reasons why this text needed to be written now. Although less than 1% of babies are currently born in birth centers in the United States, the model is expanding to meet the recent increased demand. Health care reform and the desire of women for an alternative to institutionalized birth have brought this model to the attention of many who are interested in learning more about the benefits of freestanding birth centers. Health professionals and students in disciplines including nursing, midwifery, medicine, public health, public policy, and business administration can learn a great deal about this effective model of care, shown to improve outcomes of care, consumer satisfaction, and cost.

In passages that are woven throughout the text, the reader will be introduced to "exemplar birth centers." These centers stand out as shining examples of integration into health systems, different providers working together, enhanced services, the franchise model, and innovative educational opportunities. Finally, the last chapter, "Launching a Birth Center," brings the history and current status of birth center knowledge into the future by introducing readers to the possibility of starting a birth center of their own. It is our hope that these inspiring centers and the information contained in the chapters of this book, written by expert authors, will encourage readers to support the continued growth of this model and contribute to the improvement in maternity care in the United States.

Linda J. Cole
Melissa D. Avery

Acknowledgments

During my 22 years of practicing in a freestanding birth center, I watched the growth of the birth center model of care sweep the country. One day, while spending some time browsing the library at Frontier Nursing University, a book nearly fell off the shelf into my hands, *Birth Centres: A Social Model for Maternity Care,* by Mavis J. Kirkham, PhD, RN, RM, published in 2003 in the United Kingdom. It occurred to me that we were long overdue for a book dedicated to the inception and development of the birth center model in the United States.

This book came about with the guidance and contribution of many people. I want to thank Barbara Anderson, DrPH, CNM, FACNM, FAAN, for assisting me early on to understand the process of organizing this project, and for making the introduction to Margaret Zuccarini at Springer Publishing Company. I will be forever grateful to Melissa D. Avery for joining me as coeditor, not only for her keen ability to shape ideas, but also for the friendship we found through our collaboration on this book.

Linda J. Cole

It is indeed time for the freestanding birth center to be more widely adopted as a preferred care model for healthy childbearing women and their families. Linda J. Cole had the foresight to envision this book, and I am grateful for her invitation to partner in its development and for the friendship that developed from our work together. I am awed by having learned so much more about the development of the earliest birth centers including all the midwives, physicians, nurses, women and their families, and others who persevered to bring this high-quality, high-value care model to the present time. Many thanks to all who shared their personal stories with us.

Melissa D. Avery

Without the chapter authors' willingness to contribute to this book, it would not have come to be. As coeditors, we thank all of the authors and contributors to this text, experts in their fields of midwifery, obstetrics, public health, and policy, for their important contributions. The historical contribution to the book brings a special perspective shared through the stories of those who worked so hard to create and advance the birth center model of care. We want to thank Kathryn Schrag for her expertise and passion in gathering these stories and weaving them into the first chapter in this book, coauthored with Kate E. Bauer. If not for the interest and trust in birth centers from women and families, there would be no need for this book to be written. We are grateful to these families, to the midwives and other clinicians who serve them, and to the students and professionals who will read this text and follow in their path.

Lastly, we want to thank our life partners and our families for lending us to this project. Their support of our passion for this book has been unwavering.

Linda J. Cole and Melissa D. Avery

SECTION I

The History and Development of the Freestanding Birth Center Model

CHAPTER 1

Organizing for Change: History, Pioneers, and the Formation of a National Organization

KATHRYN M. SCHRAG AND KATE E. BAUER

LEARNING OBJECTIVES

Upon completion of this chapter, the reader will be able to:

1. Describe the social and health care landscape in the United States that led to the development of the birth center concept
2. Identify early pioneers of the birth center movement
3. Describe the formation and development of the birth center trade association
4. Discuss the opportunities and challenges for birth centers

OVERVIEW AND CONTEXT

The birth center idea is not new. We know about the earliest "freestanding birth centers" in our time established by nurse-midwives caring for the poor and underserved: La Casita in Santa Fe, New Mexico (1944) and Su Clinica Familiar in Raymondville, Texas (1970). We do not know how many physicians, nurses, or traditional midwives have, over the years, responded to the needs of women and families in their communities, providers such as the family physician who shared the following example with me in the late 1990s.

> Several years into organizing to assist providers responding to women seeking an alternative to the medical model of birth in the acute care setting of the hospital, a family physician in the Midwest called the American Association of Birth Centers and asked me, "What is this birth center thing I'm hearing about?" After a brief description he replied, "Well then, I have a birth center." He went on to explain that the euphemism "recession" is really a full-fledged "depression" when it hits your town. When it hit his town, pregnant women began asking him to attend their birth at home for they only had enough money to pay him or the hospital, not both. With his busy practice it was not possible to give the time required for attending home births so he offered the only alternative he could. He would fix up the spare room in the back of his office. His wife would take care of them before and after he attended the birth. If they birthed there they would pay him. If he had to take them to the hospital for help, he would forgo his fee and they could pay the hospital. That worked until his malpractice insurer doubled his premiums when it discovered he was attending births in "his little birth center." In anger he dropped his insurance and put up a sign in his reception room that said, "If you sue me, you will get the chair you are sitting on and whatever else you see because I have no insurance." He added that he was OK with that because his son was the largest malpractice lawyer in the state.

This chapter describes the development of the model of birth center services in the United States, and its adaptation on a global scale (see the Appendix). Before proceeding, the reader must understand some basic circumstances facing anyone who embarks on replication of the modern birth center. Evidence shows that it is a viable model for midwifery-led care offering a safe, cost-effective alternative to the singular medical model of service that has dominated our present system in the United States (Ernst, 1996). The challenges to innovation and replication of any model of care in the United States, however, are vastly different from those facing most other developed countries in terms of geography, size, population distribution, access to care, economies, the positioning of professions, the role of government in regulations, and our multiple insurance mechanisms of payment for services. Among the major challenges are the following:

- Unlike most other developed countries with universal, single payer, and government-organized health care, the United States is made up of

50 individual states, each with the power to establish its own rules and regulations for both professional providers and health care institutions or facilities. Trying to replicate a promising innovation is like taking it to 50 different countries.

- These challenges of 50 states are compounded by the need for intensive education of providers, regulators, and multiple health insurance programs, each with their own increasingly complex terms for eligibility and payment for services and lack of knowledge about midwifery and out-of-hospital birth.
- One must recognize the difference between authoritative pronouncements (opinions) and research-based evidence. During the first half of the 20th century, most births were attended at home by physicians and midwives. In spite of evidence from research showing that the care provided by midwives was as good as physicians attending births at home, many obstetricians, seeking recognition for their specialization in the profession of medicine, argued that childbirth was "a pathological process from which only a small minority of women escape damage. If the profession (obstetrics) would realize that parturition viewed with modern eyes is no longer a normal function, but that it has imposing pathological dignity, the midwife would be impossible even to mention" (DeLee, 1915, p. 407). Thus, unlike in other developed countries, midwifery was gradually eliminated and the acculturation of childbirth to the medical model of care became the accepted norm in the United States.
- Key to the acceptance of the shift from the home to the acute care hospital and medical model of care was the promulgation of fear about birth—fear of pain and all the "what if" complications that *could* happen. There was no attempt to separate women with medical complications that needed that medical specialist from the majority of women anticipating a healthy, uncomplicated labor and birth—women who would be better cared for by midwives.
- Critical to understanding the importance of the development of the freestanding birth center is acknowledging that midwifery and birth centers represent a different philosophical view of childbirth from the existing dominant medical acute care view, and that these views are rooted in the education and socialization of each practitioner. Therefore, midwifery is not obstetrics, and birth centers are not acute care settings. Both are needed by the childbearing women and families seeking today's evidence-based care. Although there is an area of overlap where

collaboration and cooperation are needed to enable the provision of a system's continuum of care, the knowledge and skills of each provider and the capacities of each facility must be viewed as unique and complementary rather than competitive.

This difference in education and socialization of providers and lack of cooperation between facilities is compounded by a lack of uniformity in regulations among 50 different states that presents formidable challenges to introducing or replicating innovations, such as the freestanding birth center, nationwide (Lubic, 1979). Furthermore, the importance of payment mechanisms cannot be minimized, for without insurance reimbursement, no model of care can be sustained or replicated. Payment is a primary driver of how and by whom all health care is delivered. For example:

Birth centers, which support the start of life, can be compared to hospice care, which supports the end of life. Hospice care at the end of life was an innovation that was introduced about the same time as the freestanding birth center (National Hospice and Palliative Care Organization, 2016). The basic tenet of hospice is that the end of life cannot be cured, which is what physicians do, but it can be eased with comfort measures, which is what nurses do. Hospice has greatly relieved the burden on families at the end of life. Hospice care is now available in almost all communities nationwide, while birth centers are still struggling with obtaining legislation, regulation, and reimbursement state by state. Why? First, hospice is the provision of good old fashioned nursing care, which has always been viewed as essential and complementary rather than competitive to physician care. Second, hospice is included in the federally administered Medicare program, which is the single payer for universal health care for senior citizens.

There is no universal, single payer program for women and families at the beginning of life. The Affordable Care Act (ACA) has included midwives and birth centers under the Medicaid payment program. Time will tell if the ACA survives and, if so, whether all states will implement the ACA birth center provisions and if Medicaid reimbursement will be sufficient to meet the basic operating costs of birth centers, thus allowing women increased access to birth centers.

—Kitty Ernst.

EARLY MIDWIFE-LED MATERNITY CENTERS

La Casita

La Casita, the "little house" in Santa Fe, New Mexico, is often cited as the precursor to the modern midwife-led birth center movement (Figure 1.1). Students and midwives reflecting on their experiences at La Casita (Kroska, 2010) noted that the term *maternity home* was used then as there was no formally defined concept of a birth center. The center was initially indeed a small house, a two-room adobe structure that the midwives at Catholic Maternity Institute (CMI) opened in 1946 to complement their existing home birth practice.

Sister Theophane Shoemaker and Sister Helen Herb, both Medical Mission Sisters and nurse-midwives, came to Santa Fe in 1944 as recent graduates of the Maternity Center Association's (MCA) Lobenstine School in New York City (NYC; Varney & Thompson, 2016). The Society of Catholic Medical Missionaries had historically worked internationally providing nursing and medical care to profoundly underserved women and children. The instabilities of World War II, coupled with the lack of health care providers to address the high maternal and infant mortality rates in

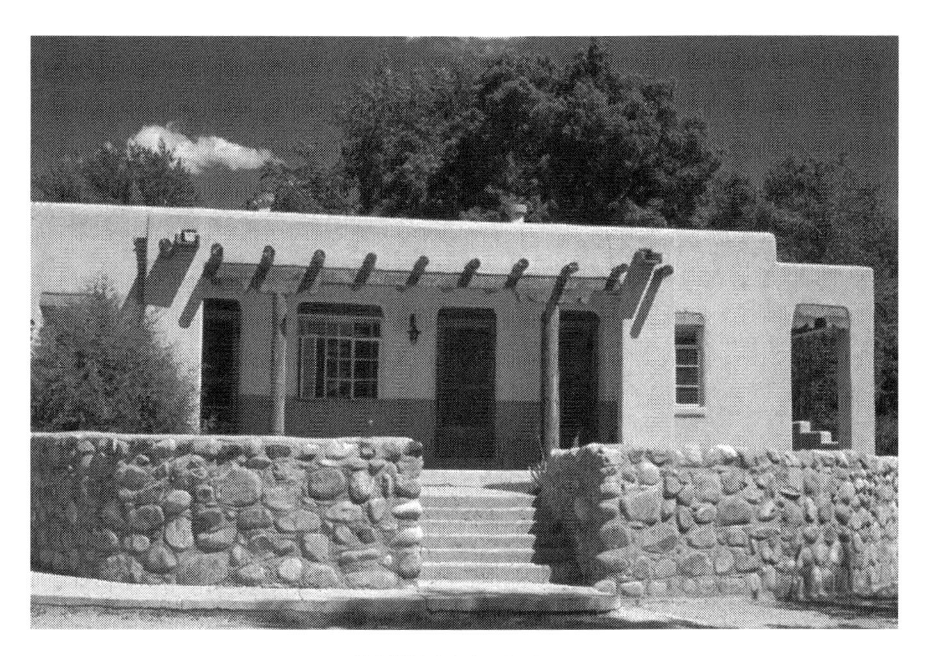

FIGURE 1.1 La Casita.

Courtesy of Elizabeth Bear.

northern New Mexico, resulted in the decision of the sisters to accept a call to Santa Fe (Cockerham & Keeling, 2010).

The midwifery practice they created, the CMI, served a primarily poor rural Spanish-American population in the Santa Fe region, which then had a county population of 30,826 (Rob Martinez, New Mexico Assistant State Historian, personal communication, June 16, 2016). The institute was originally planned as a home birth service, but responding to practical considerations, the sisters added a place where women could give birth, La Casita. Initial reasons for adding a maternity center location included proximity to a hospital for transfers and minimizing long travel times to patients' homes (Cockerham & Keeling, 2010). Soon the midwives realized that many of the women preferred to give birth at La Casita. Irene Matousek (Kroska, 2010, p. 163) commented that "only rare homes contained a shower, and the women luxuriated in the warm water, frequently shampooed their hair, and felt the therapeutic benefit of nice warm water pulsing over their lower back. Sometimes these were *long* showers!" Additional factors influencing the popularity of the maternity home were other modern conveniences, such as telephone and electricity, the ability to stay for several days free from household responsibilities, and, according to the midwives, the prestige of delivering in a medical facility (Cockerham & Keeling, 2010).

Demand for the use of La Casita grew, and by 1951 it had increased to about 20% of the births attended by CMI midwives. A new, larger facility was built across from the CMI's main building. Historians Cockerham and Keeling (2010) described CMI's mounting financial struggles and the midwives' philosophical conflict about attending a diminishing proportion of their births in the home setting. The midwives also recognized the personal advantages such as avoiding travel over poorly marked mountainous roads; the reassurance of a hospital, St Vincent, two blocks away; and the logistical simplicity for them and their midwifery students to move back and forth between the center and the clinic. By the mid-1960s, the majority of the births occurred at La Casita. The increasing expense of providing birth services at the La Casita facility, coupled with the inability of families to pay for their care, led to a growing financial strain on the organization, and in July 1969 CMI closed its doors (Cockerham & Keeling, 2010).

Student Days at CMI and La Casita

Reflections of Midwife Elizabeth (Betty) Bear

It was November 1965 when I arrived in Santa Fe and a very significant period in my life began. The city clearly showed its multicultural characteristics, but the one standout was the adobe buildings everywhere. As I arrived at CMI for the first time, it was like traveling back in time. An arched adobe entrance to the main house was inviting. The small structure to the right of CMI was predominant and its name, La Casita, most fitting. Little did I know that in the years to come it would be known as the first freestanding birth center in the United States. This "little house" became the major setting for my clinical experiences and births. I could not wait to see it and was not disappointed. I felt a warm and friendly ambience the moment I walked through the door. La Casita had all the furnishings of a home plus a large basement where prenatal classes and labor rehearsals took place.

Classes and closely supervised clinical experiences began in January 1966. My "on-call" rotation started in mid-January and was very productive. The first call came from Sister Patrick who asked me to meet her in La Casita, as one of our pregnant patients, Rosa, and her family were on their way into Santa Fe. It was a cold clear evening, so I bundled up to walk the short five blocks from my apartment to La Casita. My excitement was high as I arrived and began setting up the birthing room with Sister. The family was soon knocking at the door and Rosa, her mother, her father, and her sister all entered. Rosa was taken to the birthing room and the family settled in to the living room where José, our maintenance man, had started a fire to warm everyone.

This was Rosa's second pregnancy, so labor was well underway. Sister Patrick and I examined her, gave fluids, and helped with breathing techniques. The time had come and with Sister coaching me I delivered the most beautiful healthy girl! The family came in to see mother and baby. Rosa handed the baby to her father. It was a tradition at CMI to kneel down around the bed and have a prayer for God's blessing and a healthy baby and mother. It was spontaneous and the words came easily for me. Then we stood as the father gave his own blessing to the child and handed

(continued)

Student Days at CMI and La Casita *(continued)*

her back to Rosa. We then moved Rosa to the postpartum bedroom where her mother and sister looked after her, whereas Sister and I cleaned the birthing room and set up for the next mother. As my call time ended and I headed out the door to walk home, there were almost 4 inches of new fallen snow. It was about 5 a.m. and no one else was out on the street. The moon was full and the stars sparkled. Looking up, I deeply felt the spiritual marvel of childbirth.

Courtesy of Elizabeth Bear.

Su Clinica

Only a few years after La Casita closed, another Catholic Sister, a thousand miles away, created what historically is considered to be the second birth center in the United States: Su Clinica Familiar in Raymondville, Texas. In 1971, Su Clinica opened its doors in a rural county in the deep south of Texas. Led by Catholic Charities and the Migrant Health Division of the U.S. Department of Health, Education, and Welfare, their mission was to provide much-needed medical services to the migrant community. Sister Angela Murdaugh, a recent and enthusiastic graduate of Columbia University's midwifery program, volunteered to develop the maternity program at the clinic.

Sister Angela (personal communication, February 11, 2016) reports that the small local hospital had recently closed, and women had to travel far to give birth in the nearest hospital. Many women were attended by the community *parteras* (lay midwives) who often had a room in or behind their own homes for women to give birth, so the concept of a home-like, midwife-attended birth in another facility was familiar to women. Sister Angela was well aware of the work at La Casita, and approached the clinic administration with what to her seemed like an obvious solution to the problem: create a place within their clinic for healthy women to give birth. The administration and physicians were supportive, although initially they asked that women and their babies stay for 24 hours following the birth.

Within 3 months, Sister Angela and her support team of a licensed practical nurse (LPN) and a volunteer were attending births in Su Clinica Familiar maternity division, an eight-room area of the clinic with two exam rooms, a small office, a two-room birth area, and a two-bed postpartum room. They welcomed their first baby in July of 1972. Five months later, a much-appreciated second midwife joined the team. The midwives consulted with three obstetricians who received their transfers at the nearest hospital 25 miles away. Although the term *birth center* was not yet in common use, the philosophy and care was consistent with what we call a freestanding birth center today. The practice quickly grew and the midwives soon attended a caseload of about 150 births annually (Sister Angela, personal communication, February 11, 2016). According to the 10th anniversary report of the health center (Ramirez, 1981), the Raymondville clinic midwives had delivered more than 1,200 babies, accounting for 75% of all recorded births in Willacy County during its first 6 years.

By 1977, Su Clinica opened a second birth center, but this one was located within the walls of their transfer hospital in Harlingen. The newly formed National Health Service Corps contributed to the success of the centers with recently graduated midwives working in health care shortage areas in exchange for scholarships. Yet another national issue, the malpractice insurance crisis of the mid-1980s, resulted in the closing of both of Su Clinica's birth centers (Sister Angela, personal communication, February 11, 2016).

Sister Angela left Texas in 1981 to fulfill her responsibilities as the newly elected president of the American College of Nurse-Midwives (ACNM). While in Washington, DC, she also completed a legislative internship. Two years later, Sister Angela returned to the Rio Grande Valley. With the assistance of Catholic Charities for the first 5 years, she devoted her energy and talents toward opening a new independent birth center, Holy Family Services and Birth Center in Weslaco, Texas. Three decades later, Holy Family continues to serve women and their families (Sister Angela, personal communication, February 11, 2016).

On Influencing Political Action

Reflections of Founding Midwife Sister Angela Murdaugh

As much as I hated politics, I understood its importance and went to Washington to do a legislative internship to learn how to do it properly. In the early years of the birth center, I received an unexpected call from the office of State Representative Irma Rangel, whose Texas congressional territory included Raymondville. She

(continued)

On Influencing Political Action *(continued)*

wanted to come for a tour of the birth center and visit with me. We set up a date on a Saturday. When she arrived, I was in the midst of supporting a woman in active labor. She patiently waited in my office until the birth was accomplished. She welcomed the new baby and congratulated the mother. During our conversation, I discovered that she was there because she had gotten word from some constituents in the adjacent county that midwives were being maligned, and they had no alternative for health care. This was a case of "actions speak louder than words." What she saw sold her on birth centers and midwifery care. She remained a staunch supporter of both in the Texas legislature for her very long political career.

DEMONSTRATION AND DEVELOPMENT OF THE BIRTH CENTER CONCEPT IN THE UNITED STATES

In the 20th century, there was a cultural shift in the care of childbearing women from the midwife to the physician attending women in childbirth and a change in the place of birth from the home to the acute care hospital for more than 99% of all childbearing women. Unlike in most other developed countries with formally educated midwives, midwifery almost ceased to exist in the United States. The shift benefited the minority of women who experienced complications needing medical or surgical intervention and maternal mortality dropped dramatically. Other major influences on developing the system of care in the second half of the century included the discovery of antibiotics, medical school funding, and education under the GI Bill. Additional influences on the physician–hospital model of care were the Hill-Burton Act to establish hospitals in all eligible communities, and the beginning of employer and medical assistance insurance coverage, including maternity care. The promise to childbearing women of pain relief and the ability to deal with complications, coupled with third-party insurance, drove the shift to nearly all of childbearing women receiving physician care in hospitals (Devitt, 1977).

The singular focus on developing the specialty of obstetrics for treatment of medical complications of pregnancy and birth and the elimination of midwifery led to all birth being controlled and delivered as a medical event—an illness or an emergency waiting to happen. Identification of "low risk" and "high risk" for complications was not considered, and nurses were not trained nor hospital routines revised to meet the needs of the healthy childbearing women. Many invasive medical procedures and policies were widely accepted and routinely implemented without adequate study (e.g., pelvic shave, enema, routine episiotomy, separation of newborn from mother; Albers & Savitz, 1991). Electronic fetal monitoring, intravenous fluids, confinement to bed, and restriction of nourishment are still routine in many places in spite of the evidence that these procedures are of little value to healthy childbearing women. Epidural anesthesia became the preferred procedure for pain relief. Perhaps most important has been the promulgation of fear that eroded women's confidence in their ability to give birth.

Furthermore, the shift to hospital birth included the routine disruption of the birth experience of families without examination of the consequences: Newborns were separated from their oversedated mothers and placed in central nurseries, breastfeeding gave way to formula feeding newborns by the clock, and fathers and children were excluded and denied participation in what we are now just beginning to understand as one of the most profound teaching and "bonding" experiences of anyone's life (Johnson, 2013).

Lastly, almost all research on birth has been conducted in the acute care hospital setting where imposed routines interfered with the little understood normal physiologic process of human labor and birth. The incidences of infant mortality and low birth weight babies gradually dropped, but our rates continue to be higher than those in other developed countries where most of the care of low-risk women is provided by midwives (MacDorman, Matthews, Mohangoo, & Zeitlin, 2014).

Maternity Center Association Childbearing Center

In the early 1970s, activist, educated, insured women turned to "do-it-yourself" home birth as the only option that would guarantee the control they desired for their birth experience. Some public health and policy makers viewed this as a pending public health problem. MCA viewed it as a system's need for a safe alternative to hospital medical services that embodied the midwifery model of supportive care.

MCA was founded in 1918 with a mission to work to improve the quality of maternity care, and had been a pioneer in demonstrating solutions to pressing problems: the need for prenatal care in the 1920s, the need for nurse-midwifery education in the 1930s, and the need for formal childbirth education in the 1950s. Responding to the public demand for alternatives in care, they decided to build on the experience of the two birth centers previously described, La Casita and Su Clinica, and establish a demonstration model of a freestanding birth center in New York City. There was considerable opposition from the obstetrical community to the center being freestanding but more acceptance of the concept if located within the hospital. Based on MCA's past experience with in-hospital demonstrations, MCA decided it would only be successful if it had the autonomy to demonstrate and evaluate sustainability as primary midwifery health care for low-risk women, and pursued a freestanding model within an organized system of medical specialist collaboration and cooperation for access to acute care hospital services when indicated.

To be part of the health care system, MCA entered the complex political arenas of obtaining a certificate of need (CON) for the temporary establishment of the service, and public hearings after 2 years of operation. This required meeting all the New York codes for licensure, becoming accredited for the quality of services provided, securing liability insurance coverage, and obtaining a commitment of reimbursement from health care insurers. The development was led by Ruth Watson Lubic, CNM, general director of MCA, and in 1975 the first licensed, accredited, freestanding childbearing center (CbC) in the United States opened. The years of oppositional and redressive actions by powerful members of the medical establishment are detailed in Lubic's dissertation (Lubic, 1979).

With determination and strategic support, the center negotiated access to needed specialist and hospital services, and a contract for payment from New York's largest health care insurer, Blue Cross Blue Shield (BCBS). The contract provided that BCBS would evaluate the services for safety, client satisfaction, and costs to insurers. The published evaluation of the CbC by BCBS reported that the demonstration birth center care was safe, satisfying, and offered significant savings to payers (Canoodt, 1982), and the relationship continued.

MCA's mission was to provide services to any woman seeking a change from the conventional system, but found that the majority of families that came to the center were the upper-middle class women of Manhattan. This led to Dr. Lubic's work of the following decade: opening a birth center in a low-income NYC neighborhood. In 1988, a second MCA center, the Childbearing Center of Morris Heights Health in the South Bronx, began providing services to low-income women and their families.

EXEMPLAR
The Childbearing Center (CbC), New York, New York

Year established: 1975

Type of building/square feet/architectural features: First and garden floors of historical townhouse on the Upper East Side of Manhattan

Location (urban, suburban, rural): Urban: New York City

Business structure (for-profit, not-for-profit): Not-for-profit

Ownership: A demonstration project of Maternity Center Association (MCA)

Licensed as: Diagnostic and treatment center

Accredited by: National League for Nursing/American Public Health Association home health and community nursing services

Number of births to date/births per year: 1975–1995, the CbC births totaled 4,128 (1995 MCA Annual Report)

Services/enhanced services: Group Prenatal Care, Self-Help Education Initiated in Childbirth (SHEIC), postpartum home visits by Visiting Nurse Service of New York, and pediatric nurse practitioner (PNP) newborn and infant care

Providers: CNMs, PNPs

Client mix: Insured, well-educated, middle, and upper-middle class

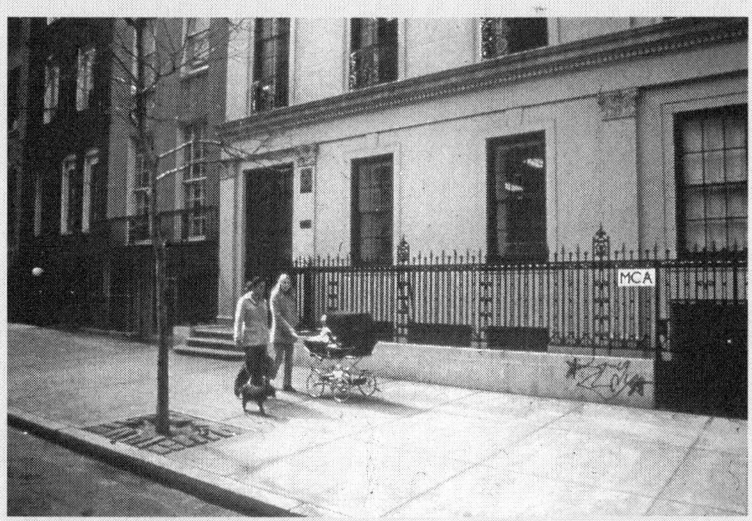

Courtesy of the American Association of Birth Centers.

(continued)

EXEMPLAR *(continued)*

The CbC in Manhattan was the first formal demonstration project of a birth center in the United States. It operated under the direction of the MCA and the skilled guidance of its general director, Ruth Watson Lubic (see narrative of the development of CbC in the text of this chapter). In 1992, MCA made the strategic decision to shift from providing direct clinical care to focus on health care system transformation, and the birth center moved location, operating as the Elizabeth Seton CbC in affiliation with St. Vincent's Manhattan Hospital. In 2003, faced with skyrocketing malpractice premiums, the birth center closed its doors, and later the same decade the hospital also closed.

In 1988, MCA opened a second NYC birth center: the Child Bearing Center of Morris Heights Health. This center, in the southwest Bronx, partnered with an existing community health center and demonstrated the application of the birth center model serving low-income families.

Ruth Watson Lubic's 1993 receipt of the MacArthur Fellowship afforded her the opportunity to replicate the model at the site of the country's worst maternal and infant outcomes: Washington, DC. The Developing Families Center (DFC) was created with Washington, DC, community partnerships, providing case management, social supports, and infant and toddler education, all under the same roof as the birth center.

The power of birth centers, recognizing pregnancy, birth, and parenting in its social context, is reflected in a letter dated February 9, 1990, and written by author Sheryl Feldman to Jennifer Dohrn, CNM, director of the Child Bearing Center of Morris Heights Health (reproduced with permission):

> *Dear Jennifer*
>
> *My first impression was fast and sure. Having spent the last several years researching birth care in the United States, today I know that the center is providing the best possible birth care available to women in America. What's really amazing is that that's only half of it. It seems to me that at the center, the community is reinventing itself.*
>
> *I understand it this way. Those of you at the center believe that mothering is significant work, that it requires a complex set of skills and that—even if you have to do it alone—you really can't do it alone. If you believe, as you seem to, that raising the young*

(continued)

EXEMPLAR *(continued)*

is a community responsibility, then what the center does, it gives women a place where they can get together and do the job. Energies join, solutions rise.

It seems to me such a contrast; that is what you are doing in comparison to what we usually do to women when they become mothers. In so many communities we squander the energy of mothers. We spill it in the waiting rooms, we dull it during labor, we destroy by the cuts we make, and we waste it afterward by sending women home alone, where they are often isolated from other mothers.

At the center all that energy goes into the intensely creative work of making the family. What I think I witnessed while I was with you was the force of that creativity. It was quite sobering and it gave me hope, so I am indebted to you.

Thank you.
Sheryl Feldman

On Connections! Connections!

Reflections of Founding Midwife Ruth Watson Lubic

In late 1969, based on my relationships with MCA as a student nurse-midwife at its school and then as a parent educator and community consultant, I had the good fortune to be offered the position of general director of that venerable not-for-profit organization, whose first executive had been Frances Perkins. There was one bothersome element for me in arriving at a decision. I knew the MCA offer represented an outstanding opportunity to advance the profession and its work over an undetermined span of time, but I had been elected by my nurse-midwife colleagues to the president-elect position of the ACNM that year and was concerned that if I accepted the position with MCA, I might be seen as abandoning my colleagues. But I felt I could not do both jobs and also knew there were many talented nurse-midwives who would make excellent ACNM leaders. So I stepped down from my elected position in favor of Carmela Cavero, who was indeed a star!

(continued)

On Connections! Connections! *(continued)*

My experience with childbearing families at MCA had taught me that new systems were needed to overcome the unacceptably impersonal in-hospital experiences of many women, some of whom were engaged in fathers "catching" babies at home because there were no other alternatives. MCA consultant Kitty Ernst and I began exploring a demonstration project for the first freestanding birth center to be a part of the health care system in the United States.

During these early years with MCA, J. Robert Willson, MD, president of the American College of Obstetricians and Gynecologists (ACOG), led a successful effort in 1971 to recognize nurse-midwives and ACNM as a partner of ACOG. It was clear that the country needed more nurse-midwives and Kitty Ernst assisted in the preparatory work for a proposal to increase midwifery education programs while I combed my community "connections!" I was able to obtain an appointment with Quigg Newton, a former mayor of Denver and at the time the president of the powerful Commonwealth Fund in New York City. When we met at the conference table to advise him on anticipated clinical matters, there was a physician named Robert Glaser. I presented MCA's concerns about the ferment in maternity services and gave our estimation of needs to increase the nurse-midwifery workforce. Shortly thereafter, MCA received a major grant to support a refresher program to "increase the preparation and utilization of nurse-midwives in the United States." A decade later, Dr. Willson agreed to serve as an officer of the inaugural board of the National Association of Childbearing Centers (NACC) under my leadership. He also served as a site visitor for accrediting early centers.

But back to more "connections"; shortly after this meeting I learned that Dr. Glaser was involved in the establishment of a medical arm of the National Academy of Sciences, the Institute of Medicine, IOM (now National Academy of Medicine). When I received a query about my willingness to serve as a member, I accepted with alacrity as one of the few nurses to be appointed; I serve to this day. From that exposure came the invitation to be a

(continued)

On Connections! Connections! *(continued)*

part of the 1973 first official American medical delegation to the People's Republic of China, which was led by John Hogness, MD, president of the IOM. One of the delegation members was George Lythcott, MD, who shortly thereafter was appointed administrator of the Health Resources and Services Administration (HRSA). It was he who offered to have HRSA fund the IOM's 1982 report "Research Issues in the Assessment of Birth Settings" (IOM, 1982), which concluded that "no setting had been adequately studied." Another delegate was Philip R. Lee, MD, who also later served on the NACC inaugural board of directors. Dr. Lee became the assistant secretary for health to the secretary of Department of Health and Human Services, Donna Shalala, in the 1990s. During those years, Dr. Lee utilized my volunteer services as a consultant to a proposed birth center on the Sioux reservation in South Dakota, and gave me an office in Washington, DC, as I used my MacArthur Fellowship stipend to work on the Developing Families Center (DFC).

I hope the reader can see that positive connections are very helpful; indeed, they are necessary to our work and we must be aware that *every* encounter has the potential for gaining, or losing, important friends for families, for midwifery, and for our health care delivery system!

Addendum

When speaking with Ruth Watson Lubic about her many contributions to birth centers, she shared what is one of my favorite stories: She had a "membership key" from Alpha Omega Alpha, the nation's most prestigious medical honor society. Dr. Glaser had nominated her for the award. Ruth would strategically wear the key on a necklace chain when she was meeting with physicians who would understand its significance—quietly making connections!

—Kathryn Schrag

THE FORMATION OF A NATIONAL ORGANIZATION

By the late 1970s, nurse-midwives and activist women across the country were responding to women seeking an alternative to hospital confinement by establishing birth centers, often in hostile environments, but without national resources and expertise. In 1979, Kitty Ernst was invited to be the graduation speaker for the nurse-midwifery program at the University of California, San Francisco (UCSF). With support from MCA, she added a tour of 14 known birth centers across the United States to assess their needs. Her findings were that, although founders were passionate about replicating the birth center model, they were all struggling with the same issues of a lack of uniform guidelines and standards needed to gain licensure and reimbursement for services and a mechanism for multisite data collection. The interviews with these pioneers further disclosed that, as a group, the founders of these centers had a common background of either social activism or missionary service that drove their passion to respond to the childbearing women seeking an alternative to the hospital medical model of care. Most were doing it alone with their own resources and support by friends. None had the support of a national voluntary health agency, such as MCA (Kitty Ernst, personal communication, August 5, 2016).

MCA responded immediately to the report of these observations by funding travel for representatives of these centers to meet in New York to determine how best to proceed. With no funding for food or hotels, participants arrived armed with sleeping bags to be housed on the couches, benches, and floors of MCA's historical, elegant townhouse on the upper east side of Manhattan in New York City (subsequently the home of Woody Allen). Cooked food for the weekend was brought in from Pennsylvania by Kitty Ernst and supplemented with fresh salad material provided by Jane Powel, an MCA board member, from her gardens on Long Island. At that meeting, the Cooperative Birth Center Network (CBCN) was formed to facilitate sharing information. The participants prioritized the need for uniform guidelines and standards necessary for gaining licensure and reimbursement for services, as well as a mechanism for multicenter data collection to evaluate the program of care they were providing.

Anita Barbey Bennetts, a nurse-midwife working on her doctorate in public health at the University of Texas School of Public Health, came prepared to gain the collaboration of the group for the first multisite study of birth centers. Jane Powel pledged $20,000 for travel to the birth centers to collect the data. The participating centers promised to open their files and provide board and room during the data collection (Kitty Ernst, personal communication, August 3, 2016). This retrospective multisite study of outcomes in 14 birth centers was published in the *Lancet* in 1982 (Bennetts & Lubic, 1982).

The NYC meeting of the midwives from the 14 birth centers represents a critical turning point for the replication of MCA's demonstration CbC through the establishment of a national organization to provide ongoing guidance for the further development and evaluation of this potentially important innovation. Funding for the establishment of the membership organization was secured by MCA from the John A. Hartford Foundation. As the work of the organization grew to meet the challenges of a changing health care marketplace, the name has changed but the founding mission has remained constant. The CBCN became the National Association of Childbearing Centers (NACC) in 1983 and the American Association of Birth Centers (AABC) in 2005 (see Table 1.1).

Throughout the 1980s, AABC laid the foundation for the promulgation of the birth center concept by developing national standards to assure quality care, fostering regulation through state licensure, securing liability insurance, establishing a mechanism for accreditation, promoting reimbursement for services, and launching a prospective multisite research study on birth center outcomes. These initiatives and the role of the birth center within the U.S. health care system are explored further in detail in Chapters 3, 8, and 9.

What Is in a Name?

What to call, and how to define, a birth center has been an ongoing discussion for the decades since the concept was introduced as a part of our health care system. The first demonstration project, MCA, used the term *childbearing center*, and this term was incorporated into the name of the professional organization in 1983, the NACC. The change to the AABC in 2005 was approved by the members to better reflect the use of the name "birth center" in public and professional parlance. In 1995, the term *freestanding* was dropped from the name of the *Birth Center Standards*, and from the title of the CABC. Without trademark protection, the name spread quickly to the hospital arena. The adoption of the name "birth center" by some hospitals to describe their medical-model labor and delivery units led to ongoing confusion regarding the model.

AABC has historically described the birth center model of care with five Ps (Ernst & Bauer, 2016b).

TABLE 1.1
Timeline of Development of the American Association of Birth Centers

Year	Event
1975	Opening of Maternity Center Association's (MCA) Childbearing Center (CbC) demonstration model in New York City (NYC)
1980	Formation of Cooperative Birth Center Network (CBCN)
1982	Publication of the first national study of outcomes of care in birth centers (Bennetts & Lubic, 1982)
1983	CBCN became the National Association of Childbearing Centers (NACC) with a multidisciplinary professional and consumer board of directors
1984	Pew Charitable Trusts Philadelphia awards grant to support drafting of national standards and birth center accreditation
1985	National standards for freestanding birth centers adopted by the membership of NACC
1985	Commission for the Accreditation of Birth Centers (CABC) established
1989	*National Birth Center Study* publication (Rooks et al., 1989)
1997	AABC Uniform Data Set collection system launched
2004	National Study of Vaginal Birth After Cesarean in Birth Centers published (Lieberman, Ernst, Rooks, Stapleton, & Flamm, 2004)
2005	NACC name changed to AABC
2013	*National Birth Center Study II* published (Stapleton, 2013)
2013	AABC received Center for Medicare and Medicaid Innovation grant to study care in birth centers
2014	AABC Position Statement on Quality published

AABC, American Association of Birth Centers.
Source: Adapted with permission from AABC (2016a).

- PEOPLE: Healthy women anticipating a low-risk pregnancy and birth, attended by qualified staff with full comprehension of midwifery practice, and qualified physician consultants
- PLACE: A maximized home rather than a minimized hospital room, which is autonomous in its management, and separate from acute obstetric/newborn care, and is equipped to provide routine care and initiate emergency procedures

- PROGRAM: Clinical services that include education, antepartum, intrapartum, postpartum, and newborn care, with informed consent and family involvement
- PRACTICE OF MIDWIFERY: Primary care that emphasizes support for pregnancy and birth as a natural physiologic process with emphasis on promotion of health and shared decision making, and operating within a system of delivery of health care
- PART OF THE SYSTEM: Arrangements for referral to collaborating physicians, complementary services, community agencies, and transfers to other levels of care including access to an acute care obstetrical/newborn unit

The Standards

The definition of a birth center included in the *AABC Birth Center Standards*, most recently updated and approved by the membership in August 2016, is:

> The birth center is a place for childbirth where care is provided in the midwifery and wellness model. The birth center is freestanding, or distinctly separate from acute care services within a hospital. While the practice of midwifery and the support of physiologic birth and newborn transition may occur in other settings, this is the exclusive model of care in a birth center. Birth centers are guided by principles of prevention, sensitivity, safety, appropriate medical intervention, and cost effectiveness. The birth center respects and facilitates a woman's right to make informed choices about her health care and her baby's health care based on her values and beliefs. The woman's family, as she defines it, is welcomed to participate in the pregnancy, birth and postpartum period. (AABC, 2016b, Birth Center Standards. Reprinted with permission)

Regulatory Definitions

In 1982, AABC published a legal description of a birth center within its Recommendations for the Regulation of Birth Centers, which the American Public Health Association (APHA) used for its *Guidelines for Licensing and Regulating Birth Centers.* Since that time, 39 states and Washington, DC, have adopted specific definitions of and regulations for birth centers, many based on the APHA *Guidelines.* The 2010 ACA added a statutory definition of a "freestanding birth center." Definitions are also found in industry organizations, such as the National Fire Protection Association, Facility Guidelines Institute, North American Industry Classifications System, National Uniform Billing Committee, and Ambulatory Health Care Facilities (Kate E. Bauer, personal communication, August 1, 2016).

On Conducting the National Birth Center Study

Reflections of Founding Midwife Kitty Ernst

Conducting the first National Birth Center Study was fraught with challenges from the beginning, but I felt deep down that the birth center concept could not survive without significant and credible evidence to support it. The first national, retrospective study voluntarily conducted by Anita Barbey Bennetts was not enough. With the voluntary help of a premier nurse-midwife researcher and epidemiologist, Judith Rooks, a plan for a large, multicenter prospective study was developed and proposed to MCA's Research Advisory Committee. Their response was "Your proposal is ambitious and laudable but, my dear, you have $20,000 to conduct a $1,000,000 study?" and "I could not get nurse-midwives to complete a one-page data form—they will never complete a twelve-page data collection form." I was crushed but without thinking responded to their challenge with, "These are birth center midwives. They will complete the forms and the study will be published in the *New England Journal of Medicine.*"

With the support and connections of Ruth Watson Lubic, director of MCA, Judith Rooks and I approached the Penn Science Center to provide the computer services necessary to proceed. They recommended the latest technology of scanned computer forms and connected us with a printer 50 miles away in Lancaster, Pennsylvania, who, upon hearing our story, also consented to print the 20,000 booklets with perforated pages of forms at their cost, which was nearly our full $20,000 budget. I was convinced that if we could get the data into a computer, someone would pay to get it out, but the challenges were just beginning.

(continued)

On Conducting the National Birth Center Study
(continued)

When the 25 boxes of printed forms arrived, we found that only the first page was perforated instead of all pages as stated in the contract. I felt that even the smallest glitch in the process of data collection would be a deterrent to busy practitioners collecting data. They were returned and reprinted.

The mid-1980s was a turbulent time for nurse-midwives and birth centers. After cataloguing and shipping the forms to the centers, the major liability insurance carrier for both the nurse-midwives and the birth centers withdrew from the market. About 25% of centers returned the unopened boxes informing us that, without liability coverage, they were forced to close. The remaining centers stayed the course, determined to provide evidence that the birth center was a concept that could become part of the solution to the problems we faced in the delivery of care to childbearing families. The returned 2,000 forms were distributed to nurse-midwives practicing in hospitals and analyzed for practice and outcome comparisons. "When you get handed a lemon, make lemonade."

The next major challenge came with the need to "clean the data" on-site at the science center. Susan Rutledge Stapleton spent months driving 65 miles from her birth center in Reading, Pennsylvania, to Philadelphia, Pennsylvania, for an untold number of nights to complete this extraordinary task for what amounted to travel reimbursement.

Now we were at the tipping point for finding and funding a credible research base for analysis and publication of the data. Dr. Alan Rosenfeld, dean of the Columbia University Mailman School of Public Health and member of MCA's Medical Advisory Board, consented to participating in the project if the funding was secured. Ruth Watson Lubic, director of MCA, after a touch and go meeting with the Kellogg Foundation, secured their consent to fund the project. Judith Rooks signed on to the staff of the Columbia University Mailman School of Public Health to work with statistician Norman Weatherby to complete the project.

The article was submitted to the *New England Journal of Medicine* and, after a year of reviews, was scheduled to be published in the

(continued)

Conducting the National Birth Center Study
(continued)

late December issue, 1989. Mission accomplished, right? Not by a long shot.

When the MCA board was informed of the success, one of the women on the board who worked for a large advertising firm exclaimed, "Wait a minute. The end of the year issue is a dead issue for any marketing of the study. If you want any coverage it will have to be prepared and disseminated immediately. I'll talk to my firm." The firm agreed to do the marketing for $16,000 and it was up to the birth centers to raise it. When informed, an urgent request went out to all centers that 32 birth centers each contribute $500, which secured the funding. Some even borrowed the money to do it. The payoff was that the nationwide coverage was extraordinary from newspapers, radio, and TV.

Only then was the mission accomplished, and it was worth every month and dollar spent to produce what came to be called "a landmark study."

Reprinted with permission from Eunice (Kitty) Ernst.

Reflections of Founding Midwife Susan Rutledge Stapleton

Kitty called me and said, "I need some help on a little project—you're not very busy, are you?" Well, no, except for running a birth center. The "little project" was the First National Birth Center Study, and it consumed a staggering amount of time for everyone involved for more than 3 years—the NACC/AABC staff, Judith Rooks (primary investigator), and, most of all, the birth center midwives and staff who spent untold hours marking little circles on thousands of scanable data forms. Kitty and I would work all day in our respective offices, and then would work on the study data into the wee hours of the morning. I spent weeks sitting on the floor in the data center in Philadelphia, surrounded by boxes of forms, cleaning data and entering corrections from the birth centers. It was a herculean effort, an unprecedented accomplishment, and remains a landmark study of birth center care.

Reprinted with permission from Susan Stapleton.

The Early Years of Birth Centers: Founding Midwives' Reflections and Birth Center Stories

The dynamic years following the opening of the CbC in New York saw birth centers opening across the country, several of which are still in operation today. Their creators tell the stories of two birth centers. Birth Care in Pennsylvania, founded in 1979, is the longest continuously operating birth center in the United States. Birth and Women's Health Center (BWHC) in Arizona, opened in 1982, is the oldest birth center in the United States that was accredited in the first group of CABC accreditations (CABC, 2016). The story of Edie Wonnell's vision in opening centers in Delaware and Pennsylvania, and reflections from Founding Midwives Perkins, Stapleton, and Gilmore about their experiences in early birth centers in Pennsylvania and New Mexico, are also included.

Two historic direct-entry midwifery practices that provide birth services on site also deserve acknowledgment. The Midwifery Center in Summertown, Tennessee, is a clinic at The Farm Community, an intentional community founded in 1971 by Stephen and Ina May Gaskin. Ina May Gaskin is an internationally recognized leader within midwifery: an author, lecturer, and advocate for midwifery and women's health. Although known primarily for their work in home birth, The Farm provides "birthing cabins" where families who travel from a distance can live for weeks or months and give birth in their temporary homes (The Farm Midwifery Center, n.d.). Maternidad la Luz, in El Paso, Texas, is a birth center that opened in 1987. Located on the border with Mexico, the center serves primarily low-income Spanish-speaking women with limited access to health care. There have been more than 15,000 births at the center, and a privately owned school for direct-entry midwives is included (Maternidad La Luz, 2016).

Birth Care and Family Health Services in Rural Pennsylvania

Reflections of Midwife Rita Rhoads

I graduated from the Frontier School of Midwifery and Family Nursing in 1977. On returning to my home in Lancaster County, Pennsylvania, I felt that God wanted me to deliver babies outside

(continued)

Birth Care and Family Health Services in Rural Pennsylvania *(continued)*

the hospital. That meant home births; however, if someone lived too far away from my home for me to attend their home birth, they still needed somewhere to deliver, so I built a building! I met Kitty Ernst at an ACNM chapter meeting. She told me my concept was called a birth center!

The building was not my biggest stumbling block as I could build on family land, on our farm in Bart, Pennsylvania. The biggest hurdle was a consulting physician. I talked to several doctors who also had home birth practices, but they all felt taking a midwife on board would alienate them further within the medical community.

I went back to my alma mater, St. Joseph Hospital School of Nursing, in Lancaster, Pennsylvania, and talked with the chief executive officer (CEO), a nun who was very sympathetic and told me that women should have safe options open to them. I used statistics showing at least 100 births/year with unlicensed providers to show the need. She agreed and asked a doctor on staff to be my consulting physician.

We opened on March 3, 1978, the first birth center in Pennsylvania and one of the first 10 in the nation. I felt very "green" with only 23 births under my belt, although I had worked labor and delivery prior to midwifery/NP school. I started with only myself and one employee whom I trained to be my aide/assistant and jack-of-all-needs. There were no licensing or written standards in 1978. I based my protocol on that of Frontier Nursing Service for its midwives and NPs.

It was the days before cell phones, but I did have a beeper and convinced the phone company that I needed a big box radio phone so my patients would not die while awaiting care. It worked by call letters similar to a ham radio. My car phone honked when the phone rang and I would dash to the car to answer it.

At first I wondered how I would deliver without electric lights in Amish homes, but we had gas lights, with dim, baby-friendly lighting. And powerful flashlights if stitching was needed. The

(continued)

Birth Care and Family Health Services in Rural Pennsylvania *(continued)*

first 10 months I did about 60 births. We grew rapidly to 140 per year. If I needed to go away, midwives from outside the area would come and give me a few days' break, but most of the time I was on call 24/7.

In 1993, I felt as if I was getting overwhelmed with the administrative side of a birth center. In order to continue the longevity of the birth center beyond my work life, I converted it to a not-for-profit with a board made up mostly of patients who were very committed to the concept and were also business owners or had worked in not-for-profit, or had other specific skills we needed.

I feel one reason the board has worked well is that I asked couples to serve together, discuss the vote, and then cast one vote per couple. They were more willing to give of their time if their spouse was present. We did have a couple of professional women who served without a partner being on the board.

As of 2016, we have delivered thousands of babies, 600+/year in three settings: birth center (60%), home (20%), and hospital (20%—vaginal birth after cesarean [VBAC], transfers). Initially we did equal home and hospital births, but the trend has been moving to more birth center births for years as we had more non-Plain clients (Plain = Amish and Mennonite).

We have grown from one midwife to seven full-time employees (9–10 persons) and one assistant to a staff of nurses (4–5 full time and 4 part time). We have also gone from no secretary to many support staff.

I attribute financial stability to the board, the executive director that was hired in 1994 and is still with us, and to the high rate of self-pay patients, which is cash flow pay-in-advance money. I have never been sorry that I worked through the lean and difficult years to reach where we are today. We are now the longest continually open birth center in the United States.

Bart Pennsylvania told by Rita Rhoads, MPH, CRNP, CNM. Reprinted with permission.

The Story of Edie Wonnell and Two Birth Centers.

Reflections of Edie Wonnell (as told to Kitty Ernst)

The story of Edith Baldwin Wonnell (Edie) and the two birth centers she founded is a story about two of the most basic characteristics of all successful leaders: passion about their work and willingness to take calculated risks. It is also a story of the importance of relationships, resilience, and reflection for achieving success in one's chosen profession. Her early years as a midwife included work with the home birth service of MCA and the establishment of a hospital-based practice at Kings County.

In the 1960s, Edie was recruited by a Wilmington hospital system to develop an innovative childbirth education program, where the staff of 20 addressed the growing demand of parents seeking more control in their birth experience. By the early 1970s, the medical staff with whom she worked became concerned about the transfers to their services from uneducated and unregulated lay midwives attending home births. Listening to concerns from the consumers in her education program coupled with those of the obstetricians at the hospital, Edie decided to become part of the solution. She enrolled in the refresher program for nurse-midwives at Booth Maternity Center in Philadelphia to update her clinical skills, while back at home, upon learning of her plans to return to midwifery, the hospital system terminated her employment.

At about the same time, she learned that a consumer and her obstetrician in Philadelphia had begun to develop a plan for a birth center. Edie joined them in their endeavor and, with a small inheritance from her mother, purchased a house located a few blocks from the Bryn Mawr Hospital. She, her husband, and her friends renovated the house that in 1978 opened as the Bryn Mawr Birth Center.

Edie lived and schooled her four children 40 miles away in Wilmington, Delaware, as did many of the first women who followed her to the birth center. One night she was driving behind a laboring couple from Wilmington to Bryn Mawr in a blinding snowstorm. She thought, "This is crazy. I have to do a birth center in Wilmington no matter what it takes." And it did take more

(continued)

The Story of Edie Wonnell and Two Birth Centers (*continued*)

to introduce midwifery and an out-of-hospital birth facility in Delaware. Kitty Ernst relates how she and Edie typed up the required state Certificate of Need (CON) application in a tent on Assateaque Island while their kids played together on the beach. The CON hearing was a public display of medical opposition, but a large consumer turnout coupled with a nurse on the panel who told of the improvement in outcomes at the Frontier Nursing Service midwife-attended home births persuaded the panel to approve the application.

Physician collaboration came more easily than expected from an obstetrician resident Edie had counseled while in his residency on how he could build a successful practice by simply listening to women and meeting their beyond-medical needs for a positive birth experience. His position on support for the birth center was, "I don't know anything about birth centers but I do know Edie Wonnell." However, when he agreed to collaborate he did ask, "Now what do I say to the woman being transferred?" Edie replied with something like, "Understand first that she is scared and disappointed so take her hand (touch is important), look into her eyes and tell her you know she is disappointed that giving birth at that wonderful birth center has not turned out as she hoped or planned but, that is why you are here, to fix the problem. You will explain everything as you go along. In doing this you will have helped her to transfer the months of trust she has given us at the birth center to trusting you and the hospital. Script your partners and the nurses to do the same; look at it as a one minute opportunity to build a positive relationship for risk management purposes."

When Edie arranged to meet with the transfer hospital's chief administrator, the man who had previously fired her when he learned of her intentions to return to clinical midwifery, she brought with her a leading woman in the community, a supporter of the birth center with DuPont heritage. This clearly upper-class woman strolled into the office, sat down, and leaned over to ask, "Now Richard, how long is this going to take?" He quickly replied that it

(*continued*)

The Story of Edie Wonnell and Two Birth Centers (*continued*)

would only take a few minutes; that he could not write a formal agreement but would write up a memo of understanding that the birth center will have access to the hospital like every other medical service or nursing facility in the community. The meeting was over.

Edie had incorporated both birth centers as not-for-profit. When the 1985 liability insurance crisis hit, the Wilmington birth center board of directors moved to close the center. Since she owned the birth center property and rented it to the center, Edie instead chose to reincorporate the birth center as a privately owned business, and temporarily operated without malpractice coverage as the center transitioned to its new organizational structure.

The birth center in Wilmington, Delaware, and the birth center in Bryn Mawr, Pennsylvania, operate at full capacity today. The story of Edie Wonnell is one of extraordinary resilience in the face of adversity, but she has always stated, "I have no regrets" (Edie Wonnell, personal communication, August 16, 2016). Her full story is chronicled in the book *Women, Power, and Childbirth: A Case Study of a Free-Standing Birth Center* (Turkel, 1995).

Arizona's First Birth Center

Reflections of Kathryn Schrag, MSN, CNM, FNP

The story of Arizona's first birth center is probably most remarkable for the resiliency and determination of the midwives and the families they served. Opened in Tucson in 1982, and still thriving today, the center adapted to the dynamic health care environment of its first three decades by reorganizing six times. More than 11,000 births later, our story is a reflection of the turbulence of the dysfunctional health care system in the United States.

- 1982–1986: Tucson Birth Center opened as a midwife-owned practice, founded by my colleague Mariann Shinoskie and

(*continued*)

Arizona's First Birth Center *(continued)*

myself. We were the classic small business start-up: borrowing money, exploring regulations, remodeling a building, working endless hours without pay the first year, and feeling exhilaration and terror as we navigated new waters. A key to our success was the good fortune of meeting obstetrician-gynecologist John Vrtiska, who worked with the center for the next 20 years.

- 1986–1990: In response to the lack of availability of malpractice insurance in the private sector, we sold the practice to Thomas Davis Medical Center, a multispecialty physician practice, where Dr. Vrtiska was a shareholder. We stayed in our same location, remained the directors of the center, and received a welcomed pay raise. During this period, we received our CABC accreditation.
- 1990–1998: With the support of our admitting hospital, Tucson Medical Center, we had the opportunity to leave the multispecialty practice and form a small private practice owned by both physicians and midwives. This practice was re-named Birth and Women's Health Center. We designed a new building adjacent to the hospital property that included offices, classroom and the birth center facility. Women had three choices for care: a midwife attended birth at the birth center, a midwife attended birth at the hospital, or a physician attended birth at the hospital.
- 1998–2002: In an attempt to have the power to negotiate with falling reimbursement from managed care organizations, we reincorporated into a limited liability company (LLC) with the addition of three obstetricians, and grew to a large women's health care practice including physicians and other advanced practice nurses. BWHC retained 25% ownership and remained in the same location, as the other providers opened other offices to provide geographic coverage across the city.
- 2002–2006: Financial difficulties of this large practice resulted in the decision for the certified nurse-midwives (CNMs) and birth center practice to leave the practice and form their own independent not-for-profit birth center. The birth center and

(continued)

Arizona's First Birth Center *(continued)*

midwives again remained in the same location, and Dr. Vrtiska and his partners continued to provide collaborative services for several more years.

- 2007–present: Malpractice insurance crises once again required a new organizational model, as premiums rose to financially untenable rates in spite of a 25-year history of not a single malpractice claim against the midwives. The solution was to become a department within the well-respected local Federally Qualified Health Center (FQHC), El Rio Health Center. Once again, the midwives and their birth center stayed in the same location. Four years later, in response to growing demand for their services, they moved to a new and larger facility.

From the beginning, the birth center has enjoyed a reputation for quality within the community. Strong relationships with physicians, hospital-admitting privileges for the midwives, reimbursement by all major insurance payers, and national accreditation from CABC contributed to the success. When forces beyond control of the birth center arose, the midwives and the clients of the birth center responded with creativity and the determination to survive.

On Hiring Your Own Collaborating Physicians

Reflections of Founding Midwife Elizabeth Gilmore (as told by Carl Gilmore, Elizabeth Gilmore's widower, and Marcy Andrew, CPM, Elizabeth's colleague and president of the National College of Midwifery)

Finding a highly qualified and sympathetic collaborating physician is sometimes a challenge for independently owned birth centers. When the Taos Birth Center was faced with limited options for a supportive obstetrician in its rural New Mexico community, it thought "outside the box" and hired its own!

(continued)

On Hiring Your Own Collaborating Physicians *(continued)*

> Elizabeth understood that in order for midwifery care to be sustainable and to provide any long-term effects on our health care system, it needed to be recognized as a viable profession. Her gift was to be able to keep midwifery care intimate and individualized at the same time that she worked to standardize it just enough for the outside world to be able to understand and help validate it. She saw professionalization as necessary to creating the relationships with the medical community that would develop a more holistic and integrated healthcare system. She knew it was essential for gaining Medicaid and insurance reimbursement and thus being able to serve families of all incomes. She saw this not only in the realm of midwifery practice but also midwifery education, and eventually founded the National College of Midwifery. (Marcy Andrew, personal communication, June 14, 2016)

In 1998, the birth center hired a husband–wife team, Drs. Heidi Rinehart and Rudy Fedrizzi, to be part of their practice. The physicians had given birth to one of their own children with the midwives at The Farm in Tennessee and truly embraced the midwifery model of care. At the time of their arrival, the midwives were operating out of the home of one of the midwives that had been converted into a "Birth Cottage" while the new birth center was being built, and for a moment in time three midwives, two students, two doctors, and a receptionist were all sharing three desks. Carl and Marcy recall it being an intimate experience!

When the construction was complete, one wing was dedicated to the physician offices and exam room, and the other to the midwifery practice, with a shared waiting room. All clients who saw the doctors for their initial visits were referred to the midwives for a consultation if they were good candidates for out-of-hospital care. Often care shifted back and forth depending on how the pregnancy progressed. Some clients chose to have their prenatal

(continued)

On Hiring Your Own Collaborating Physicians
(continued)

care with the physicians, but then decided to have their birth at the birth center. The midwives were the primary providers for all births at the birth center, and for their own patients the physician would also attend.

There were other examples of true collaborative practice: weekly chart reviews of clients who shared care with both the midwives and physicians, a certified professional midwife (CPM) who taught a group prenatal program with clients of both practices, physician assistance at the birth center for minor complications such as the repair of a third-degree laceration, CPM invitation to the hospital obstetrical committees, and the physicians participating in a teaching role at the National College of Midwifery.

In 2001, another obstetrician couple, Drs. Shanti Mobling and Scott Resnick, joined the birth center practice. Three years later, Heidi and Rudy moved from New Mexico, and Shanti and Scott moved their practice from the birth center and started a private practice, Women's Health Institute. They continued to provide friendly collaboration with the midwives, and hired their own team of CNMs to provide hospital-based care. At the time of this writing, these same CNMs are planning to reopen the recently closed birth center (Carl Gilmore and Marcy Andrew, personal communication, June 15, 2016).

On Opening My Own Birth Center
Reflections of Founding Midwife Susan Rutledge Stapleton

No one does anything alone. The women and families we served provided the encouragement to carry on. Their feedback about the impact we had on their lives continues today, and the honor of sharing such an important time in their lives has been humbling and rewarding.

(continued)

On Opening My Own Birth Center *(continued)*

I opened Reading Birth and Women's Center, with very limited personal funds and resources, 2 years after a national malpractice insurance crisis caused the closure of McTammany Nurse-Midwifery Center. As we planned for renovating the tiny, old home we had purchased, my husband was skeptical that it could be done. I told him that we would do it with volunteers, to which he replied, "Why would people volunteer to do all the work for this?" Then families came out every day for months, bringing their skills and energy to accomplish what we could have never afforded or done alone. They did everything—demolition, wiring, carpentry, hanging drywall, painting, hauling trash, designing sign and logo, landscaping—all for pizza and beer. A father served as general contractor, making detailed lists of the materials that we needed to buy for the next weekend's work crew. One woman commented, "I'm not having any more babies. I'm doing this for womankind." Their enthusiasm was infectious and uplifting when I felt overwhelmed or discouraged. It was really their support that convinced me that my crazy dream was important and possible. Once open, the talented and dedicated birth center staff, my husband and family, and Kitty Ernst and Ruth Watson Lubic gave me strength to carry on.

As was true of all midwives at the time, my education included absolutely nothing about running a business. Few midwives went into the field because they wanted to run a business or be a political activist, although both turned out to be critical. After a few years of operating my birth center, and working 80 or more hours per week, my tax accountant husband noted that I had made a grand total of $4,000 income the previous year. He asked, "Do you want to do this as a business or as a hobby? Because if you don't want to do it as a hobby, then you need to start running it like a business." With his help, I began to learn business skills and implemented good business practices that resulted in the birth center becoming profitable and sustainable beyond my wildest dreams.

Reprinted with permission from Susan Stapleton.

On Working With Entrepreneurs

Reflections of Founding Midwife Sandra Perkins

If you are ready for it, life will come to you, with a challenge. That was certainly true when obstetrician entrepreneur Robert McTammany recruited me to Reading, Pennsylvania. He asked me to join a team of practitioners who would play a critical role in bringing about a new generation of care that pregnant women were asking for. The word that would energize this major effort was "CHOICE." Just being able to give women ownership of their body and pregnancy would turn the status quo for current maternity care on its ear.

We couldn't sit around waiting for lightning to strike. Failure was not an option. I think, rather than sit around, we developed a "working" list of doable things to get started.

When women win, it would be our win. This analogy expresses what I see, what I felt when a stranger said to me, "I want you to bake a cake . . . oh, and I forgot to tell you, there is no kitchen, no stove or microwave or sink. Worst of all, you have to create your own recipe." Kind of like getting a big something out of a little nothing. Then, our next steps became clearer and clearer. I believe that things change when people of like minds have work that is bigger than themselves.

OPPORTUNITIES AND CHALLENGES FOR BIRTH CENTERS

Liability Insurance

Birth centers were dealt an almost fatal blow by the liability insurance industry in the mid-1980s when the insurance carrier for nurse-midwives and birth centers withdrew from the liability market, and many centers closed. Today, rather than the lack of availability of insurance, the issues include skyrocketing costs and midwives' and collaborating physicians' fear of being sued. Despite these challenges, the number of birth centers in the United States increased 60% between 2008 and 2016 (Figure 1.2).

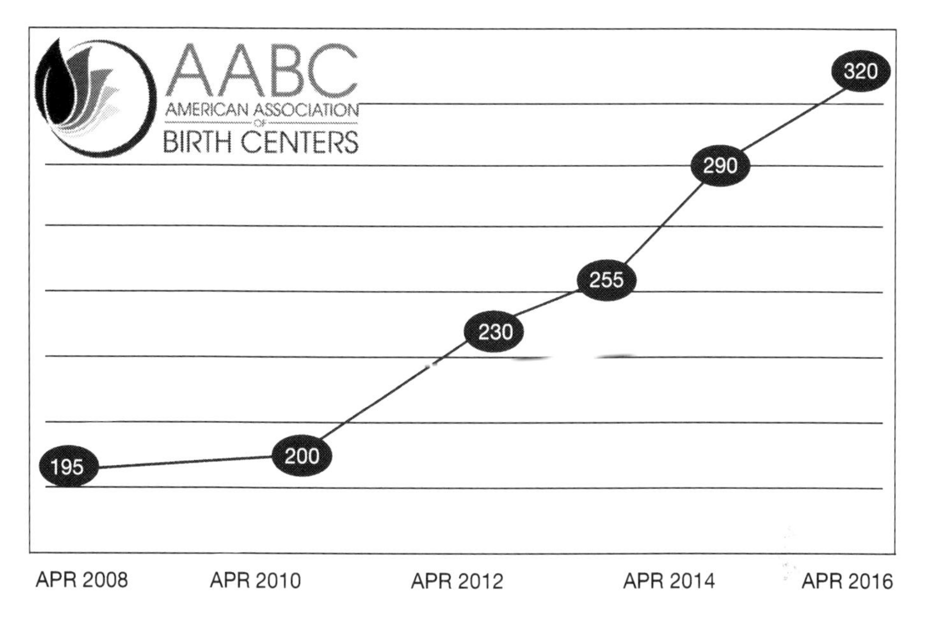

FIGURE 1.2 Growth in the number of midwifery-led birth centers in the United States from 2008 to 2016.

Source: AABC, American Association of Birth Centers.

Evaluation of the Birth Center Model

Key to the success of the development of the birth center model was the evaluation of the concept. AABC recognized that research had been a pillar in the foundation of birth centers. In 1982, the IOM published its report *Research Issues in the Assessment of Birth Settings* (IOM, 1982). Based on the IOM recommendations for the research and using the Centers for Disease Control and Prevention (CDC) data collection methodology, AABC launched a national multisite study of physiologic birth in birth centers. Results of this study, the *National Birth Center Study* (Rooks et al., 1989), demonstrated that modern birth centers can identify women who are low risk for obstetrical complications and can care for them in a way that provides benefits. The year following the publication of Rooks' study, AABC launched a prospective study on the controversial issue of the safety of out-of-hospital birth for women seeking a trial of labor after cesarean (TOLAC). Published in 2004 (Lieberman et al., 2004), the study determined that there were risks associated with TOLAC in the birth center. In 1995, AABC began development of a national registry, now named the

Perinatal Data Registry (PDR), as a means to continue to collect clinical and utilization data on the birth center model of care. This large prospective data set includes data on all maternity providers in all settings, and will continue to be a critical source of information for both individual birth centers and researchers. The *National Birth Center Study II* (Stapleton et al., 2013), a second AABC-funded multisite study, reaffirmed the safety and cost savings of the birth center model of care.

Consumers

Increased consumer access to scientific information through the Internet and social media has led individual women to seek more personal birth experiences and stronger, more activist consumer movements for "evidence-based" care, such as ImprovingBirth, Where's My Midwife?, and Evidence Based Birth. Childbirth Connection's (formerly MCA) 2013 Listening to Mothers III national survey reports that only 35% of mothers rate the U.S. maternity care system as excellent, and that in the future two thirds of respondents would definitely consider a freestanding birth center for care (Declercq et al., 2013).

Although still a small minority in absolute number, there has been a near doubling of the out-of-hospital birth rate in the last decade, from 0.87% to 1.50%. Sixty-four percent of the out-of-hospital births have been at home, but the percent of birth center births is trending upward (MacDorman, Matthews, & Declercq, 2014; Martin, Hamilton, Osterman, Driscoll, & Mathews, 2017). In spite of these trends, progress in changing hospital and medical routines in pregnancy and birth continue to prove disappointing.

Reimbursement

It should be recognized that reimbursement has always been a driving force in hospitalization for birth. From the beginning of the birth center movement, there has been a consciousness about the cost-effectiveness of the model. In spite of demonstrated cost-effectiveness, birth centers often struggle to receive compensation sufficient to cover their actual costs. As a time-intensive single service unit, there is little opportunity to cost shift, to increase productivity volume, or to scale up ancillary services to increase revenue. The costs of providing care and the payment for services have been and will continue to be a critical factor in sustaining birth centers and integrating them into the mainstream of the health care system (see Chapters 6 and 10).

Professional Midwifery

Although the development of the birth center concept was led by CNMs, the growth of direct-entry midwifery in the United States has been an important contributor to birth centers. Certification for CPMs began in 1994. As of 2014, there have been more than 2,400 certificates awarded and approximately one in six midwives in the United States today is a CPM (National Association of Certified Professional Midwives [NACPM], 2014). The CDC issues annual birth certificate data with categorization of birth site and provider in its National Vital Statistics Reports. According to the latest data, although CNMs/certified midwives (CMs) attend 91% of the total midwife-attended births in the United States, a CNM/CM is the birth attendant in 54% of birth center births and an "other midwife," including CPM, in 40% of those births (Martin et al., 2017). The CPMs' clinical foundation in the out-of-hospital setting coupled with the broader scope of practice of the CNM creates opportunities for collaborative models.

Organizational Models

The majority of the early birth centers were the direct result of a community need and passionate midwives. Most of today's AABC member centers continue to share those same origins and organize as an independent for-profit structure. Over the years, there have been other organizational models including birth centers that are not-for-profit corporations, centers that are owned by hospitals or universities or large medical practices, centers that operate under the umbrella of a FQHC, birth centers that are publicly owned, and some with hybrid corporate structures. There have been and will continue to be attempts at franchising, experimentation with one organization having several centers in a metropolitan area, and the business model of one organization with operating centers across a state or across the country. The lack of a national health care system provides opportunity and barriers to determining the best organizational structure for the birth center model.

Birth Centers in Contemporary Health Care Reform

In the 21st century, we live with a new set of issues in our health care system. There is a welcome national drive to collect data for accountability and conduct research to make all practice evidence based. Very large data sets can be mined for discoveries that would not be possible by traditional research methods. Cost has greatly escalated, and many childbearing women continue to be uninsured, underinsured, or are participating in a patchwork of care services. The majority of health insurance is provided in some kind of managed system. Yet, care is still billed on a fee-for-service basis, which results in challenges for the business of health care. Providers are often subject to productivity schedules, complicated coding to bill for services, reduced reimbursements from insurance companies, and delayed or denied payments. A number of hospitals have downsized or closed their obstetrical units. Midwifery is growing and collaborative practice between nurse-midwives and physicians is increasingly accepted, while enrollment in obstetrical residency has remained constant, and hospitalist physicians have been introduced into hospital settings (Ernst & Bauer, 2016b).

Midwifery in the birth center setting is increasingly recognized by many as part of the solution to what has been called the "perinatal paradox" (Sakala & Corry, 2008): The United States spends more money, and does more interventions in perinatal care, than any country but accomplishes less. The 2013 report of the IOM (2013) and recent publications by Alliman, Jolles, and Summers (2015), Romano (2013, 2015), and Stone, Ernst, and Stapleton (2016) address the system-level solutions that birth centers offer. In 2015, birth centers were recognized by the ACOG and the Society for Maternal Fetal Medicine by their inclusion in the consensus document Levels of Maternal Care (ACOG, 2015). In the most recent Committee Opinion on Planned Home Birth (ACOG, 2016), ACOG acknowledged the woman's right to make an informed choice about site of birth, and states that "hospitals and accredited birth centers are the safest settings for birth." In an era of a rapidly changing health care environment, health care futurists tell us that entrepreneurialism will be encouraged, innovation will be rewarded, traditional models will be passé, and that customer-centered care will be imperative (Federal Trade Commission, 2004). From the earliest publications of AABC, the consistent message is that the determining factors in the survival of the birth center concept have been and continue to be "safety, satisfaction, and savings." This same message is at the core of the Institute for Healthcare Improvement's Triple Aim initiative (Berwick, Nolan, & Whittington, 2008). Birth centers, an example of needed "disruptive innovation" (Christensen, 2000), are uniquely positioned to address the vision of health care reform for maternity care in the United States. Professional organizations supporting birth centers are listed in Table 1.2.

TABLE 1.2
Professional Organization Publications and Statements Supporting Birth Centers

1982	American Public Health Association's (APHA) "Guidelines for Regulating and Licensing Birth Centers"
1982	The Institute of Medicine's (IOM) report *Research Issues in the Assessment of Birth Settings*
1988	CHAMPUS (Civilian Health and Medical Program of the Uniformed Services) reimbursement of birth center services
1989	Pilot study of the Frontier Nursing Service "Community-Based Nurse-Midwifery Education Program," done by the American Association of Birth Centers (AABC) in Perkiomenville, Pennsylvania
1999	"The Future of Midwifery" report by the Pew Health Professions Commission and the University of California Center for Health Professions
2008	Milbank Report: "Evidence-Based Maternity Care: What It Is and What It Can Achieve"
2010	Medicaid Birth Center Reimbursement Act passed; part of the Affordable Care Act
2010	IOM's report *The Future of Nursing: Leading Change, Advancing Health,* which describes the Family Health and Birth Center (FHBC) in Washington, DC as an exemplar model of care
2012	Cochrane Pregnancy and Childbirth Group's report on institutional settings for birth
2013	IOM's second *Research Issues in the Assessment of Birth Settings*
2012	American College of Nurse-Midwives (ACNM), Midwives Alliance of North America, and National Association of Certified Professional Midwives's "Consensus Statement on Physiologic Birth"
2012	ACOG/American Academy of Pediatrics (AAP) "Guidelines for Perinatal Care"
2013	Truven Report: "The Cost of Having a Baby in the United States"
2015	American College of Obstetricians and Gynecologists (ACOG)/Society for Maternal–Fetal Medicine (SMFM) "Obstetric Care Consensus: Levels of Maternity Care"
2014	The Lancet Series on Midwifery
2014	National Institute for Health and Care Excellence: "Guidelines on Site of Birth" (United Kingdom)

BIRTH CENTER PIONEERS

Birth Centers in the United States: Founding Midwife Eunice Kitty Ernst, CNM

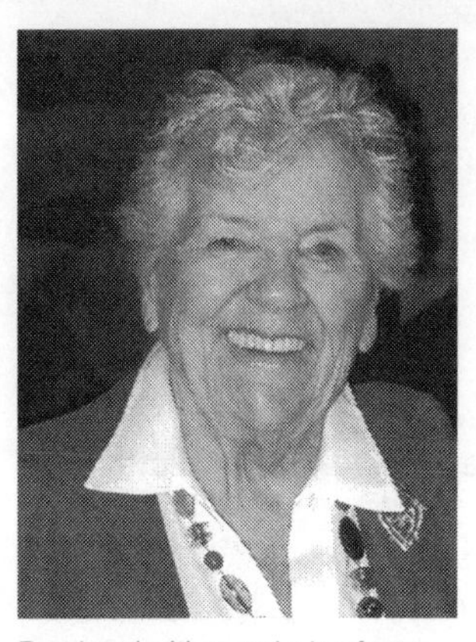

Reprinted with permission from Eunice (Kitty) Ernst

Birth date and place: 1926, Weston, Massachusetts

Current residence: Perkiomenville, Pennsylvania

Professional education:

- 1947: Diploma, Waltham Hospital School of Nursing, U.S. Cadet Nurse Corps Waltham, Massachusetts
- 1951: Certificate, Frontier Graduate School of Midwifery, Kentucky
- 1957: BS in Education, Hunter College, New York
- 1959: MPH, Columbia University Mailman School of Public Health and Administrative Medicine, New York
- 1971: Refresher course in nurse-midwifery, Downstate Medical Center, State University of New York, New York

Selected professional work and honors:

- 1951–1954: CNM, Frontier Nursing Service, Beech Fork District Nursing Center, Kentucky
- 1954–1958: CNM at MCA, New York
- 1959–1961: Faculty at Columbia University Department of Nursing, New York
- 1960–1963: President-elect, then president, American College of Nurse-Midwives (ACNM)
- 1962–1970: Parent educator, lecturer, consultant
- 1971–1976: Transitioned Salvation Army's Booth Maternity Center to midwifery-led maternity hospital
- 1982–1983: Vice president, ACNM

(continued)

- 1981–1983: Founder/director of Cooperative Birth Center Network (CBCN), Perkiomenville, Pennsylvania
- 1982: Recipient of Martha May Elliot Award, American Public Health Association (APHA)
- 1983–1993: Director of National Association of Childbearing Centers (NACC), Perkiomenville, Pennsylvania
- 1984: Recipient of John B. Franklin Memorial Award, Salvation Army Philadelphia
- 1998: Recipient of Hattie Hemschemeyer Award, ACNM
- 1988–1991: Launched Community-Based Nurse-Midwifery Education Program, Perkiomenville, Pennsylvania
- 1991–present: Mary Breckenridge Chair of Midwifery, Frontier School of Midwifery, Hyden, Kentucky
- 1992: Recognition of Outstanding Service, NACC
- 1993: MCA Medal for Distinguished Service
- 1993–2007: Coordinator of American Association of Birth Center's (AABC) Consulting Group
- 2001: Doctor of Science *honoris causa,* Case Western Reserve University, Ohio
- 2003: Recipient of Carola Warburg Rothschild Award, MCA, New York
- 2007–2008: President, ACNM
- 2010: Recipient of Living Legend Award (Midwives Alliance of America)
- 2011: Doctor of Humane Letters—Frontier Nursing University
- 2014–present: Member, board of directors, Frontier Nursing University

Personal involvement with the development of birth centers:

- 1971–1976: Assisted in planning and implementation of the childbearing center (CbC), New York
- 1976–1978: Consultation and evaluation of McTammany Nurse-Midwifery Center, Reading, Pennsylvania
- 1981–1983: Founder and director of CBCN; investigator in national survey of birth centers

(continued)

- 1983–1991: Executive director of NACC, Perkiomenville, Pennsylvania
  - Drafted first Recommendations for the Regulation of Birth Centers
  - Developed and presented "How to Start a Birth Center" workshops
  - Project director and author: National Study of Birth Centers
  - Coauthor: Results of the National Study of Vaginal Birth After Cesarean in Birth Centers
  - Directed pilot program to establish national standards and mechanism for accreditation
- 2006–2009: President of AABC
- Author, board member, advisor, speaker, and consultant on birth centers and the health care system

Birth Centers in the United States: Founding Mother
Elizabeth Gilmore, CPM
Information provided by
Carl Gilmore, husband, and Marcy Andrew, colleague

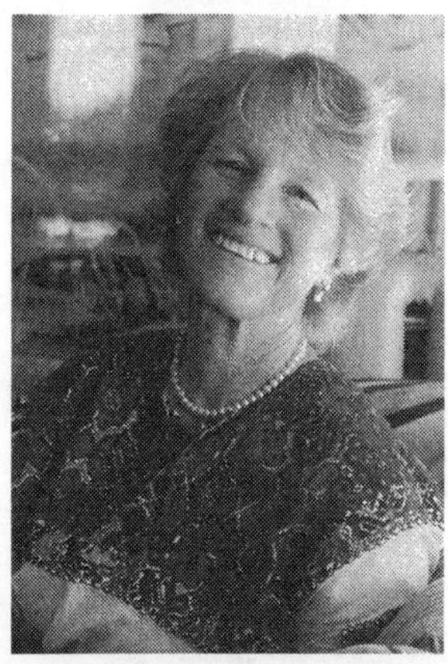
Courtesy of Carl Gilmore

Birth date and place: 1947, Mt. Kisco, New York. Grew up in Mexico City, Mexico

Death date and place: August 2011, Taos, New Mexico

Professional education:
- 1969: BA, English, University of Wisconsin, Madison
- 1979: New Mexico Licensed Midwife
- 2000 (approximate date): MS, Midwifery, Midwives College of Utah

(continued)

Professional work life and honors:

- 1979–1982: Founder, Taos Midwives Group Practice
- 1983: Founder, New Mexico Midwives Association
- 1983–2007: Founder, Northern New Mexico Midwifery Center (birth center)
- 1989: Founded National College of Midwifery
- 1989–2010: President and faculty at National College of Midwifery
- 1991: Cofounded Midwifery Education Accreditation Council (MEAC); served on board of directors
- 2001–2001: Recipient of Professional Achievement Award, American Association of Birth Centers (AABC)
- 2001: Northern New Mexico Midwifery Center received National Model Award from the WHO Safe Motherhood Initiative—USA
- 2002: Northern New Mexico Midwifery Center named first Mother Friendly Birth Service in the nation by Coalition for Improving Maternity Services
- 2015: Recipient of Sage Femme Award, Midwives Alliance of North America
- Speaker on midwifery, nationally and internationally

Personal involvement with the development of birth centers:

- Cofounder of New Mexico's first independent birth center
- Director of the first CPM birth center accredited by the Commission for the Accreditation of Birth Centers (CABC)
- CABC's site visitor

Birth Centers in the United States: Founding Midwife Ruth Watson Lubic, CNM

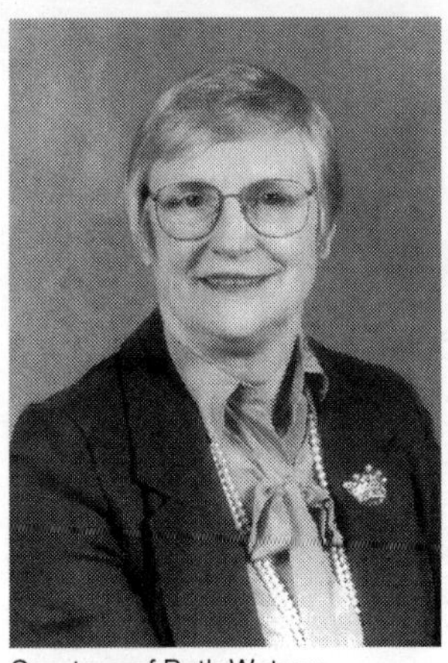

Courtesy of Ruth Watson Lubic, CNM

Birth date and place: 1927, Bristol, Pennsylvania

Current residence: Washington, DC

Professional education:

- 1955: Nursing diploma, Hospital of the University of Pennsylvania
- 1959: BS in Nursing, Teachers College, Columbia University, New York
- 1961: MA, Teaching of Medical-Surgical Nursing, Columbia University
- 1962: Midwifery Certificate, Maternity Center Association (MCA)/Downstate Medical Center, State University of New York, New York
- 1979: EdD, Applied Anthropology, Teachers College, Columbia University, New York
- 1980: Certificate, Columbia University School of Business, Institute of Not-for-Profit Management, New York

Selected professional work life and honors:

- 1962: Clinical instructor, Downstate Medical Center, State University of New York, New York
- 1963–1997: Maternity Center Association: Patient educator (1993–1997), General Director (1970–1995), Director of Clinical Projects (1995–1997)
- Mid-1960s: American College of Nurse-Midwives (ACNM) executive director, New York City (NYC)

(continued)

- 1971: Elected as member of Institute of Medicine (IOM)
- 1973: Participant in the first official American medical delegation to the People's Republic of China
- 1992–2009: Developing Families Center: Founder and president (1992–2002); Founder and President of Family Health & Birth Center (1992–2009)
- 1993: Recipient of MacArthur Foundation Fellows award; award used to launch the DFC, Washington, DC
- 2001: Recipient of National Academy of Medicine Gustav O. Lienhard Award
- 1995–1997: Adjunct professor, Georgetown and New York Universities
- 1997: Recipient of Carola Warburg Rothschild Award, MCA
- 2001: Living Legend designation, American Academy of Nurses
- 2003–present: DFC and FHBC founder and president emerita, Washington, DC
- Honorary doctorates from seven universities, including University of Massachusetts School of Medicine

Personal involvement with the development of birth centers:

- 1975: Founder and director of the first U.S. demonstration project birth center, New York City
- 1979: Dissertation: Barriers and Conflict in Maternity Care Innovation
- Director of MCA Birth Centers: The CbC (Manhattan, 1975–1995) and Child Bearing Center of Morris Heights Health (South Bronx, 1988–1992), and FHBC, Washington, DC (1998–2003)
- 1983: Cofounded National Association of Childbearing Centers (NACC)
- 1983–1991: NACC's president of board of directors
- 1996–1998: NACC's foundation project director

Birth Centers in the United States: Founding Midwife Sister Angela Murdaugh, CNM

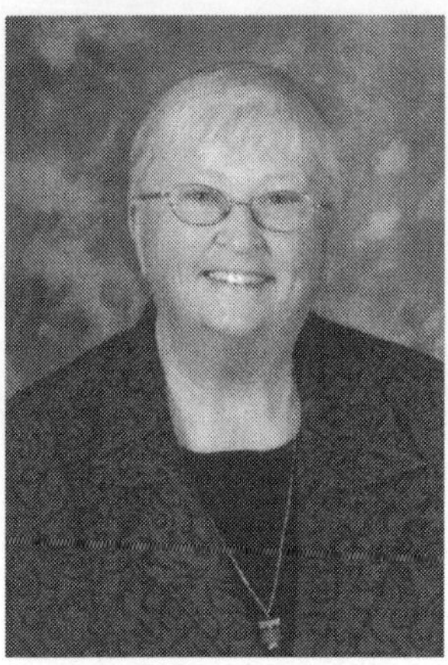

Courtesy of Sister Angela Murdaugh, CNM, FACNM

Birth date and place: September 1940, Little Rock, Arkansas

Current residence: San Antonio, Texas

Professional education:

- 1969: BSN, St. Louis University, Missouri
- 1970: FSM, Franciscan Sisters of Mary, St. Louis, Missouri
- 1971: MSN, Columbia University, New York
- 1981: Legislative internship with NETWORK, Washington, DC

Professional work life and honors:

- 1972–1980: Founded and directed a birth center within Su Clinica Familiar, Raymondville, Texas
- 1981–1983: President of American College of Nurse-Midwives (ACNM)
- 1984–2006: Founded and directed Holy Family Services and Birth Center, Weslaco, Texas
- One of the founders of Midwives Alliance of North America
- 1986–2002: Various offices (including president) within Consortium of Texas Certified Nurse-Midwives
- 1992: Recipient of Professional Achievement Award, National Association of Childbearing Centers (NACC)
- 2004–2006: Chair of the Texas ACNM chapter
- Midwifery faculty for many nurse-midwifery educational programs

(continued)

Personal involvement with the development of birth centers:

- Founded two of first birth centers in the United States
- NACC: Board member, 1983–1985, 1991–1993, 2001–2003; secretary, 1986–1987
- Participated in original development of NACC and the Birth Center Standards
- Site visitor for Commission for the Accreditation of Birth Centers (CABC)
- Chair of Birth Center Committee of the Consortium of Texas Certified Nurse-Midwives
- Worked with Texas Department of Public Health to write regulations for birth centers (1986), and revisions in 1997 and 2002

Birth Centers in the United States: Founding Midwives
Sandra Mae Perkins, CNM

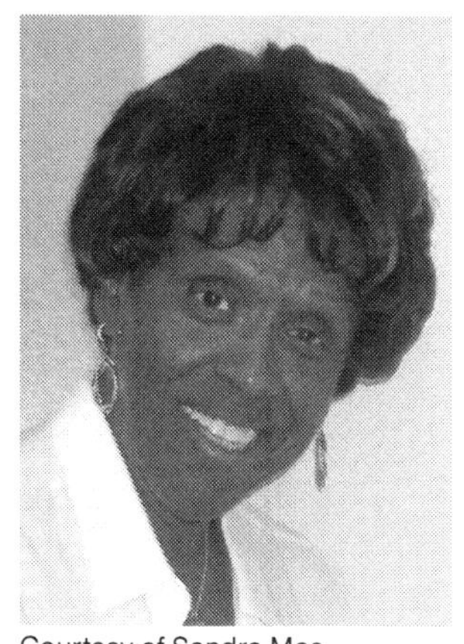

Courtesy of Sandra Mae Perkins, CNM

Birth date and place: 1944, Newport, Rhode Island

Current residence: Sacramento, California

Professional education:

- 1966: Diploma in Nursing, Newport Hospital School of Nursing, Rhode Island
- 1971: Diploma in Christian Education, Zion Bible Institute, Rhode Island
- 1974: Certificate in Nurse Midwifery, University of Mississippi
- 2003: AS in Pharmacy Technician, Western Career College, California

(continued)

Professional work life and honors:

- 1966–1968: RN, Sutter Memorial Hospital, California
- 1968–1971: RN, Sacramento County Hospital, California
- 1971–1973: RN, Newport Hospital, Rhode Island
- 1974–1976: Staff midwife, Delta Health Center, Mound Bayou, Mississippi
- 1975–1980: Mission work trips to various countries in Africa
- 1977–1982: Cofounder and director, McTammany Nurse-Midwifery Center, Reading, Pennsylvania
- 1982–1985: Assistant director of Cooperative Birth Center Network (CBCN)/National Association of Childbearing Centers (NACC), Perkiomenville, Pennsylvania
- 1988–2000: Project coordinator, University of California Davis Medical Center, OB/GYN Clinic, Sacramento, California
- 2015: Doctor of Humane Letters, Frontier Nursing University, Kentucky

Personal involvement with the development of birth centers:

- Director of one of the first birth centers in Pennsylvania
- Leadership role in the early development of the American Association of Birth Centers (AABC)
- Faculty: NACC's "How to Start a Birth Center" workshop
- Investigator: CBCN's birth center survey: The freestanding birth center (Bennetts & Lubic, 1982)
- Commissioner: CABC inaugural board

Birth Centers in the United States: Founding Midwife Susan Rutledge Stapleton, CNM

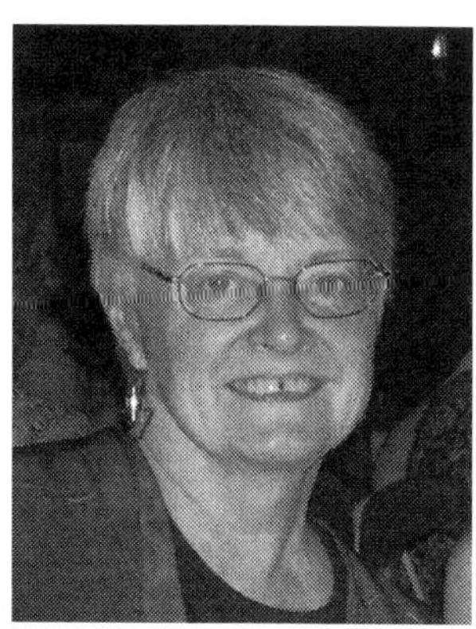

Courtesy of Susan Rutledge Stapleton, CNM

Birth date and place: 1947, Portland, Tennessee

Current residence: Kennebunk, Maine

Professional education:

- 1971: BSN, The Ohio State University
- 1975: MSN, Marquette University, Wisconsin
- 1984: Certificate in Midwifery, University of Medicine and Dentistry of New Jersey
- 2008: DNP, Frontier Nursing University

Professional work life and honors:

- 1984–1985: Staff midwife, McTammany Nurse-Midwifery Center, Pennsylvania
- 1985–2007: Founder, owner, director, Reading Birth and Women's Center, Pennsylvania
- 1988–1991: Development of curriculum for Community-Based Nurse-Midwifery Education Program, Frontier Nursing Service, Kentucky
- 1990–1993: Founder, director, St. Joseph Hospital Nurse-Midwifery Service, Reading, Pennsylvania
- 2000: Recipient of Professional Achievement Award, American Association of Birth Centers (AABC)
- 2008–2009: Director, Frontier School of Midwifery and Family Nursing Faculty Practice, Kentucky
- 2013–present: Data coordinator, Strong Start for Mothers and Newborns Initiative, AABC

(continued)

Personal involvement with the development of birth centers:

- Founded private practice birth center
- National Association of Childbearing Centers (NACC)/AABC
  - 1995–1999: President
  - 2005: Chair of Data Registry Task Force; development and monitoring of Perinatal Data Registry
  - 2005–present: Chair of Research Committee
  - Data coordinator, Strong Start for Mothers and Newborns Initiative
  - Author, *AABC Quality Assurance Manual*
  - Chair of Standards Committee
- The Commission for the Accreditation of Birth Centers (CABC)
  - 2004–2016: Commissioner
  - 2009–2015: President
  - 2015–2016: Clinical vice chair
- Research investigator
  - 1986–1989: National Study of Birth Centers, coinvestigator
  - 1994–2004: National Birth Center Vaginal Birth After Cesarean Study
  - 2007–2010: National Study of Birth Centers II, primary investigator

Other Champions of Birth Center Development

Boxes 1.1 and 1.2 present words of wisdom from founding midwives Ruth Watson Lubic and Kitty Ernst. Although this chapter has highlighted their accomplishments, and those of four other founding midwives of the birth center movement, their success did not happen in isolation. The history of the development of birth centers in the United States is one that rests on the work done by hundreds of people donating countless hours of their time and expertise: creating businesses, risking personal financial and political security, cultivating community relationships, changing state and federal regulations, creating and revising standards, serving on

BOX 1.1
Principles for a Successful Professional Life: Ruth Watson Lubic

- Begin with the needs of the people you serve, not your own needs or those of your profession, but those of the people
- Take care of all the people of the nation
- Trust your caring instincts
- Learn to tolerate uncertainty
- Choose your professional colleagues for their caring philosophy, not their professional preparation
- Be aware that the medical model has failed to serve all the people of the nation
- Avoid anger; it consumes energy and clouds your vision
- Avoid bitterness against political opponents
- Value the giving and receiving of truth
- Strengthen your sense of humor; it can neutralize opposition and brighten the darkest days
- Recognize the importance of persistence
- Base a design for change on the best science possible; then test your performance
- Overcome the fear associated with leadership
- Remember, the people you serve are your strength. Listen to them! You will be rewarded

Source: Lubic (1997)

BOX 1.2
Partial Transcript From Kitty Ernst's Acceptance Speech for the 1981 Martha May Elliot Award
American Public Health Association Convention
The Martha May Elliot award is granted annually in honor of exceptional and unusual achievement in the field of maternal child health

Most of what we know we have learned from parents. The subtle but critical differences between midwifery and obstetrics, between giving birth and being delivered, was taught to me by independent, clear thinking courageous Kentucky mountain women in the eloquent simplicity of their humble surroundings. . . .

Childbearing families are seeking a system of maternity care that is measured by the intellect but controlled by the heart. How do we keep what is good in the present system while we shed the unnecessary or even harmful parts as we move forward into new understandings? How do we bring together the interests of those who now have a monopoly on the maternity care dollar with those who should

(continued)

BOX 1.2 *(continued)*

be included in sharing that dollar? And how do we keep childbearing families from being caught in the crunch? How do we negotiate these components into a system that will continue to move forward to comprehensive maternity care for all . . . for all childbearing families? Everyday that we delay, we lose. Our delay has already created a desperation in an increasing number of families. I say desperation because *their* childbirth experience cannot wait. Their hopes and aspirations, for the most part derived from their personal investigations of scientific evidence supporting their desire for a natural birth and their careful weighing of benefits and hazards; *their* experience cannot wait for professions, politicians, products, profits, or processes to change.

Today a small but significant number of parents are taking responsibility of the management of care during pregnancy and birth into their own hands, they are making demands on the system, which if unmet by the system, they manage on their own with whatever help they can get. This is viewed by some to be very bad, even to the point of being declared child abuse. Yet all to whom we have spoken around the world, with whom we have worked across the nation, from whom we have learned in developing obstetrically safe and personally satisfying services, the absolute opposite is true. Universally, parents and the providers who have worked with them to take more responsibility in making their own decisions about their pregnancy, birth, and parenting speak in terms of greater knowledge, deeper understanding, profound experiences, intense positive interactions, accomplishments, achievements, acceptance, miracles, unifying forces at work, a sense of family. How can institutions and professions have such a dim view of birth that occurs outside of their setting and control, while those who are participating in it report such an exhilarating, light-filled experience? Could it be that we are missing something? We have before.

One of my most negative recollections in my experience in my work as a nurse-midwife is of the mothers who refused to have their boy babies circumcised. I was forced to force back the foreskin on their little penises a day or so after birth, all in the high and mighty name of cleanliness and science and whatever. But they knew better than I, for most of them didn't continue the procedure. But I, in the name of good care, intimidated them into allowing me to teach them to do it. And now we know that wasn't right at all. . . .

There is no real evidence that the place of birth in itself is a factor contributing to higher morbidity and mortality. We moved all birth into the disease-oriented setting of the hospital for the sake of the minority of women who might become obstetrically complicated. . . . We made this movement without ever studying the home as the place of birth, and we created new problems; *iatrogenic* and *nosocomial* are new words in our vocabulary. Could it be that we seize this opportunity to go with these parents who are opting for alternatives, and study the human

(continued)

BOX 1.2 *(continued)*

species in its natural habitat? It amazes me that we are threatened rather than thrilled that some young people view birth as a healthy normal life experience.

To me, if for no other reason, we should be interested in home birth and birth centers for reasons of science. In every other species known to man, naturalists of all disciplines go to extraordinary lengths to observe—not interfere, but observe—the reproduction of organisms from snails to elephants in their natural habitat, and many of these studies are federally funded! Yet the human species has never been so observed. In the name of science and the need for standardization, we have interfered with such delicate dynamics as maternal–newborn attachment. . . . It is no wonder parents are in protest; they understood. Every woman who ever asked or reached out for her baby at birth and was denied and intimidated by those who cared for her and knew so much about what was right, she understood that something died within her at that moment. Drs. Kennell and Klaus, under great stress and harassment from their colleagues, dared to look objectively and describe that consistent human attachment behavior that we now pedal as a commodity and call "bonding." What else do we not understand?

So although change is almost always presented as a process of simple evolution, it is never simple. It is never a single faceted activity. It is, however, frozen, forced, or facilitated by those in control. We, the providers, the planners, the protectors of the public health and welfare—in short, the professionals—we share to some extent the control that has the power to free the changes that are being explored, changes that hold the promise of humanistic principles of care, needed to control the temptation to technologicalize this little understood but definitely profound human experience. We have the power, for now at least, to force the masses of childbearing families to accept our mumbo jumbo whether it relates to pushing back a foreskin or putting on a fetal monitor, or we have the power to facilitate the ushering in of a new era in maternity care where we counsel rather than control and educate rather than intimidate. . . .

boards, and much, much more (see Table 1.3). Every state and many communities have their unsung heroes who were not acknowledged in this chapter; they too deserve celebration and honoring.

Before there was the evidence to demonstrate the safety of birth center care, before standards and quality assurance mechanisms were in place, and before the concepts of collaboration and interdisciplinary teams were popular, there were brave families who came to the birth centers, and colleagues who supported them. These people understood the commonsense approach that was the foundation of the early birth centers and are to be commended.

TABLE 1.3
Other Champions of the Birth Center Movement

Inaugural Board of Directors: National Association of Childbearing Centers (NACC); 1983

Name, Title	State	Notable Professional Work
Ruth Watson Lubic, CNM, EdD	New York	General Director, Maternity Center Association's (MCA) Childbearing Centers NYC
Philip Randolph Lee, MD, FACP	California	Director, Health Policy Program, School of Medicine, University of California, San Francisco
J. Robert Willson, MD, FACOG	New Mexico	Adjunct Professor, Obstetrics and Gynecology, University of New Mexico School of Medicine; Past President, American College of Obstetricians and Gynecologists
Anne Strickland Squadron, JD	New York	President, MCA board of directors
Phyllis R. Farley	New York	Chairman, MCA board of directors
Ann Anderson Legget	New York	MCA board of directors
Jane Leigh Powell	New York	Vice President, MCA board of directors
Louise H. Stephaich	New York	MCA board of directors
Alexandra Lally Peters	New York	MCA board of directors
George Silver, MD, FAAP	Connecticut	Professor of public health, Yale University
Edith Baldwin Wonnell, CNM	Pennsylvania	Founder, the birth center in Bryn Mawr, Pennsylvania, and the nurse-midwifery birthing center in Wilmington, Delaware
Paul A. Branca, MD, FAAP	Pennsylvania	Director of the Nurseries, Jefferson Medical College
Charles S. Mahan, MD, FACOG	Florida	Professor of Obstetrics and Gynecology, University of Florida, College of Medicine

(continued)

TABLE 1.3
Other Champions of the Birth Center Movement *(continued)*

Name, Title	State	Years of Service
Inaugural Board of Directors: National Association of Childbearing Centers (NACC); 1983		
Sister Angela Murdaugh, CNM	Texas	Founder, Su Clinica Familiar, Raymondville, Texas
Leon Warshaw, MD, FACP	New York	Founder and Executive Director, New York Business Group on Health

Name, Title	State	Years of Service
Presidents, Board of Directors: NACC/American Association of Birth Centers (AABC)		
Ruth Watson Lubic, CNM	New York	1983–1991
Marion McCartney, CNM	Maryland	1992–1994
Susan Rutledge Stapleton, CNM	Pennsylvania	1994–1998
Henry Maicki, MD	Michigan	1999–2002
Lylaine Gavette, CNM	Arizona	2003–2004
Jill Alliman, CNM	Tennessee	2004–2006
Cynthia Flynn, CNM	Washington	2007–2008
Linda Cole, CNM	Tennessee	2008–2012
Lesley Rathbun, CNM	South Carolina	2013–2017
Amy Johnson-Grass, ND, CPM	Minnesota	2016–2017 President Elect

Name, Title	State	Professional Work
Inaugural Board of Directors: Commission for the Accreditation of Birth Centers (CABC); 1987		
Eunice Cole, RN, Chair	Washington	President, American Nurses Association

(continued)

TABLE 1.3
Other Champions of the Birth Center Movement *(continued)*

Inaugural Board of Directors: Commission for the Accreditation of Birth Centers (CABC); 1987

Name, Title	State	Years of Service
Ann Scupholme, CNM	Florida	Director of Women's Health Services, Jackson Memorial Health Systems; founder of the first public hospital birth center
Gregory Lang, Obstetrician	Pennsylvania	Clinician, Allentown Birth Center Consultant
Jamie Bolane	Colorado	Childbirth educator/artist/owner, Childbirth Graphics
Mary Lou Longeway, RN	Michigan	Administrator, Southfield Birth Center
Richard Walker, Obstetrician	Texas	Clinician, organized first plan for franchise
Stanley Fisch, Pediatrician	Texas	Clinician, consultant to Holy Family Services
Solbritt Murphy, Pediatrician	New York	Director, Bureau of Maternal and Child Health
Sandra Perkins, CNM	Pennsylvania	Founder, McTammany Nurse-Midwifery Center

Inaugural Advisory Council: CABC; 1987

Name, Title	State	Professional Work
H. Robert Cathcart	Pennsylvania	President of Pennsylvania Hospital, chairman of the American Hospital Association, commissioner for Joint Commission on Accreditation of Hospitals
George Collentine, MD	Wisconsin	Surgeon
Carolyn Davis, RN PhD	Ohio	Administrator of Health Care Financing Administration, U.S. Department of Health and Human Services (HHS)

(continued)

TABLE 1.3
Other Champions of the Birth Center Movement *(continued)*

Inaugural Advisory Council: CABC; 1987		
Name, Title	**State**	**Years of Service**
Claire Fagin, RN PhD	Pennsylvania	Dean, University of Pennsylvania School of Nursing
Phyllis Leppert, MD, PhD	North Carolina	Director, Perinatal Research, Duke University Consultant to Rochester NY Birth Center
Vince Hutchins, MD	Maryland	Deputy Director of Maternal and Child Health Bureau, HHS
Stanley Peck	Washington, DC	Vice President, Health Insurance Association of America
George Reader, MD	New York	Professor of public health, Cornell University
Elizabeth Sharp, CNM, DrPH	Georgia	Professor of midwifery, Emory University

Chairperson or President: CABC		
Name, Title	**State**	**Years of Service**
Eunice Cole, RN	Washington, DC	1987–1990
Ann Scupholme, CNM	Florida	1991–1992
MaryLou Longeway, RN	Michigan	1993–1995
Catherine Head, CNM	Pennsylvania	1996–2000
Jean Douglas-Smith, RN	Iowa	2000–2002
Denise Roy, CNM	Pennsylvania	2003–2008
Susan Rutledge Stapleton, CNM	Pennsylvania	2009–2015
Dana Brown, CPM	Alaska	2015–2016
Ashton Osborne, RN	South Carolina	Newly elected chairperson
Jamie Hauser	Louisiana	Newly elected president

CNM, certified nurse-midwives; CPM, certified professional midwife; ND, naturopathic doctor.

Among this group of heroes are the inaugural boards and advisory councils of NACC and CABC, and the leadership within those organizations that continues to this day. They include powerful consumers and professionals who volunteered their time and expertise to the cause. This interdisciplinary foundation of the beginnings has remained a defining feature of both organizations and the national adoption of the birth center model.

The International Application of the Model

An unanticipated benefit of the origination of the birth center concept occurring in the United States, a country without a national health care system, was the independent creation of standards, policies, and systems of care for birth centers. What was rapidly developed by the birth center movement in the United States during the dynamic 1970s and 1980s provided guidance for other countries to adapt as part of or parallel to their national health care systems. The reader is referred to the Appendix in this book to learn about the history and current status of birth centers across the globe.

CONCLUSION AND LOOKING FORWARD

The history of the development of the birth center in the United States is worthy of an entire textbook or published doctoral dissertation. There are so many stories untold and individuals unsung. From the very beginning, there was a commitment to quality assurance and improvement, the provision and demonstration of cost-effective care and to providing extraordinary patient satisfaction, all long before these concepts became trendy as they are in today's health care arena. The small but mighty birth center movement is a demonstration of successful disruptive innovation.

The birth of innovation is a perceived need. The birth of the birth center concept in this country is rooted in local communities, where women seeking more control over their childbirth experience found health care providers who responded to that need. It has been a story of resiliency, a movement that often grew from a small group of passionate and dedicated people in communities across the nation. Parallel to the unfolding of birth centers locally was the national development of a professional trade organization. The AABC created standards and a mechanism for ensuring quality, secured payment for services, conducted research, and promoted legislation for appropriate regulation. Parallel to the development of birth centers in the United States has been the response of communities to similar needs in countries around the world. Across all of these spheres, the birth center model is a success story of interdisciplinary and interagency collaborations and commitment to the challenging work of initiating a cultural change. A chapter on history may suggest that the work has been done, but it has only begun.

REFERENCES

Albers, L., & Savitz, D. (1991). Hospital setting for birth and use of medical procedures in low risk women. *Journal of Midwifery, 36*, 327–333.

Alliman, J., Jolles, D., & Summers, L. (2015). The innovation imperative: Scaling freestanding birth centers, centering pregnancy and midwifery led-maternity homes. *Journal of Midwifery and Women's Health, 60*(3), 244–249.

American Association of Birth Centers. (2016a). An historical timeline. Retrieved from http://www.birthcenters.org/?page=history

American Association of Birth Centers. (2016b). Birth center standards. Retrieved from http://www.birthcenters.org/?page=Standards

American College of Nurse-Midwives, Midwives Alliance North America, & National Association of Certified Professional Midwives. (2013). Supporting healthy and normal physiologic childbirth: A consensus statement by ACNM, MANA, and NACPM. *Journal of Perinatal Education, 22*(1), 14–18.

American College of Nurse-Midwives. (2015). Leading midwifery organization releases updated clinical bulletin on home birth. Retrieved from http://www.midwife.org/Home-Birth-Clinical-Bulletin-Press-Release

American College of Obstetricians and Gynecologists. (2015). Obstetric care consensus: Levels of maternal care. Retrieved from http://www.acog.org/Resources-And-Publications/Obstetric-Care-Consensus-Series/Levels-of-Maternal-Care

American College of Obstetricians and Gynecologists. (2016). Committee opinion no. 669: Planned home birth. Retrieved from https://www.acog.org/-/media/Committee-Opinions/Committee-on-Obstetric-Practice/co669.pdf?dmc=1&ts=20160727T0416202794

Bennetts, A., & Lubic, R. W. (1982). The free-standing birth centre. *Lancet, 319*(8268), 378–380.

Berwick, D. M., Nolan, T. W., & Whittington, J. (2008). The triple aim: Care, health, and cost. *Health Affairs, 27*(3), 759–769. doi:10.1377/hlthaff.27.3.759

Canoodt, L., Sieverts, S., & Schachter, M. (1982). Alternatives to the conventional in-hospital delivery: The childbearing center experience. *Acta Hospitalita, 22*(4), 324–339.

Christensen, C. M., Bohmer, R., & Kenagy, J. (2000). Will disruptive innovators cure health care? *Harvard Business Review*. Retrieved from https://hbr.org/2000/09/will-disruptive-innovations-cure-health-care

Cockerham, A., & Keeling, A. (2010). Finance and faith at the Catholic Maternity Institute, Santa Fe, New Mexico, 1944–1969. *Nursing History Review, 18*, 151–166. doi:10.1891/1062–8061.18.151

Commission for the Accreditation of Birth Centers. (2016). Accredited birth centers. Retrieved from https://www.birthcenteraccreditation.org/find-accredited-birth-centers

Declercq, E., Sakala, C., Corry, M., Applebaum, S., & Herrlich, A. (2013). Listening to Mothers 111, New Mothers Speak Out. Retrieved from http://transform.childbirth-connection.org/wp-content/uploads/2013/06/LTM-III_NMSO.pdf

DeLee, R. (1915). Progress towards ideal obstetrics. *American Journal of Obstetrics, 73*, 407.

Devitt, N. (1977). The transition for home to hospital in the United States, 1930–1960. *Birth and Family Journal, 4*(2), 47–58.

Ernst, E. (1996). Midwifery, birth centers, and health care reform. *Journal of Obstetric, Gynecologic, and Neonatal Nursing, 25*, 433–439.

Ernst, K., & Bauer, K. (2016a). Birth centers in the United States. Retrieved from http://www.birthcenters.org/?page=history

Ernst, K., & Bauer, K. (2016b). The birth center experience. Retrieved from http://c.ymcdn.com/sites/www.birthcenters.org/resource/collection/028792A7-808D-4BC7-9A0F-FB038B434B91/1.TheBCExperience.pdf

Federal Trade Commission. (2004). Improving health care: a dose of competition: A report by the Federal Trade Commission and the Department of Justice. Retrieved from https://www.ftc.gov/reports/improving-health-care-dose-competition-report-federal-trade-commission-department-justice

Institute of Medicine. (1982). *Research issues in the assessment of birth settings*. Washington, DC: National Academies Press.

Institute of Medicine. (2013). An update on research issues in the assessment of birth settings-workshop summary. Retrieved from http://iom.nationalacademies.org/Reports/2013/An-Update-on-Research-Issues-in-the-Assessment-of-Birth-Settings.aspx

Johnson, K. (2013). Maternal-infant bonding: A review of the literature. *International Journal of Childbirth Education, 28*(3), 17–22.

Kroska, R. (2010). *History of nurse-midwifery in Santa Fe, New Mexico*. Self-Published.

Lieberman, E., Ernst, E. K., Rooks, J. P., Stapleton, S., & Flamm, B. (2004). Results of the national study of vaginal birth after cesarean in birth centers. *Obstetrics & Gynecology, 104*(5), 933–942.

Lubic, R. (1979). *Barriers and conflict in maternity care innovation* (Doctoral dissertation). Teacher's College Columbia University. Retrieved from http://www.worldcat.org/title/barriers-and-conflict-in-maternity-care-innovation/oclc/11347650/editions?referer=di&editionsView=true

Lubic, R. W. (1997). Principles for a successful professional life. *Journal of Midwifery & Women's Health, 42*(1), 53–58.

MacDorman, M. F., Matthews, M. S., & DeClercq, E. (2014). Trends in out-of-hospital births in the United States, 1990–2012. iNCHC Data Brief, No 144. Retrieved from https://www.cdc.gov/nchs/data/databriefs/db144.pdf

MacDorman, M. F., Matthews, T. J., Mohangoo, A. D., & Zeitlan, J. (2014). International comparisons of infant mortality and related factors: United States and Europe, 2010. *National Vital Statistics Reports, 63*(5), 1–6. Retrieved from https://www.ncbi.nlm.nih.gov/pubmed/25252091

Martin, J. A., Hamilton, B. E., Osterman, M. J., Driscoll, A. K., & Matthews, T. J. (2017). Births: Final data for 2015. *National Vital Statistics Report, 66*(1). Hyattsville, MD: National Center for Health Statistics.

Maternidad La Luz. (2016). History, Maternidad La Luz. Retrieved from http://www.maternidadlaluz.com/history.sstg

National Association of Certified Professional Midwives. (2014). Who are CPMs? Retrieved from http://nacpm.org/about-cpms/who-are-cpms/

National Hospice and Palliative Care Organization. (2016). Hospice: A historical perspective. Retrieved from http://www.nhpco.org/history-hospice-care

Ramirez, X. (Ed.). (1981). *10 years of health care: Su Clinica Familiar and family health services program*. Self-Published.

Romano, A. (2013). New opportunities for birth centers in transforming the health care system. *Journal of Midwifery and Women's Health, 58*(5), 492–493.

Romano, A. (2015). Why invest in maternity care innovation? Retrieved from http://maternityneighborhood.com/whitepapers/why-invest-in-maternity-care-innovation/

Rooks, J., Weatherby, N., Ernst, E., Stapleton, S., Rosen, D., & Rosenfeld, A. (1989). Outcomes of care in birth centers: The National Birth Center Study. *New England Journal of Medicine, 321*(26), 1804–1811.

Sakala, C., & Corry, M. (2008). Evidence-based maternity care: What is it and what can it achieve. *Milbank Memorial Fund report*. Retrieved from https://www.cdc.gov/nchs/data/databriefs/db144.pdf

Stapleton, S., Osborne, C., & Illuzzi, J. (2013). Outcomes of care in birth centers: Demonstration of a durable model. *Journal of Midwifery and Women's Health, 58*(1), 3–14.

Stone, S., Ernst, E., & Stapleton, S. (2016). The freestanding birth center: Evidence for change in the delivery of healthcare to childbearing families. In B. A. Anderson, J. P. Rooks, & R. Barroso (Eds.), *Best practice in midwifery: Using the evidence to implement change* (2nd ed., pp. 261–282). New York, NY: Springer Publishing.

The Farm Midwifery Center. (n.d.). Accommodations. Retrieved from http://www.thefarmmidwives.org/accommodation

Turkel, K. D. (1995). *Women, power, and childbirth: A case study of a free-standing birth center.* Westport, CT: Greenwood Publishing Group.

Varney, H., & Thompson, J. B. (2016). *A history of midwifery in the United States: The midwife said* fear not. New York, NY: Springer Publishing.

CHAPTER 2

Meeting the Need for Innovation in Maternity Care

DIANA R. JOLLES AND
PAULA PELLETIER-BUTLER

LEARNING OBJECTIVES

Upon completion of this chapter, the reader will be able to:

1. Evaluate the concepts of innovation and disruptive innovation as they relate to freestanding birth centers as the normative, Level 1 model of care for childbearing families in the United States
2. Explore how contemporary birth centers use the nine standards of the American Association of Birth Centers (AABC) as the basis for disruptive innovation

Innovation refers to new ideas, devices, or methods, or the acts or processes of introducing new ideas, devices, or methods. *Disruptive innovation* is the term used to explain how "complicated, expensive products and services are eventually converted into simpler, affordable ones" (Hwang & Christensen, 2007, p. 1329). Birth centers have been demonstrated to be a disruptive innovation, capable of enhancing population health, consumer experiences, and value (Alliman & Phillippi, 2016; Rooks et al., 1989; Stapleton, Osborne, & Illuzzi, 2013). Drivers of innovation within birth centers include adversity, social crisis, and necessity. Throughout this book, readers will explore how the context of care in the United States has driven the birth center as an innovation.

ADVERSITY DRIVES INNOVATION

Innovation is inspired by adversity. Beginning with the landmark Institute of Medicine's (IOM) reports *Crossing the Quality Chasm* (2001) and *To Err Is Human* (2000), the national quality movement in the United States is aligned around the Triple Aim to improve the patient experience of care and improve population health, while reducing per capita cost (Berwick, Nolan, & Whittington, 2008; IOM, 2000, 2001). The mounting pressure to improve quality and decrease waste while reducing costs and increasing value is coming from multiple sectors of the health care system: consumers, providers, administrators, policy makers, and third-party payers (Carter et al., 2010; Howard & Jolles, 2015; Sakala & Corry, 2008).

The staggering U.S. outcome statistics for newborns and women who give birth is inspiration enough to unearth alternative solutions. In many parts of the United States, a woman has essentially one in three chances of having a cesarean birth just by walking through the hospital door, and in a few places almost one in two chances (Table 2.1; Kozhimannil, Law, & Virnig, 2013). Cesarean section is an endorsed quality measure capable of detecting system-level quality defects (Main et al., 2006). The World Health Organization and *Healthy People 2020* both place cesarean benchmarks well below our current national rate. Birth centers have demonstrated the ability to exceed benchmarks across geographical, political, and contextual barriers over the past 40 years (Table 2.1; Alliman & Phillippi, 2016; Rooks et al., 1989; Stapleton et al., 2013).

Significant variation in the quality of health care in the United States is driven by nonmedical determinants rather than the needs and preferences of the population (Fisher, Goodman, Skinner, & Bronner, 2009). Facilities are independent drivers of cesarean and decreased breastfeeding rates (Clark, Belfort, Hankins, Meyers, & Houser, 2007; Corallo et al., 2014; Gregory, Ramicone, Chan, & Kahn, 1999; Howell, Richardson, Ginsburg, & Foot, 2002; Kogan, Singh, Dee, Belanoff, & Grummer-Strawn, 2008; Kozhimannil et al., 2013; Dartmouth Atlas Project, 2007). Variation in provider type is a known driver of cesarean birth (Clark et al., 2007; Sandall, Soltani, Gates, Shennan, & Devane, 2015). Healthy childbearing women at low medical risk have demonstrated a greater sensitivity to unwarranted variations in care that decrease quality and drive cost increases (Kozhimannil et al., 2013).

TABLE 2.1
Disparities in Health Equity

Race	U.S. Birth Certificates 2013[1] 3,957,577	All AABC Strong Start Site Births 2012–2014 3,036 total	AABC Strong Start Site Births Low Medical Risk at Onset of Labor 2012–2014 2,082 total
Nulliparous Term Vertex Singleton Cesarean			
Non-Hispanic White	1,025,012 (25.9%)	110 (13.4%)	34 (6.9%)
Non-Hispanic Black	1,218,933 (30.8%)	19 (16.2%)	9 (10.8%)
Hispanic	1,052,715 (26.6%)	33 (13.7%)	21 (11.1%)
Any Breastfeeding			
Race	**CDC National Immunization Survey 2012[2] *n* = 15,141**	**AABC PDR Medicaid Births *n* = 3,136**	**Low Medical Risk *n* = 2,082**
Hispanic	2,788 (82.4%)	374 (94.7%)	271 (96.1%)
Non-Hispanic White	8,811 (83.0%)	1,221 (95.8%)	781 (95.8%)
Non-Hispanic Black	1,476 (66.4%)	130 (92.2%)	112 (97.4%)
Non-Hispanic Asian	683 (83.2%)	16 (94.1%)	20 (100%)
Non-Hispanic American Indian Alaska Native	217 (71.5%)	16 (94.1%)	13 (100%)

AABC, American Association of Birth Centers; CDC, Centers for Disease Control and Prevention; PDR, Perinatal Data Registry.

[1]Martin et al. (2015).

[2]CDC (2011, 2016).

SOCIAL CRISIS DRIVES INNOVATION

Throughout history, the solving of a crisis has always been a tangible driver of innovation. The ongoing, persistent promulgation of racial and ethnic disparities coupled with unreliable quality of the health care system takes the urgency of the call for innovation to a critical level. Lack of equity in maternity care and the resulting disparity has reached epic proportions (see Table 2.1). Institutionalized racism and the privilege of the medical system is a known driver of racial disparity and inequity (Agency for Healthcare Research and Quality, 2015; Markus & Rosenbaum, 2010; Robbins et al., 2014).

Preliminary data from the AABC's Strong Start for Mothers and Newborns initiative project demonstrates a protective effect of birth center care against racial disparity, demonstrating superior outcomes on core national quality measures, including nulliparous term vertex singleton cesarean and breastfeeding (Jolles, 2016; Table 2.1). The data out of the AABC Strong Start sites is important because it demonstrates a diverse population, which mirrors the national sociodemographic profile. AABC's Strong Start is a free program funded by Centers for Medicare and Medicaid Services (CMS) providing support and services to women who qualify. Statistically significant racial variations of intention to breastfeed occurred upon entry to care within the Strong Start site birth centers, with significantly more non-Hispanic White women intending to breastfeed upon entry to care. However, on admission in labor, these differences in breastfeeding intention disappeared as a result of the model of care. There were no statistically significant racial variations in breastfeeding on discharge. Women and newborns cared for within the AABC Medicaid sample used less formula among breastfed infants in the first 2 days of life; the rate of exclusive breastfeeding was increased on discharge, 18% higher than national benchmarks and 52% higher than the national average. When compared to the nationally reported data on breastfeeding from the Centers for Disease Control and Prevention (CDC) National Immunization Survey, birth center Strong Start sites far exceeded national performance across racial groups. The perinatal episode of care within the birth center model has been demonstrated to produce superior outcomes for breastfeeding, decrease disparity, increase equity, and improve population health.

There is agreement among many midwifery organizations that birth center care may be one of the most plausible solutions to the racial disparities surrounding birth, particularly when providers of the same race and ethnicity serve their communities. Midwives and birth workers of color and members of the National Association of Birth Centers of Color are working hard to employ innovative solutions to address these disparities with encouraging results. The AABC's own Strong Start program is also documenting progress in the 40+ birth centers that are providing this level of care. Racial disparities surrounding birth require a strong call to action with a variety of innovative approaches, and although there is no quick fix, the tangible crusade for solutions on a national level is a reason for hope.

NECESSITY DRIVES INNOVATION

Innovation is also born out of necessity. According to the American Association of Medical Colleges (AAMC), the total demand for physicians is projected to grow up to 17% with significant shortages projected by 2025 due to the aging population and overall population growth. The AAMC projects that by 2025 there will be a shortage of up to 12,300 "medical specialists" and up to 20,200 "other specialists" (Dall, West, Chakrabarti, & Lacobucci, 2016). At first glance, we can correlate this information to conclude that we need more midwives. In addition, consumers will be forced to look beyond the more traditional approach to the physician/inpatient-based health care system due to the projected lack of physicians. The outpatient, often home-like environment of the birth center provides communities with specialty provider care in a proven safe environment.

DISRUPTIVE INNOVATION: LEVEL 1 CARE FOR ALL

Birth centers are poised to fulfill the Triple Aim as the demonstration model for "Level 1" care for childbearing families in the United States. In 2014, the American College of Obstetricians and Gynecologists (ACOG) and Society for Maternal-Fetal Medicine released an Obstetric Care Consensus statement, detailing "Levels of Maternal Care" (Obstetric Care Consensus no. 1: Safe Prevention of the Primary Cesarean Delivery, 2014). One of the purposes of the statement was to foster the development and equitable distribution of maternal care systems, which promote risk-appropriate care.

According to the latest evidence, the majority of childbearing women in the United States are at low medical risk, suggesting that the health care delivery system should reliably provide access to integrated, evidence-based, Level 1 care (Carter et al., 2010; Robbins et al., 2014). Rather than having access to family-centered, home-like environments, it is well known that the predominant model of labor and delivery in the United States resembles "an intensive care unit" (Shah, 2015, p. 2182). In 2016, the conversation regarding "risk-appropriate" care has been largely predominated by the appropriate care for high-risk women (Korst et al., 2015). The lack of risk-appropriate care for the majority of childbearing women, who are at low medical risk, is not well appreciated (Institute of Medicine [IOM] and National Research Council [NRC], 2013).

Level 1 care is a high-value care model, although commonly presented within the hierarchical description of the levels of care as a "low" level of care (Korst et al., 2015; Menard et al., 2015). Instead, birth centers offer enhanced care services, family-centered care, and a system well designed to refer to a higher level of care when appropriate. The birth center model of care is designed to engage consumers in life-course care, addressing the social determinants of health that are understood to influence 80% of health outcomes (Howell, Palmer, Benatar, & Garrett, 2014; Lubic & Flynn, 2010).

THE STRUCTURE AND PROCESS OF INNOVATION

In order for the birth center model to spread, it must maintain the effective components of the model of care, while adapting to the requirements of the local political and professional community: adherence to the nine American Association of Birth Center standards (Table 2.2; see Chapter 8). Midwife and nonmidwife entrepreneurs recognize the social and economic imperative of introducing the birth center innovation to more and more communities across the United States. Adherence to the model is best preserved through achieving accreditation through the Commission for the Accreditation of Birth Centers (CABC). Accreditation is an essential component of the structure of innovation, moving the birth center model to scale and the innovative and normative Level 1 care for the majority of childbearing families in the United States (Alliman, Jolles, & Summers, 2015).

Throughout the book, readers will be exposed to innovation within the AABC standards (Table 2.2). Birth centers are using community participatory design to engage communities in the planning of services, evaluation of care, and design of culturally humble care delivery. Community-based planning is an ongoing and continuous process and the root of disruptive innovation. Readers will explore a variety of legal entities and business and administrative structures used to support birth center growth. From sole proprietors through partnerships with federally qualified health centers, birth centers have adapted to the unique opportunities within each community to support viable and creative business models. Birth facilities and staff drive cost in the United States. Throughout the book, readers will explore how birth centers provide an

TABLE 2.2
Innovation Exemplars Linked to AABC Birth Standards

American Association of Birth Centers Standard	Innovation Exemplars
Planning: The birth center assesses the needs of the childbearing community in developing services and programs.	Community participatory design, "Friends of the Birth Center," community advocacy partnerships, ongoing and regular needs assessments, community owners, community board of directors
Organization: The birth center is a legally constituted organization with a governing body that establishes policy, lines of responsibility, and accountability.	Various business entities: Sole proprietors, LLC, Inc., 501 (c) 3, federally qualified health centers
Administration: The birth center is administered according to the mission, goals, and policies of the governing body in a manner that assures financial viability while producing high-quality services responsive to the needs of the population being served.	Small business, large community health center, and corporate models; centralized and decentralized administration; varied financing models including 100% of revenue based on billed services and blended models of billed revenue and grants; cash only models
Facility, equipment, and supplies: The birth center establishes and maintains a safe, home-like environment for healthy women with space for furnishings, equipment, and supplies.	Homes to office buildings; rented and owned; Jacuzzi spas prevalent; accessible kitchens and family space, traditional beds, necessary medical supplies readily available and not immediately visible
Quality of services: The birth center provides high-quality, family-centered, maternal and newborn services.	Evidence-based care, benchmarking, guidelines, and protocols; Commission for the Accreditation of Birth Centers; consumer satisfaction surveys; team quality improvement meetings, drills, quarterly reviews

(continued)

TABLE 2.2
American Association of Birth Centers Standards and Innovation *(continued)*

American Association of Birth Centers Standard	Innovation Exemplars
Staffing and personnel: High-quality, family-centered maternal and newborn care is provided by qualified professional and clinical staff with access to and availability of consulting clinical specialists.	Midwifery-led, CPMs, CMs, CNMs, RNs, doulas, community health workers, massage therapy, acupuncture, naturopaths, collaborative perinatologists, obstetricians, family practice physicians; certified coders and billers; outsourced billing specialists
The health record: Health records of the birth center provide a format for continuity and documentation of maternal and newborn information readily accessible to health care practitioners.	Midwifery-designed programs, such as Maternity Neighborhood, Private Practice, and Mobile Midwife; consumer portals and education, interoperable data systems; patient portals; shared decision-making tools
Evaluation of quality of care: There is an established program for evaluating the quality of direct care services to childbearing families, with an organizational plan to identify and resolve problems.	Quality assurance and quality improvement structure, use of the AABC Perinatal Data Registry, regular team quality meetings and debriefings, simulation, rapid cycle improvement, and root cause analysis programs

AABC, American Association of Birth Centers; CMs, certified midwives; CNMs, certified nurse-midwives; CPMs, certified professional midwives.

innovative, high-value alternative to hospital facilities offering enhanced access to interprofessional and diverse staff as well as aesthetically pleasing, nonmedicalized environments. These innovations increase consumer opportunities for holistic, noninterventive care while providing increased access to therapeutic hydrotherapy, family spaces, kitchen access, and outdoor space, all while saving money.

In 2011, the IOM hosted a series of workshops on innovation, "The Healthcare Imperative: Lowering Costs and Improving Outcomes: Workshop Series Summary" (Yong, Saunders, & Olsen, 2010). The document provides a road map for birth centers on the road to disruptive innovation. According to the IOM, innovation will occur only by decreasing unnecessary services (e.g., services beyond the evidence base) and inefficient delivery of services (e.g., inappropriate use of provider specialties). Some highlights of appropriate use of providers include the following examples.

Midwife-Led Care

Midwifery care, by its very design, is an innovative approach that utilizes person-centered care; longer prenatal visits providing time for questions, emotional support, and continuity of care; increased satisfaction by the woman and her family; and lower costs. Midwives of all credentials have been the slow and steady innovators of a better birth experience for decades no matter the birth setting: hospital, birth center, or home. Midwives are the pioneers of birth innovation that continues to happen every single day, one birth at a time across the United States.

Collaborative Staffing Models

More and more birth centers are using the talents and expertise of midwives with various credentials for an innovative collaborative practice. Neither the Accreditation Commission for Midwifery Education nor the American Midwifery Certification Board, the educational accreditation body and the regulatory board responsible for CNM/CM education and practice, requires out-of-hospital birth clinical experience. Out-of-hospital births require a different skill set that is distinct from hospital or obstetric practice protocols; there are nuances to that care that can only be learned through regular out-of-hospital experience. Conversely, most licensed midwives (LMs)/CPMs have not attended hospital births or experienced higher risk births, providing an increased awareness of emergent conditions and a broader perspective on what is normal. Also, most LMs/CPMs do not learn clinical pharmacology, leading to a limited formulary, and do not currently have prescriptive authority in any state.

There are certain elements in the education of these two different-but-similar clinicians that have the potential to be complementary to one another. Blending these two credentials in a birth center allows for interdisciplinary partnerships that benefit the providers professionally as well as the families they serve. Adding physicians, whether allopathic or naturopathic, can add yet another collaborative element to the team (see Chapter 7).

Doulas

Ancient innovation in modern times is one way to describe the doula. Some birth centers employ doulas, whereas others simply have a referral network for their clients to seek out if desired. Doulas are known to lower cesarean rates, decrease use of anesthesia, influence labor duration, and increase women's satisfaction with the birthing experience.

Complementary Practitioners

In many parts of the United States, integrative care providers such as naturopathic physicians, chiropractic physicians, acupuncturists, massage therapists, aromatherapists, and more are specializing in women's health and pregnancy/postpartum. Many of these practitioners are seeking referrals or collaborations from the birth center community. There is still a paucity of research on the efficacy of some of the methods used by these practitioners, but interest is growing and the well-informed provider can give some insight and recommendations to the birth center client, particularly when the other practitioners are a part of the birth center practice (see Chapter 11).

Acupuncture during pregnancy has been shown to decrease musculoskeletal pain, nausea, and other digestive disorders such as constipation or heartburn. Acupuncture and moxibustion have also been studied in relationship to fetal presentation, with the most notable success in shifting breech to cephalic presentation. Many also turn to acupuncture for labor induction or augmentation. Although the research remains inconclusive, having an acupuncturist as a part of the team can be utilized as another potential tool in the toolbox for women who may be open to this integrative therapy.

CONCLUSION

Crisis, necessity, and disruption lead to creativity and innovation. Urgent quality issues coupled with a health care financing system at the breaking point will force a restructuring of the maternity care system in the United States. Real innovation will come when health care systems broadly adopt the community-based birth center model of care for the majority of pregnant women. Integrating birth centers in the health care system can provide high-quality, individualized services that lead to better birth outcomes for all women in the United States.

REFERENCES

Agency for Healthcare Research and Quality. (2015). *2014 national healthcare quality and disparities report* (No. 15-0007). Rockville, MD: Author.

Alliman, J., Jolles, D., & Summers, L. (2015). The innovation imperative: Scaling freestanding birth centers, CenteringPregnancy, and midwifery-led maternity health homes. *Journal of Midwifery and Women's Health, 60*(3), 244–249. doi:10.1111/jmwh.12320

Alliman, J., & Phillippi, J. C. (2016). Maternal outcomes in birth centers: An integrative review of the literature. *Journal of Midwifery and Women's Health, 61*(1), 21–51. doi:10.1111/jmwh.12356

American College of Obstetricians and Gynecologists, Society for Maternal Fetal Medicine. (2014). Obstetric Care Consensus No. 1. Safe prevention of the primary cesarean delivery. *Obstetrics and Gynecology, 123*(3), 693–711. doi:10.1097/01.AOG.0000444441.04111.1d

Berwick, D. M., Nolan, T. W., & Whittington, J. (2008). The Triple Aim: Care, health, and cost. *Health Affairs, 27*(3), 759. doi:10.1377/hlthaff.27.3.759

Carter, M. C., Corry, M., Delbanco, S., Foster, T. C., Friedland, R., Gabel, R., . . . Simpson, K. R. (2010). 2020 vision for a high-quality, high-value maternity care system. *Women's Health Issues, 20*(1), S7–S17. doi:10.1016/j.whi.2009.11.006

Center for Disease Control and Prevention. (2014). Breastfeeding report card, United States 2014. Retrieved from https://www.cdc.gov/breastfeeding/pdf/2014breastfeedingreportcard.pdf

Center for Disease Control and Prevention. (2016). NIS survey methods. Retrieved from http://www.cdc.gov/breastfeeding/data/nis_data/survey_methods.htm

Clark, S. L., Belfort, M. A., Hankins, G., Meyers, J. A., & Houser, F. M. (2007). Variation in the rates of operative delivery in the United States. *American Journal of Obstetrics & Gynecology, 196*(6), 526.e1–526.e5. doi:10.1016/j.ajog.2007.01.024

Corallo, A. N., Croxford, R., Goodman, D. C., Bryan, E. L., Srivastava, D., & Stukel, T. A. (2014). A systematic review of medical practice variation in OECD countries. *Health Policy (Amsterdam, Netherlands), 114*(1), 5–14. doi:10.1016/j.healthpol.2013.08.002

Dall, T., West, T., Chakrabarti, R., & Lacobucci, W. (2016). IHS Inc., *The Complexities of Physician Supply and Demand: Projections from 2013 to 2025.* Washington, DC: Association of American Medical Colleges.

Dartmouth Atlas Project: Center for Evaluative Clinical Sciences. (2007). Effective care: A Dartmouth Atlas Project topic brief. Retrieved from http://www.dartmouthatlas.org/downloads/reports/effective_care.pdf

Fisher, E. S., Goodman, D. C., Skinner, J., & Bronner, K. (2009). *Health care spending, quality and outcomes: More isn't always better.* The Dartmouth Institute for Policy and Clinical Practice. Retrieved from http://www.dartmouthatlas.org/downloads/reports/Spending_Brief_022709.pdf

Gregory, K. D., Ramicone, E., Chan, L., & Kahn, K. L. (1999). Cesarean deliveries for Medicaid patients: A comparison in public and private hospitals in Los Angeles county. *American Journal of Obstetrics & Gynecology, 180*(5), 1177–1184. doi:10.1016/S0002-9378(99)70613-7

Howard, E., & Jolles, D. (2015). Navigating the perinatal quality landscape. *Journal of Perinatal and Neonatal Nursing, 29*(2), 116–129. doi:10.1097/JPN.0000000000000092

Howell, E., Palmer, A., Benatar, S., & Garrett, B. (2014). Potential Medicaid cost savings from maternity care based at a freestanding birth center. *Medicare and Medicaid Research Review, 4*(3), 1–13. doi:10.5600/mmrr.004.03.a06

Howell, E. M., Richardson, D., Ginsburg, P., & Foot, B. (2002). Deregionalization of neonatal intensive care in urban areas. *American Journal of Public Health, 92*(1), 119–124. doi:10.2105/AJPH.92.1.119

Hwang, J., & Christensen, D. M. (2007). Disruptive innovation in health care delivery: A framework for business-model innovation. *Health Affairs, 27*(5), 1329–1335.

Institute of Medicine. (2000). *To err is human: Building a safer health system.* Washington, DC: National Academies Press.

Institute of Medicine. (2001). *Crossing the quality chasm: A new health system for the 21st century.* Washington, DC: National Academies Press.

Institute of Medicine and National Research Council. (Ed.). (2013). *An update on research issues in the assessment of birth settings: Workshop summary.* Washington, DC: National Academies Press.

Jolles, D. (2016). *Care processes and outcomes of childbearing Medicaid beneficiaries* (Unpublished doctoral dissertation). Texas Woman's University, Denton, TX.

Kogan, M. D., Singh, G. K., Dee, D. L., Belanoff, C., & Grummer-Strawn, L. (2008). Multivariate analysis of state variation in breastfeeding rates in the United States. *American Journal of Public Health, 98*(10), 1872–1880. doi:10.2105/AJPH.2007.127118

Korst, L. M., Feldman, D. S., Bollman, D. L., Fridman, M., El, H. I., Fink, A., & Gregory, K. D. (2015). Cross-sectional survey of California childbirth hospitals: Implications for defining maternal levels of risk-appropriate care. *American Journal of Obstetrics & Gynecology, 213*(4), 527.e1–527.e12. doi:10.1016/j.ajog.2015.07.014

Kozhimannil, K., Law, M. R., & Virnig, B. A. (2013). Cesarean delivery rates vary tenfold among US hospitals; reducing variation may address quality and cost issues. *Health Affairs, 32*(3), 527–535. doi:10/1377/hlthaff.2012.1030

Lubic, R., & Flynn, C. (2010). The family health and birth center: A nurse-midwife-managed center in Washington, DC. *Alternative Therapies in Health and Medicine, 16*(5), 58.

Main, E. K., Moore, D., Farrell, B., Schimmel, L. D., Altman, R. J., Abrahams, C., . . . Sterling, J. (2006). Is there a useful cesarean birth measure? Assessment of the nulliparous term singleton vertex cesarean birth rate as a tool for obstetric quality improvement. *American Journal of Obstetrics & Gynecology, 194*(6), 1644–1651. doi:10.1016/j.ajog.2006.03.013

Markus, A. R., & Rosenbaum, S. (2010). The role of Medicaid in promoting access to high-quality, high-value maternity care. *Women's Health Issues: Official Publication of the Jacobs Institute of Women's Health, 20*(1 Suppl.), S67–S78. doi:10.1016/j.whi.2009.11.012

Martin, J. A., Hamilton, B. E., Osterman, M. J. K., Curtin, S. C., & Mathews, T. J. (2015). Births: Final data for 2013. *National Vital Statistics Reports, 64*(1). Retrieved from http://www.cdc.gov/nchs/data/nvsr/nvsr64/nvsr64_01.pdf

Menard, M. K., Kilpatrick, S., Saade, G., Hollier, L. M., Joseph, G. F., Jr., Barfield, W., . . . Conry, J. (2015). Levels of maternal care. *American Journal of Obstetrics & Gynecology, 212*(3), 259–271. doi:10.1016/j.ajog.2014.12.030

Robbins, C. L., Zapata, L. B., Farr, S. L., Kroelinger, C. D., Morrow, B., Ahluwalia, I., . . . Barfield, W. D. (2014). Core state preconception health indicators—pregnancy risk assessment monitoring system and behavioral risk factor surveillance system, 2009. *Morbidity and Mortality Weekly Report. Surveillance Summaries, 63*(3), 1–62. Retrieved from https://www.cdc.gov/mmwr/preview/mmwrhtml/ss6303a1.htm

Rooks, J. P., Weatherby, N. L., Ernst, E. K. M., Stapleton, S., Rosen, D., & Rosenfield, A. (1989). Outcomes of care in birth centers: The national birth center study. *New England Journal of Medicine, 321*(26), 1804–1811. Retrieved from doi:10.1056/NEJM198912283212606

Sakala, C., & Corry, M. P. (2008). Achieving the Institute of Medicine's six aims for improvement in maternity care. *Women's Health Issues: Official Publication of the Jacobs Institute of Women's Health, 18*(2), 75–78. doi:10.1016/j.whi.2007.12.001

Sandall, J., Soltani, H., Gates, S., Shennan, A., & Devane, D. (2015). Midwife-led continuity models versus other models of care for childbearing women. *The Cochrane Database of Systematic Reviews, 9,* CD004667. doi:10.1002/14651858.CD004667.pub4

Shah, N. (2015). A NICE delivery—the cross-Atlantic divide over treatment intensity in childbirth. *New England Journal of Medicine, 372*(23), 2181–2183. doi:10.1056/NEJMp1501461

Stapleton, S. R., Osborne, C., & Illuzzi, J. (2013). Outcomes of care in birth centers: Demonstration of a durable model. *Journal of Midwifery and Women's Health, 58*(1), 3–14. doi:10.1111/jmwh.12003

Yong, P. L., Saunders, R. S., & Olsen, L. (2010). The healthcare imperative: Lowering costs and improving outcomes: Workshop series summary. Washington, DC: National Academies Press. Retrieved from https://www.nap.edu/read/12750/chapter/1

CHAPTER 3

The Contemporary Birth Center as Part of an Integrated Care Model

LINDA J. COLE

LEARNING OBJECTIVES

Upon completion of this chapter, the reader will be able to:

1. Describe two models of categorizing perinatal care
2. Explain how the birth center model fits into an integrated care model
3. Discuss the ideal transfer of care from the birth center setting

Freestanding birth centers began to open in the 1970s, largely in response to women's desire for more control in their birth environment. Publications such as *Our Bodies Ourselves* (Boston Women's Health Book Collective, 1976), *Immaculate Deception* (Arms, 1979), and *Spiritual Midwifery* (Gaskin, 1980) brought new inspiration and awareness to women who desired to play a larger role in their own health decisions. These decisions intersected with a wave of antiestablishment sentiment among youth who were actively rejecting war as well as the overarching political, educational, and medical systems. Emerging from the counterculture of this time period was a model of care for birth that sought to take birth out of the medical model in the hospital and embrace a social model for birth in a new kind of facility called the freestanding birth center.

The increase in the number of birth centers in recent years has brought this model of care to the attention of more health care providers, legislators, policy makers, and consumers. In the decade between 2004 and 2014, the number of births occurring in freestanding birth centers doubled from 23% of all out-of-hospital births in 2004 to 46% in 2014 (MacDorman & Declercq,

2016). The expansion and success of this innovative model of care has led to health care systems and birth centers working together in ways that are mutually beneficial. More importantly, the integration of health systems and birth centers ultimately benefits families and communities by placing the woman at the center of care and providing the most appropriate level of care for each individual woman.

In this chapter, two models for defining levels of care are introduced. The first model, risk-based care, has been the prevalent model for decades. A more recent model based on appropriate levels of care, including birth center care, is also explored. Coordination of services between levels of care, and integrating the birth center into a larger system of care delivery, is examined. Within this framework, it is possible to understand how creating and maintaining a cooperative environment and facilitating efficient and safe transfer of patients between levels and systems can be achieved.

DEFINING THE FREESTANDING BIRTH CENTER

The American Association of Birth Centers (AABC), the nation's foremost authority on birth centers, defines the freestanding birth center as a "home-like facility existing within a health care system with a program of care designed in the wellness model of pregnancy and birth. Birth centers are guided by principles of prevention, sensitivity, safety, appropriate medical intervention, and cost effectiveness. Birth centers provide family-centered care for healthy women before, during and after normal pregnancy, labor and birth" (AABC, n.d.). The U.S. federal government defines the freestanding birth center as "a health facility that is not a hospital or physician's office, where childbirth is planned to occur away from the pregnant woman's residence that is licensed or otherwise approved by the state to provide prenatal, labor and delivery, or postpartum care and other ambulatory services that are included in the plan" (Patient Protection and Affordable Care Act, 2010).

A freestanding birth center is a facility separate from acute obstetric/newborn care with autonomy in formulation of policy and management of operation (AABC, n.d.). A birth center may be located in a house, a medical office setting, or within a hospital, as long as it functions separate and apart from the acute care setting traditionally housed in the labor and delivery unit, with accoutrements such as labor inductions, epidurals, and surgical capability. Various providers deliver primary care within the birth center facility including licensed midwives (LMs), certified professional midwives (CPMs), certified nurse-midwives/certified midwives (CNMs/CMs), and physicians.

More important than the physical setting, or who provides care in freestanding birth centers, are the elements of the model of care. A recent consensus document defines birth center care as "peripartum care of low-risk women with uncomplicated singleton term pregnancies with a vertex presentation who are expected to have an uncomplicated birth" (Menard et al., 2015, p. 261). Additionally, philosophical elements of the birth center model of care include care of the low-risk woman and infant, support for pregnancy and birth as a normal physiologic process supported within the midwifery model of care, and high value placed on family-centered care. Inclusion of the woman's family and chosen support person(s) is an important element of birth center care. The birth center is a place where partners and children are welcomed regularly at prenatal visits, as well as during birth and the postpartum period. There are provisions made for the family's comfort during labor and birth, including a family room or living room and a food preparation area or kitchen. Common hospital policies limiting nutritional intake and freedom of movement are starkly absent in the birth center setting. The woman does not lose her identity by trading in her clothing for a hospital gown, and is able to transform the environment of the birth room—through decorations, pictures, music, and aromas—into a space that brings her a sense of comfort and safety. In Chapter 11, the impacts of these elements of birth center care on physiologic birth are explored in more depth.

MODELS OF CATEGORIZING CARE

Two models that categorize the care of pregnant women in the United States are the risk model and the levels of maternal care model. The purpose of categorizing the levels of care of pregnant women is to make the best effort to deliver the most appropriate care for the individual patient based on health status, care provider, and facility capabilities. Treatment intensity can then be tailored to the clinical presentation of each patient. The focus of the risk model is toward the fetus and newborn, whereas the focus in the levels of care model is on the parturient, or woman receiving care, and the most appropriate facility for her perinatal care, given her unique set of medical and social circumstances.

Risk Assessment

Risk assessment, or the practice of assigning a level of risk to an individual patient, has become a routine practice in the care of pregnant women over the past century. This has led to a more medicalized model of childbirth for the majority of childbearing women in this country, regardless of actual health status (Jordan & Murphy, 2009). Although no uniformly applied assessment tool exists, this systematic practice helps providers in decision making regarding antepartum testing and fetal surveillance. Routine testing, such as screening for gestational diabetes, and obtaining the patient's blood pressure and weight at every visit are ways in which providers identify risk in pregnancy. Certain disease states in pregnancy such as gestational diabetes or preeclampsia place women and their fetuses at risk for poorer outcomes than women identified to have an absence of disease, and risk assessment can help to identify the appropriate provider and place of birth.

It is generally accepted that only women without significant risk factors should be under the care of midwives in birth centers, although in some birth centers there is a collaborative care model allowing for a portion of the pregnancy or birth experience to be under the care of a midwife with some level of physician collaboration (Stevens, Witmer, Grant, & Cammarano, 2012). This arrangement is most likely to occur where midwives have hospital privileges, in addition to their birth center practice, giving them the opportunity to remain integrally involved with patients' care in cases where a higher level of care is warranted. The purpose of risk assessment is to predict which women and their fetuses or neonates are most likely to experience adverse events, to assign resources to those most in need, and to avoid unnecessary interventions (Institute of Medicine [IOM] and National Research Council [NRC], 2013).

Maternity care providers and the women they serve can interpret risk very differently (Bryers & Van Teijlingen, 2010; Stahl & Hundley, 2003). Risk assessment and assignment can have the effect of fostering fear and uncertainty in women throughout their pregnancy and delivery. For this reason, birth center providers focus on the normalcy of pregnancy and birth and encourage healthy lifestyle choices to optimize the pregnancy outcome. It is suggested that one of the roles of the midwife in this climate of fear, risk, and intervention is to help women build confidence in their ability to have a healthy pregnancy and give birth normally (Neerland, 2013). The *Guidelines for Licensing and Regulating Birth Centers* (American Public Health Association [APHA], 1982) advocated for birth centers to set their own risk identification criteria to assist in identifying appropriate low-risk clients for birth center care. This assessment was meant to be applied throughout pregnancy and delivery and focused on reducing perinatal risk with attention toward the fetus and newborn. A simple definition of low-risk pregnancy is "singleton, term, vertex pregnancies and the absence of any other medical or surgical conditions" (IOM and NRC, 2013, p. 32). A cornerstone of the risk model is the avoidance of intervention in the low-risk pregnancy. Any intervention in the normal physiologic process must be shown to do more good than harm, as adverse events can occur when low-risk women are treated in high-intervention sites (Carter et al., 2010; IOM and NRC, 2013; Jordan & Murphy, 2009). Women identified as high-risk feel a loss of control and have lower expectations for their birth, causing them increased stress during the pregnancy (Jordan & Murphy, 2009). Clearly, a change in how pregnancy is viewed in our society is needed, since the vast majority of pregnancies are normal and uncomplicated.

Levels of Maternal Care

In 2015, the American College of Obstetricians and Gynecologists and the Society for Maternal-Fetal Medicine created a consensus document delineating five levels of obstetric care including birth center care as a distinct level of care appropriate for the care of normal, singleton pregnancy of women with term, vertex presentation expected to have an uncomplicated labor and delivery (Menard et al., 2015). Complementary to but distinct from the neonatal focus of the widely known risk-based model, this document was based on current evidence and sought to standardize care definitions and begin to encourage the distribution of equitable services in a system with wide geographic variances. It was endorsed by AABC, the American College of Nurse-Midwives (ACNM), the Association of Women's Health, Obstetric and Neonatal Nurses, and the Commission for the Accreditation of Birth Centers (CABC; Menard et al., 2015). The document represents the first time that freestanding birth centers have been recognized by the larger mainstream obstetrical organizations in the United States as an entity included in the framework of a larger system of integrated care. This document followed a publication from the United Kingdom's National Institute for Health and Care Excellence (NICE), which concluded that healthy women with normal pregnancies are safer giving birth at home or in a midwife-led unit than under the supervision of an obstetrician in a hospital (National Institute for Health and Care Excellence [NICE], 2014). One of the stated objectives of the U.S. document was "to foster the development and equitable geographic distribution of full-service maternal care facilities and systems that promote proactive integration of risk-appropriate antepartum, intrapartum, and postpartum services" (Menard et al., 2015, p. 259). This consensus document recognized primary maternal care providers in birth centers including CNMs, CMs, CPMs, and LMs who are legally recognized to practice within the jurisdiction of the birth center, family physicians, and OB/GYNs. Such an inclusive recognition of providers of maternity care was unprecedented.

In many geographic areas of the country, women lack access to perinatal care, and approximately half of U.S. counties lack an OB/GYN (Rayburn, Klagholz, Murray-Krezan, Dowell, & Strunk, 2012). Therefore, it makes perfect sense to continue to grow the birth center model so that every community has access to care at this basic level. Additionally, every region of the country should have an integrated system to provide appropriate care based on the acuity of the patient and transfer to a higher level of care when needed. Staff at every freestanding birth center must have a clear understanding of their capability to handle more complex maternal and newborn cases than originally planned for, and have a well-defined threshold for transferring patients to a higher level of care (Menard et al., 2015).

INTEGRATED HEALTH SERVICES

Integrated service delivery is "the organization and management of health services so that people get the care they need, when they need it, in ways that are user-friendly, achieve the desired results, and provide value for money" (World Health Organization, 2008). Freestanding birth centers cannot exist in a vacuum, and depend on the larger health care system for referrals both into and out of the birth center practice. Physicians in support of this midwifery-led care model have proposed building freestanding birth centers on a large scale in association with hospitals, where women with uncomplicated pregnancy can give birth. Similar to the way outpatient surgical centers served the purpose of moving less complex surgeries out of the hospital, this scaling of the integrated birth center model could improve the experience, and safely decrease the cost of birth (Woo, Milstein, & Platchek, 2016).

Not all women who access antepartum care at a birth center are eligible, or remain eligible, for birth center care throughout their pregnancy, delivery, or postpartum periods. In addition, there are instances where a newborn exhibits symptoms suggesting the need for transfer to a higher level of care. In these cases, a referral arrangement needs to be in place so that patients may quickly be transferred to a different level of care appropriate to their condition. Figure 3.1 illustrates how the birth center, as the point of primary care, fits into the larger integrated health care system.

Birth center providers and consumers rely on ancillary services, such as laboratory, social services, and nutritional services, to provide the full complement of perinatal care. Additionally, the availability of specialists located under the umbrella of hospital or acute care is crucial to maintaining the safety of birth center practice through consultation, collaborative management, or referral, depending on the clinical situation. Ideally, there is fluid movement back and forth between the different levels of integrated care. For instance, a woman may be referred to a specialist by a birth center midwife for evaluation of a suspected deviation in fetal growth. Fetal surveillance may ensue for a period of time with normal findings, in which case the patient may return to birth center care, anticipating a normal birth center delivery. The common goal within an integrated health system should always be that a patient receives the right care from the right provider at the right time and the right place to do the most good and the least harm (Carter et al., 2010).

An example illustrating how a patient can move in and out of birth center care in an integrated health care system is explored in Figure 3.1 and the following case study.

CASE STUDY: Transfer Between Birth Center and Hospital Care Locations

Rachel is a 36-year-old primigravida who has done some research on her birth options, would like to have an unmedicated birth, and has chosen a birth center for her care. The birth center is located in a mid-sized city with a university hospital 2 miles away. Rachel attends an orientation at her first prenatal visit and learns that she is a candidate for prenatal genetic testing because of her age. The midwife refers Rachel to the genetic counselor at the hospital, and after discussing her risks and testing options, Rachel makes the decision to forego any testing. The pregnancy continues normally until 27 weeks, when it is discovered that she has gestational diabetes. While she continues regular prenatal care at the birth center, she is also referred to the diabetes center at the hospital for teaching and management. After 4 weeks, she has gained excellent control of her gestational diabetes with diet and exercise, and she is released

(continued)

CASE STUDY: Transfer Between Birth Center and Hospital Care Locations *(continued)*

from the diabetes center still able to receive birth center care. Rachel goes into spontaneous labor at 40 weeks and is admitted to the birth center in active labor with a singleton, vertex pregnancy. She dilates rapidly to 8 centimeters, but then becomes very fatigued and her contractions slow down significantly. The midwife consults the hospital physician to make her aware of this patient's current status and the possibility of transfer. Using the situation, background, assessment, recommendation (SBAR) format, the midwife presents information in a brief, organized, and predictable fashion to the physician (Thomas, Bertram, & Johnson, 2009). The midwife proposes the plan that Rachel and the midwife have created to rest, and then attempts to augment her labor with breast pump stimulation. This proves to be unsuccessful, and after several more hours, the decision is made by Rachel and the midwife to move to the hospital setting. The hospital and physician are notified, again using the SBAR format. The patient prefers to go in her car that is driven by her husband rather than an ambulance, since there is no fetal distress, and her labor has stopped progressing with no concern for delivery en route. Records are electronically transferred to the hospital labor and delivery unit. The nurses readily receive Rachel onto their unit with the midwife continuing to care for Rachel, since she has privileges to practice at the hospital. The nurses know and trust the midwife, and treat Rachel with kindness, even acknowledging her disappointment with having to transfer from the birth center. With pitocin augmentation, Rachel has a beautiful birth in the hospital with a healthy newborn. She is released home the following day. A home visit is arranged at 3 days postpartum as well as 2-week and 6-week visits at the birth center. The patient is referred to the physician at 6 weeks postpartum for a desired tubal ligation.

Creating the Cooperative Environment Through Collaborative Practice

The airline industry and national security and intelligence communities are all examples of teams that have created cooperative environments in response to crises (Thomas, Sexton, & Helmreich, 2004). Cooperative environments are created when more than one party enters into a shared vision

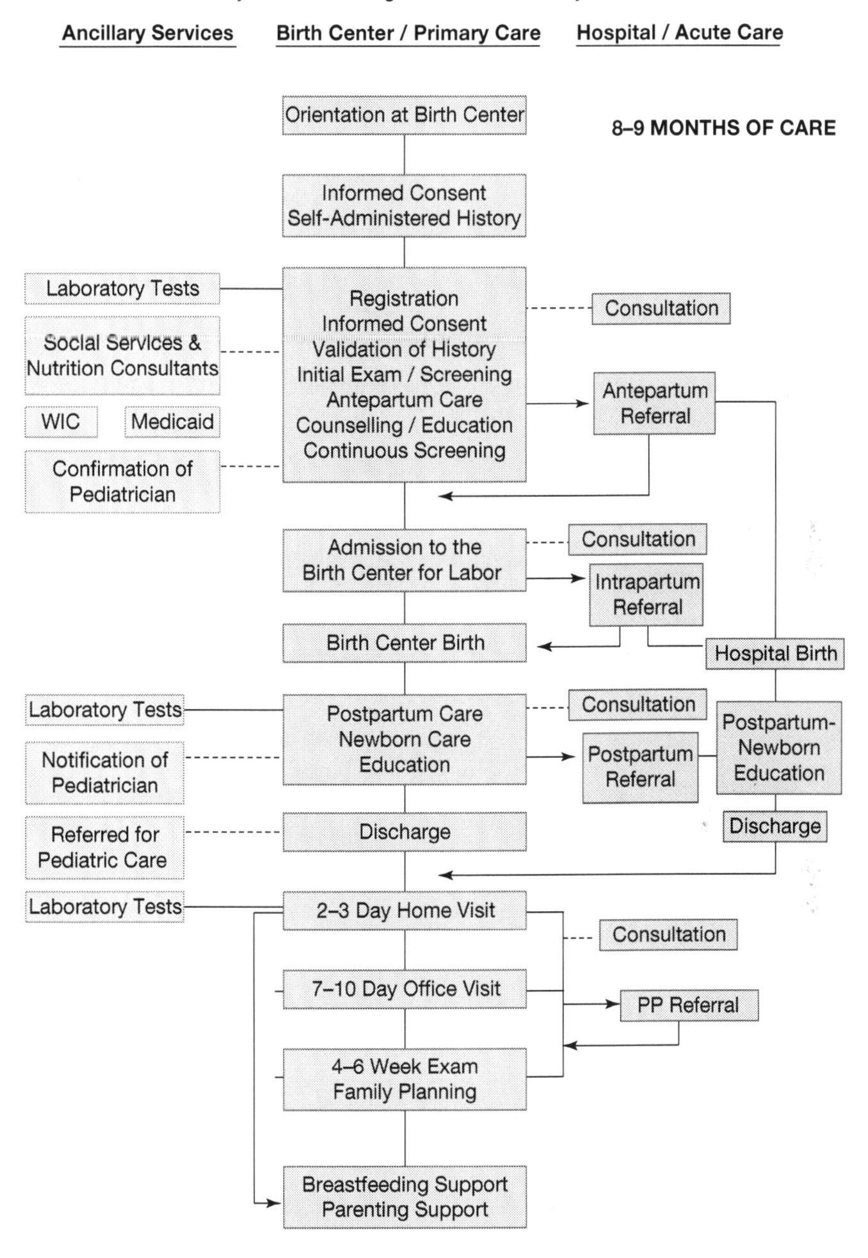

FIGURE 3.1 Algorithm showing the role of primary care birth centers in an integrated health system.

WIC, Women, Infants, and Children; PP, postpartum.

Source: AABC (2017).

through collaboration and consensus building. Solutions to the most difficult problems can be found if leaders and individuals representing different organizations or levels of care have the ability to listen to one another and reach a workable solution in an environment of mutual respect. "Good collaboration is an additive, bringing together a team that is greater than the sum of its parts through capitalization on strengths" (Waldman, Kennedy, & Kendig, 2012, p. 436). Within hierarchical health care systems, and between those systems and other organizations that wish to work toward successful collaboration, it is imperative that individuals are willing and able to permeate the boundaries created by the specialized silos of institutions and educational disciplines. Situational leadership, whereby the provider who is closest to the patient and whose scope of practice best matches the clinical picture, replaces hierarchical leadership in highly effective interdisciplinary teams (King, Laros, & Parer, 2012).

In 2010, the IOM published *The Future of Nursing: Leading Change, Advancing Health,* which advocated for interdisciplinary cooperation and full practice authority for nurses, defined as practicing to the full extent of their education and training (Institute of Medicine of the National Academies, 2010). Since this landmark report, others have continued to question the status quo. Barriers to effective collaborative practice still exist, restricting the practice of midwifery. These are primarily restrictions on independent practice including physician surcharges, reimbursement rates, admitting privileges, and the flawed notion of vicarious liability (King et al., 2012). Slowly, and state by state, many of these restrictions are being removed through improved legislation due to the vision and hard work of many people who care deeply about health care. Waldman et al. (2012) summarized some of the most important questions to ask when considering regulatory authority, formal agreements, provider responsibilities, and limitations and restrictions on practice in Table 3.1. More recently, the need to design practice models to address health care shortages has initiated a focus on team-based care. Guiding principles of team-based care are:

- The patient and families are central to and actively engaged as members of the health care team
- The team has a shared vision
- Role clarity is essential to optimal team building and team functioning
- All team members are accountable for their own practice and to the team
- Effective communication is key to quality teams
- Team leadership is situational and dynamic (ACOG, 2016)

TABLE 3.1
Regulatory Issues in Collaborative Practice

Regulatory Authority	Required Agreement	Provider Responsibilities	Limitations/Restrictions
• Who regulates CNM/CM/NP practice? • What does the regulatory board require? • How is scope of practice defined? • Does the CNM/CM/NP have prescriptive authority? If so, what type? • Does the CNM/CM/NP have the legal authority to prescribe legend drugs? Controlled drugs? • Is special certification, education, or other documentation necessary for delegation of prescriptive authority?	• Are there requirements for a written agreement or protocols? • What must be included in the writing? • What should be excluded in the writing?	• What are each party's legal responsibilities within the agreement? • Must the parties practice at the same site for a designated period of time? • Must the parties participate in a documentation review process? • Do the regulatory entities require reports or audits? • Are disclosure statements related to the type of providers in practice required to be posted? • What is the delegation of backup coverage when the physician is unavailable?	• Is there a limit on the number of CNMs/CMs/NPs with whom a physician may collaborate or supervise? • Is there a limit on the number of physicians with whom a CNM/CM/NP may collaborate? • Are there geographical limitations on the distance between parties when care is provided?

CMs, certified midwives; CNMs, certified nurse-midwives; CPMs, certified professional midwives; NPs, nurse practitioners.

Reprinted from Obstetrics and Gynecology Clinics of North America 39 by Richard Waldman, Holly Powell Kennedy and Susan Kendig, pages: 435–444, 2012 with permission.

Interprofessional education is a relatively new area of focus in many medical, nursing, and other health profession schools across the country and may lend more to interdisciplinary practice. The terms *interprofessional* and *interdisciplinary* are often used interchangeably. Interdisciplinary practice has been defined as "collaborative practice that combines the insights of several professional disciplines, consumers, and community members in designing care or programs" (Margolis, Rosenberg, Umble, & Chewning, 2013, p. 950). The Interprofessional Education Collaborative (IPEC), started in 2009, developed core competencies that assist health professions working collaboratively to have a broader impact on individual and population health. These core competencies integrate key concepts of knowledge, skills, values, and attitudes into interprofessional education and resulting interprofessional collaboration (IPEC, 2016). As our health care system navigates change to serve more patients, improve quality, expand geographic reach, and deliver care in more cost-effective ways, interprofessional collaboration and innovative practice become increasingly necessary (Alliman, Jolles, & Summers, 2015; Avery, Montgomery, & Brandl-Salutz, 2012; King et al., 2012).

Transfer of Care

Transfer from birth center care may become necessary during the antepartum period when complications arise. Stevens et al. (2012) propose that the antepartum referral rate in a birth center with a collaborative care model can also be referred to as the "collaborative rate." In this model, "the patient stays within the practice for joint management of care with the midwives and obstetrician. The most common antepartum cases, which were referred to the physician and jointly managed, included gestational diabetes, hypertensive disorders, nonreassuring fetal testing, postdate inductions, hypothyroidism, multiple gestation, and other conditions" (Stevens et al., 2012, p. 354).

Though it is assumed that a healthy woman receiving birth center care will embark on a normal, physiologic journey in her efforts to give birth, it is not uncommon for women and newborns to need to be transported to a hospital due to unforeseen complications. In these cases, there needs to be a clear understanding of the capability of the level of care a birth center offers and the acuity of the woman or newborn. Agreements, policies, and procedures need to be in place with the sending and receiving facilities; communication between the birth center, transport team, and receiving hospital must be efficient and clear. Quality improvement programs should be in place to ensure patient safety (American College of

Obstetricians and Gynecologists [ACOG], 2012; Menard et al., 2015). Interdisciplinary team communication is a guiding principle in creating a culture of safety in midwifery care (ACNM, 2006). A notable consensus statement emerged from the Home Birth Summit, to which this author was a delegate in 2011. The summit, held in Warrenton, Virginia, brought together many disciplines, representing all stakeholder groups with an interest in homebirth. Many of the concepts explored were pertinent to out-of-hospital birth in general, including the following consensus statement:

> We believe that collaboration within an integrated maternity care system is essential for optimal mother-baby outcomes. All women and families planning a home or birth center birth have a right to respectful, safe, and seamless consultation, referral, transport, and transfer of care when necessary. When ongoing inter-professional dialogue and cooperation occur, everyone benefits. (Reprinted by permission from Home Birth Summit, n.d.)

The majority of transfers from a birth center to a hospital are for nonemergent clinical situations, including labor dystocia, maternal fatigue, or premature rupture of membranes with lack of ensuing labor. More than 80% of women with these conditions are primigravidas (Stapleton, Illuzzi, & Osborne, 2013). Emergency transfers from a birth center to a hospital are rare, but do occur. These can include fetal malpresentation, prolapsed umbilical cord, placental abruption, fetal distress, postpartum hemorrhage, or retained placenta. In addition, occasionally an unstable newborn requires transfer to a higher level of care.

When transfer of a patient becomes necessary, it is not just the patient requiring transfer. Patient information, authority, and responsibility for patient care also need to be transferred from one provider to another. Many midwives who practice in birth centers also maintain hospital privileges, allowing them to continue providing care to the transferred woman in a higher acuity setting. Certain elements of a transfer, when properly executed, can optimize the safety and experience of everyone. These include immediate access to the receiving provider, interactive and respectful communication, organized presentation of historical and current clinical information, involvement of the transferring provider to the degree of her/his scope of practice, and privileges at the receiving facility. If these privileges are not in place, the midwife may remain to provide continuity and support, if the woman desires (Home Birth Summit, n.d.). In addition, there are activities after the episode of care that contribute to a successful transfer, and can contribute to continuous process improvement. Relevant documents such as a discharge summary should be sent to the referring provider. Follow-up care between providers can be coordinated; in many cases, the care can revert back to the birth center provider upon discharge from the hospital. Debriefing the case with providers and with the woman prior to hospital discharge allows all parties to have a common understanding of why the transfer was needed. A defined process to regularly review transfer cases with a goal of safety and quality improvement should be in place, and include all stakeholders (Home Birth Summit, n.d.). Some states have formed collaborative perinatal groups that have created quality improvement initiatives pertaining to safe transfers of care when needed from community-based birth centers to hospitals. These initiatives focus their attention on creating the safest process for transfer, with the woman at the center of care.

CONCLUSION

The freestanding birth center model is an option for women and families in many more communities every year. As an enduring model with data demonstrating safety, satisfaction, and cost-effectiveness (see Chapters 4, 5, and 6), integration into larger health care systems is happening and will become even more common in years to come. Applied risk screening and movement of patients between appropriate levels of care naturally lend to care delivery within an integrated system, made even stronger by applying the concepts of collaboration and interprofessional practice. The birth center will continue to gain the attention of the medical community, no longer as an outsider, but as a key component of an integrated system of care.

REFERENCES

Alliman, J., Jolles, D., & Summers, L. (2015). The innovation imperative: Scaling freestanding birth centers, CenteringPregnancy, and midwifery-led maternity health. *Journal of Midwifery and Women's Health, 60*, 244–249. doi:10.1111/jmwh.12320

American Association of Birth Centers. (2017). *How to start a birth center workshop manual* (25th ed.). Perkiomenville, PA: Author.

American Association of Birth Centers. (n.d.). What is a birth center? Retrieved from http://www.birthcenters.org/?page=bce_what_is_a_bc

American College of Nurse-Midwives. (2006). Creating a culture of safety in midwifery care [Position Statement]. Retrieved from http://www.midwife.org/ACNM/files/ACNM

LibraryData/UPLOADFILENAME/000000000059/Creating%20a%20Culture%20of%20Safety%20in%20Midwifery%20Care%2012.06.pdf
American College of Obstetricians and Gynecologists. (2012). *Communication strategies for patient handoffs* [Committee opinion]. Retrieved from http://www.acog.org/Resources-And-Publications/Committee-Opinions/Committee-on-Patient-Safety-and-Quality-Improvement/Communication-Strategies-for-Patient-Handoffs
American College of Obstetricians and Gynecologists. (2016). Collaboration in practice: Implementing team-based care [Executive Summary]. *Obstetrics and Gynecology, 127*(3), 612–617.
American Public Health Association. (1982). APHA guidelines for licensing and regulating birth centers (Policy Statement Adopted by the Governing Council of The American Public Health Association, November 17, 1982) Retrieved from https://c.ymcdn.com/sites/www.birthcenters.org/resource/collection/028792A7-808D-4BC7-9A0F-FB038B434B91/9.APHA_Guidelines.pdf
Arms, S. (1979). *Immaculate deception*. New York, NY: Bantam Books.
Avery, M. D., Montgomery, O., & Brandl-Salutz, E. (2012). Essential components of successful collaborative maternity care models. *Obstetrics and Gynecology Clinics of North America, 39*, 423–434. doi:10.1016/j.ogc.2012.05.010
Boston Women's Health Book Collective. (1976). *Our bodies ourselves* (1st ed.). New York, NY: Simon & Schuster.
Bryers, H., & Van Teijlingen, E. (2010). Risk, theory, social and medical models: A critical analysis of the concept of risk in maternity care. *Midwifery, 26*, 488–496. doi:10.1016/j.midw.2010.07.003
Carter, M. C., Corry, M., Delbanco, S., Foster, T. C., Friedland, R., & Gabel, R. (2010). 2020 vision for a high quality, high value maternity care system [Special issue]. *Women's Health Issues, 20*(1 Suppl.), S7–S17. doi:10.1016/j.whi.2009.11.006
Gaskin, I. M. (1980). *Spiritual midwifery*. Summertown, TN: The Book Publishing Company.
Home Birth Summit. (n.d.). Common ground statements. Retrieved from http://www.homebirthsummit.org
Institute of Medicine and National Research Council. (2013). *An update on research issues in the assessment of birth settings*. Washington, DC: National Academies Press.
Institute of Medicine of the National Academies. (2010). *The future of nursing: Leading change, advancing health*. Washington, DC: National Academies Press.
Interprofessional Education Collaborative. (2016). *Core competencies for interprofessional collaborative practice*. Washington, DC: Author.
Jordan, R. G., & Murphy, P. A. (2009). Risk assessment and risk distortion: Finding the balance. *Journal of Midwifery and Women's Health, 54*(3), 191–200. doi:10.1016/j.jmwh.2009.02.001
King, T. L., Laros, Jr., R. K., & Parer, J. T. (2012). Interprofessional collaborative practice in obstetrics and midwifery. *Obstetrics and Gynecology Clinics of North America, 39*, 411–422. doi:10.1016/j.ogc.2012.05.009
MacDorman, M., & DeClercq, E. (2016). Trends and characteristics of United States out-of-hospital births 2004-2014: New information on risk status and access to care. *Birth, 43*(2), 116–124. doi:10.1111/birt.12228
Margolis, L. H., Rosenberg, A., Umble, K., & Chewning, L. (2013). Effects of interdisciplinary training on MCH professionals, organizations and systems. *Maternal Child Health Journal, 17*, 949–958. doi:10.1007/s10995-012-1078-8
Menard, M. K., Kilpatrick, S., Saade, G., Hollier, L., Joseph, G. F., Barfield, W., . . . Conry, J. (2015). Levels of maternal care. *American Journal of Obstetrics & Gynecology, 125*, 259–271. doi:10.1016/j.ajog.2014.12.030

National Institute for Health and Care Excellence. (2014). Intrapartum care for healthy women and babies. Retrieved from https://www.nice.org.uk/guidance/cg190/chapter/recommendations

Neerland, C. E. (2013). A supportive approach to prenatal care. In M. D. Avery (Ed.), *Supporting a physiologic approach to pregnancy and birth* (pp. 29–47). Ames, IA: Wiley-Blackwell.

Patient Protection and Affordable Care Act. (2010). Nondiscrimination amendment to the PPACA. 42 U.S.C. § 300gg-5.

Rayburn, W., Klagholz, J., Murray-Krezan, C., Dowell, L., & Strunk, A. (2012). Distribution of American Congress of Obstetricians and Gynecologists Fellows and Junior Fellows in practice in the United States. *Obstetrics and Gynecology, 119*(5), 1017–1022. doi:10.1097/AOG.0b013e31824cfe50

Stahl, K., & Hundley, V. (2003). Risk and risk assessment in pregnancy: Do we scare because we care? *Midwifery, 19*, 298–309. doi:10.1016/S0266-6138(03)00041-X/

Stapleton, S. R., Osborne, C., & Illuzzi, J. (2013). Outcomes of care in birth centers: Demonstration of a durable model. *Journal of Midwifery & Women's Health, 58*(1), 3–14. doi: 10.1111/jmwh.12003

Stevens, J. R., Witmer, T. L., Grant, R. L., & Cammarano, D. J. (2012). Description of a successful collaborative birth center practice among midwives and an obstetrician. *Obstetrics and Gynecology Clinics of North America, 39*, 347–357. doi:10.106/j.ogc.2012.05.003

Thomas, C., Bertram, E., & Johnson, D. (2009). The SBAR communication technique: Teaching nursing students professional communication skills. *Nurse Educator, 34*(4), 176–180. doi:10.1097/NNE.0b013e3181aaba54

Thomas, E. J., Sexton, J. B., & Helmreich, R. L. (2004). Translating teamwork behaviours from aviation to healthcare: Development of behavioural markers for neonatal resuscitation. *Quality and Safety in Health Care, 13*(Suppl. 1), i57–i64.

Waldman, R., Kennedy, H., & Kendig, S. (2012). Collaboration in maternity care: Possibilities and challenges. *Obstetrics and Gynecology Clinics of North America, 39*, 435–444. doi: 10.1016/j.ogc.2012.05.011

Woo, V., Milstein, A., & Platchek, T. (2016). Hospital affiliated outpatient birth centers: A possible model for helping to achieve the triple aim in obstetrics. *Journal of the American Medical Association, 316*(14), 1441–1442.

World Health Organization. (2008). Technical brief no. 1. Retrieved from http://www.who.int/healthsystems/technical_brief_final.pdf

SECTION II

Birth Center Outcomes: The Triple Aim

CHAPTER 4

Clinical Outcomes in Birth Centers

JULIA C. PHILLIPPI AND
KATHLEEN DANHAUSEN

LEARNING OBJECTIVES

Upon completion of this chapter, the reader will be able to:

1. Compare maternal and neonatal outcomes in birth center and hospital settings
2. Explain difficulties with data aggregation across birth center studies
3. Identify common indications for antepartum, intrapartum, postpartum, and neonatal transfers from birth center care
4. Identify risk factors for complications while receiving birth center care

The effect of the location of birth on perinatal outcomes is an essential component of informed consent for women. In this chapter, we synthesize data from a variety of trials to provide an overview of clinical outcomes in birth centers. These studies are international in scope and include data from birth centers located in the United States, Europe, and Australia. Most of the birth centers studied in the United States are freestanding or not located within or adjacent to a hospital. However, the international birth center studies also include birth centers that function as independent units within a hospital. We rely primarily on four well-designed, large, and recent studies of birth center care with samples that allow clear inferences to today's clinical practice. In the *National Birth Center Study II*, Stapleton, Osborne, and Illuzzi (2013) analyzed data from 22,403 U.S. women planning birth center birth, including 15,574 who were admitted to a freestanding birth center in labor. In the Birthplace Study,

Birthplace in England Collaborative Group (2011) reported on 11,666 British women planning birth center births, of which 11,282 were admitted to freestanding birth centers in labor. Waldenström and Nilsson (1997) reported on 928 Swedish women receiving in-hospital birth center care in one of the only randomized controlled trials in the birth center literature. In 2004, Gottvall, Grunewald, and Waldenström reported clinical outcomes of 3,256 pregnancies (among 2,534 women) cared for by the same birth center over a 10-year span.

In addition to this contemporary research, we examine all relevant studies of birth center care published since 1980, limiting the search to studies of birth locations with admission criteria similar to American Association of Birth Centers (AABC standards; see Chapter 8). We acknowledge that there are limitations to this approach, especially as we attempt to describe and combine studies in the distant past and those in countries with different health care systems. However, the gestalt of the literature on care in birth centers allows for evaluation of these centers for birth and practice.

SYNTHESIS OF MATERNAL OUTCOMES

Maternal Outcome Data Overview

The data used to describe maternal outcomes in birth centers were gathered from 23 publications using 14 total data sets. Manuscripts were initially identified through a search of Google Scholar, Cumulative Index to Nursing and Allied Health Literature (CINAHL), and PubMed databases using "birth center"/"birthing center", and "outcomes." Articles published in English-language, peer-reviewed journals since 1980 were selected. Forty-three articles were identified for full review and manuscripts were excluded from further analysis if the research had a singular focus (e.g., perineal integrity) and did not provide comprehensive data on maternal outcomes, if they did not define the birth center practice model, or if the practice model did not meet AABC criteria for birth center practice. For example, manuscripts were excluded if they referred to practices prohibited in AABC birth centers, including the use of misoprostol or Pitocin for labor induction or augmentation, vacuum or forceps-assisted births, or the use of continuous fetal monitoring. In addition, at least one study was excluded because its outcome data included women who would have been considered too high risk for most birth centers (e.g., women with multiple fetuses and women with a fetus in a breech presentation).

These 14 data sets included a total of 84,300 women planning to give birth in a birth center, using a variety of study designs. Nine studies involved a comparison between outcomes in birth centers and outcomes among a matched sample of women giving birth in hospitals (Benatar, Garrett, Howell, & Palmer, 2013; David, von Schwarzenfeld, Dimer, & Kentenich, 1999; Feldman & Hurst, 1987; Jackson et al., 2003; Overgaard, Fenger-Grøn, & Sandall, 2012a, 2012b; Overgaard, Møller, Fenger-Grøn, Knudsen, & Sandall, 2011; Scupholme & Kamons, 1987; Scupholme, McLeod, & Robertson, 1986). In nine studies, researchers used an observational design to describe outcomes among women utilizing birth center services without a direct comparison group (Fullerton et al., 1997; Nguyen et al., 2009; Roberts & Sward, 2001; Rooks, Weatherby, & Ernst, 1992a, 1992b, 1992c; Rooks et al., 1989; Rowe et al., 2013; Stapleton et al., 2013). Two large studies of low-risk women reported outcomes across home, birth center, and hospital births (Brocklehurst et al., 2011; Wax, Pinette, Cartin, & Blackstone, 2010). Finally, the outcomes from one randomized controlled trial of women assigned to birth center versus hospital care were reported in three publications (Waldenström & Nilsson, 1993, 1994, 1997).

These data were collected over 30 years, and from five countries. Of the 14 data sets, 10 were collected in the United States (Benatar et al., 2013; Feldman & Hurst, 1987; Fullerton et al., 1997; Jackson et al., 2003; Nguyen et al., 2009; Roberts & Sward, 2001; Rooks et al., 1989, 1992a, 1992b, 1992c; Scupholme & Kamons, 1987; Scupholme et al., 1986; Stapleton et al., 2013; Wax et al., 2010); and one each from Denmark (Overgaard et al., 2012a, 2012b), England (Brocklehurst et al., 2011; Rowe et al., 2013), Germany (David et al., 1999), and Sweden (Waldenström & Nilsson, 1993, 1994, 1997). Four of the 14 data sets included women who were attended by a diversity of intrapartum providers, including physicians, certified nurse-midwives (CNMs), and other legally practicing midwives such as certified professional midwives (CPMs) and licensed midwives (LMs); the providers in these data sets were all located in the United States (Jackson et al., 2003; Nguyen et al., 2009; Rooks et al., 1989, 1992a, 1992b, 1992c; Wax et al., 2010). The women represented in the remaining data sets were served exclusively by midwives during their birth center care, with U.S. studies specifying that these providers were CNMs.

Serious Maternal Complications

Studies utilizing comparison groups indicate that women in birth centers have no increased statistical risk of serious maternal outcomes as compared with women in hospital care. Events that constitute "serious maternal outcomes" are not defined consistently across studies. However, they generally include maternal death and severe morbidity such as the need for admission to an intensive care unit (ICU), hysterectomy, or blood transfusion. Most studies reported no serious adverse maternal events in either birth center or hospital groups. Waldenström and Nilsson report that one woman from each group (hospital and birth center) was admitted to the ICU and both had full recoveries (Waldenström & Nilsson, 1997). David et al. (1999) noted one death in the hospital group but did not report the cause. Finally, in the Birthplace Study, Brocklehurst et al. (2011) noted a statistically significant increase in the number of women requiring blood transfusion and transfer to higher acuity care among those planning hospital births as compared with those who intended birth in freestanding centers.

Mode of Birth

Women planning to give birth in a birth center at the time they begin labor are more likely to have a spontaneous vaginal birth when compared with women planning birth in a hospital. Five studies used matched cohorts of low-risk women planning to labor in a birth center or a hospital (Brocklehurst et al., 2011; David et al., 1999; Jackson et al., 2003; Overgaard et al., 2011; Scupholme et al., 1986), whereas the other studies compared their birth center sample to national averages (Rooks et al., 1989, 1992a, 1992b, 1992c; Stapleton et al., 2013). In all of the studies cited, women who started labor planning to give birth in a birth center were included in the birth center sample, regardless of whether they subsequently transferred to the hospital. All studies found higher rates of spontaneous vaginal birth in the birth center groups.

Six studies found that women receiving birth center care were significantly less likely to experience assisted vaginal birth with forceps or vacuum (Benatar et al., 2013; Brocklehurst et al., 2011; David et al., 1999; Feldman & Hurst, 1987; Jackson et al., 2003; Overgaard et al., 2011), with an additional study reporting lower rates of assisted birth without statistical significance (Scupholme et al., 1986). (Use of forceps and vacuum devices is not permitted in Commission for the Accreditation of Birth Centers [CABC]-accredited birth centers; however, they may be used following hospital transfer.) Among the five studies with matched samples of low-risk women, the cesarean rate within the birth center cohort was lower but did not reach significance (David et al., 1999; Feldman & Hurst, 1987; Jackson et al., 2003; Scupholme et al., 1986; Waldenström & Nilsson, 1997);

three additional analyses involving unmatched low-risk comparison groups found a significantly lower cesarean birth rate among women who received birth center care as compared with women who solely received hospital-based care (Benatar et al., 2013; Brocklehurst et al., 2011; Overgaard et al., 2011).

Oxytocin Use and Length of Labor

The three research teams that measured length of labor reported significantly longer labors among mothers beginning care in birth centers as compared with the hospital (Feldman & Hurst, 1987; Scupholme et al., 1986; Waldenström & Nilsson, 1997). Wax and colleagues (2010) analyzed more than 745,000 U.S. birth certificates and found that the 4,661 women who gave birth in a freestanding birth center were significantly more likely to have prolonged or precipitous labor. (The study authors did not provide a definition of prolonged labor.) Although birth center staff may have a greater appreciation for the range of normal duration of physiologic labor, this finding most likely also reflects the greater in-hospital use of oxytocin. The use of intrapartum oxytocin is prohibited in CABC-accredited birth centers, and therefore was not used in any of the birth centers in this analysis; prolonged labor and "failure to progress" is a primary indication for hospital transfer. However, birth center clients who transferred to the hospital had significantly lower rates of hospital oxytocin use during labor in all six studies reporting this outcome (Brocklehurst et al., 2011; Feldman & Hurst, 1987; Jackson et al., 2003; Overgaard et al., 2011; Scupholme et al., 1986; Waldenström & Nilsson, 1997).

Pain Management

Pain relief options vary across birth centers, countries, and time periods. Water immersion is a primary pain relief method used in birth centers; studies have also described women receiving narcotic analgesia, pudendal or paracervical blocks, nitrous oxide, and sterile water papules in birth center settings (Feldman & Hurst, 1987; Jackson et al., 2003; MacVicar et al., 1993; Roberts & Sward, 2001; Rooks et al., 1989, 1992b; Scupholme & Kamons, 1987; Scupholme et al., 1986; Waldenström & Nilsson, 1994, 1997). Moreover, additional methods are often available to women following hospital transfer, including epidural anesthesia. Women in hospitals are significantly more likely to receive an epidural (Brocklehurst et al., 2011; Feldman & Hurst, 1987; Jackson et al., 2003; Overgaard et al., 2011; Waldenström & Nilsson, 1994, 1997).

When a comparison group was included in the study design, researchers found that birth center clients were less likely to use pharmacological methods of pain relief as compared with those giving birth in a hospital (Feldman & Hurst, 1987; Jackson et al., 2003; Scupholme et al., 1986; Waldenström & Nilsson, 1994, 1997). One exception is Waldenström (1994), who found that women in birth centers were more likely to use sterile water papules than a matched group in the hospital. However, the last reported pain relief outcome data were collected in the late 1990s. This may represent declining research interest around pharmacological pain relief, fewer pharmacological options offered in birth centers, or both. In the 1980s and 1990s, when data were collected, rates of narcotic analgesia use by birth center clientele ranged from 43% to 13.1%. Rooks et al. (1989) stratified by parity and noted that 24% of nulliparas used pharmacological relief compared with 6.2% of multiparas.

Perineal Integrity

Women in birth center care experience fewer episiotomies and spontaneous perineal lacerations than women in hospital care (Brocklehurst et al., 2011; David et al., 1999; Feldman & Hurst, 1987). Although episiotomy rates have declined over the last 20 years in all settings, birth centers have consistently reported lower rates of episiotomy when compared with hospitals, and three studies found statistically significant differences (Brocklehurst et al., 2011; David et al., 1999; Feldman & Hurst, 1987). Data collected in New York City (NYC) showed a 47.2% birth center episiotomy rate compared with 78.1% in a matched, low-risk hospital cohort (Feldman & Hurst, 1987). A German study found a 15.7% episiotomy rate in the birth center compared with a 54.8% rate in area hospitals (David et al., 1999). The data from the Birthplace Study showed an episiotomy rate of 8.6% in freestanding birth centers compared with 19.3% in a hospital obstetric unit not staffed by midwives (Brocklehurst et al., 2011).

Three studies reported that women cared for in birth centers were significantly more likely to maintain intact perinea during birth. In these studies (located in Denmark, Germany, and the United States), women birthing in hospitals had significantly higher rates of first- and second-degree lacerations (David et al., 1999; Feldman & Hurst, 1987; Overgaard et al., 2011). In a likely reflection of the trend away from episiotomies, the rate of intact perinea experienced in birth centers increased over time, with 25% reported in the early 1980s versus 61.3% in the mid-2000s (Feldman & Hurst, 1987; Overgaard et al., 2011). Two studies reported differences in third- and fourth-degree lacerations; although rates in birth centers were lower, the overall incidence was too low to assess statistical significance (Brocklehurst et al., 2011; Overgaard et al., 2011).

Transfer of Care

Out-of-hospital care is primarily appropriate for low-risk women; a change in risk status requires transfer to higher level care. Maternal transfer from birth center care can occur at any time during the antepartum, intrapartum, or postpartum period, with antepartum transfers occurring for both medical and nonmedical reasons. (Examples of nonmedical reasons include the woman moving or choosing a different provider.)

Data on birth center transfers are complicated by the fact that studies define and measure transfers differently. For example, some studies divided antepartum transfer rates into medical and nonmedical, whereas others did not differentiate, and one included a separate category for women experiencing first-trimester loss (Stapleton et al., 2013). Comparing intrapartum transfer rates across studies is even more difficult. Some authors determine this rate as the number of women transferring while in labor divided by all women entering prenatal care at a birth center (Feldman & Hurst, 1987; Jackson et al., 2003; Waldenström & Nilsson, 1993, 1994, 1997), whereas others calculate rates based on a denominator of women admitted to the birth center in labor (David et al., 1999; Fullerton et al., 1997; Overgaard et al., 2011, 2012a; Roberts & Sward, 2001; Rooks et al., 1989, 1992b, 1992c; Scupholme & Kamons, 1987; Stapleton et al., 2013). Still others include in the denominator those women admitted in labor as well as women in labor who are assessed by center providers and transferred to hospital care prior to admission (Brocklehurst et al., 2011; Nguyen et al., 2009; Rowe et al., 2013; Scupholme et al., 1986).

Eighteen studies reported transfer rates. From entry to prenatal care through the postpartum period, up to 54.7% of women intending to give birth in a birth center experienced a transfer of care (Jackson et al., 2003). Across studies, the majority of transfers were for nonemergency conditions.

Antepartum Transfers

Antepartum transfer rates ranged up to 27.2% in a sample of approximately 1,800 U.S. women seeking birth center care in the mid-1990s (Jackson et al., 2003). Antepartum transfer indications include medical complications precluding birth center care (Table 4.1). In addition, preterm births and pregnancies that extend past 42 gestational weeks are not considered appropriate for out-of-hospital care in more recent studies. Some

TABLE 4.1 Common Antepartum Transfer Indications
Malpresentation
Hypertension
Prolonged rupture of membranes
Postterm pregnancy
Preterm pregnancy
Intrauterine growth restriction
Gestational diabetes mellitus
Multiple gestation
Bleeding
Isoimmunization
Fetal anomaly
Intrauterine fetal demise
Maternal preference

studies include nonmedical transfers such as maternal geographic relocation in the antepartum transfer category and have higher rates than studies that separate out nonmedical reasons for ending birth center care. Stapleton and colleagues (2013) reported a 13% antepartum transfer rate for medical reasons. Multiparous women are more likely than nulliparous women to be transferred antepartum (Waldenström & Nilsson, 1994).

Intrapartum Transfers

The most recent studies report intrapartum transfer rates ranging from 11.6% in a sample of 839 Danish women to 16.5% in the Birthplace Study (Brocklehurst et al., 2011; Overgaard et al., 2011). Similarly, the *National Birth Center Study II* (Stapleton et al., 2013) reported that 12.4% of the approximately 15,000 women admitted in labor were transferred intrapartum. The *National Birth Center Study II* also reported that 4.5% of women initially evaluated in labor were transferred prior to admission to the birth center (Stapleton et al., 2013). Studies providing information on intrapartum transfers noted that the most common indications included

TABLE 4.2
Common Intrapartum Transfer Indications

Lack of progress in labor*
Meconium*
Fetal distress*
Need for analgesia*
Hypertension*
Malpresentation*
Prolonged rupture of membranes*
Maternal infection

*More common with primigravid women.

lack of progress in labor, rupture of membranes without labor, and prolonged labor (Table 4.2).

Three studies reported rates for emergent versus nonemergent maternal intrapartum transfers and noted that the majority of transfers were nonemergencies (Rooks et al., 1992c; Rowe et al., 2013; Stapleton et al., 2013). Two of these studies were published in the last 5 years and included large samples of more than 10,000 women (Rowe et al., 2013; Stapleton et al., 2013). Of the 12.4% of women experiencing intrapartum transfer in the *National Birth Center Study II*, less than 2% were transferred emergently (Stapleton et al., 2013). Rates of emergent transfer differ by parity. In the secondary analysis by Rowe et al. (2013) of the birthplace data, 27% of all nulliparas planning a birth center birth were transferred to the hospital during labor, with 9.5% of all nulliparas transferred for a "potentially urgent" indication. In comparison, 5% of multiparous women were transferred to the hospital during labor, whereas only 1.5% of multiparous women were urgently transferred. Of note, nulliparous and multiparous women had similar rates of "potentially urgent" hospital transfer immediately following a birth. Across studies, the leading reason for emergent transfer was nonreassuring fetal heart rate (Fullerton et al., 1997; Nguyen et al., 2009; Stapleton et al., 2013).

In studies reporting intrapartum transfer rates, approximately one third of nulliparous women were transferred during labor, with rates ranging from 27.3% to 29.6% (Brocklehurst et al., 2011; Rowe et al., 2013).

Nulliparous women were transferred at approximately five times the rate of multiparous women; they accounted for 81.6% of the laboring women transferred in the *National Birth Center Study II* and 77% of women transferred from freestanding birth centers in the Birthplace Study (Brocklehurst et al., 2011; Overgaard et al., 2011; Rowe et al., 2013; Stapleton et al., 2013; Waldenström & Nilsson, 1997).

Postpartum Transfers

Eleven studies reported postpartum transfer statistics, which ranged from 0.5% to 4.5% (Brocklehurst et al., 2011; David et al., 1999; Feldman & Hurst, 1987; Overgaard et al., 2011; Roberts & Sward, 2001; Rooks et al., 1992c; Rowe et al., 2013; Scupholme et al., 1986; Stapleton et al., 2013; Waldenström & Nilsson, 1994, 1997). In the postpartum period, women were most commonly transferred for hemorrhage or retained placenta (Brocklehurst et al., 2011; Rooks et al., 1989; Stapleton et al., 2013; see Table 4.3). As with other transfer rates, various denominators were used including all women planning birth center birth, all those admitted in labor, or all those who gave birth in the center. The *National Birth Center Study II* (Stapleton et al., 2013) provides further insight into these transfers, reporting that 2.4% of women who gave birth in a birth center required postpartum transfer, and 0.5% of these women were transferred emergently.

Vaginal Birth After Cesarean

Few of the studies described provide information or analysis related to the clinical outcomes of women attempting a vaginal birth after cesarean (VBAC) in a birth center setting, primarily because many birth centers include a uterine scar as an exclusion criterion from birth center care. However, several studies have assessed attempted VBAC outcomes in birth

TABLE 4.3
Common Postpartum Transfer Indications

Hemorrhage
Retained placenta*
Laceration repair/sphincter damage†

*Condition is more common with multiparous women.
†More common with primigravid women.

centers and have found high rates of vaginal birth along with slightly increased risk to the mother and neonate, especially among women with more than one cesarean or neonates past the 42nd week of gestation. These studies were excluded from the larger analysis due to their narrow focus. Although women giving birth in birth centers have rates of uterine rupture that are similar to or less than those experienced in a hospital setting, the time between recognition of distress and expedited birth may increase the perinatal mortality rate. As with many measures of adverse perinatal outcomes, the incidence of uterine rupture and subsequent maternal or neonatal death is small across few studies, and thus conclusive statements cannot be made about the safety of VBAC in the birth center setting.

Two relatively recent German studies used a national data set with information required from all midwives practicing out of hospital (Beckmann, Barger, Dorin, Metzing, & Hellmers, 2014; David, Gross, Wiemer, Pachaly, & Vetter, 2009). These authors compared two groups of women experiencing a second pregnancy. The experimental group had a history of cesarean, whereas the control group had a vaginal birth with their first pregnancy. Both studies found a VBAC rate of approximately 75% compared with a vaginal birth rate of more than 95% among women with no history of cesarean. Both authors reported a high transfer rate (~40%) for women attempting VBAC out of hospital, compared with a 5% transfer rate for women in the control group without a previous cesarean. Women with prior cesareans were more likely than women in the control group to be transferred for arrest of labor or suspected cephalopelvic disproportion (Beckmann et al., 2014; David et al., 2009).

David et al. noted that women with prior cesareans were significantly more likely to give birth to neonates with Apgar scores less than 7 at 5 minutes; however, this may be clinically insignificant as there were no differences in rates of neonatal intensive care unit (NICU) admission or infant mortality (David et al., 2009). There were no uterine ruptures or postpartum hysterectomies/laparotomies due to birth injury. Although both David et al. (2009) and Beckman et al. (2014) observed a higher rate of postpartum transfer among women with a prior cesarean, these women did not have higher rates of retained placenta or hemorrhage, which are the most common reasons for transfer in non-VBAC–related studies.

Two studies provide insight into VBAC in U.S. birth centers. Harrington, Miller, McClain, and Paul (1997) provide data from a hospital-based birth center in Los Angeles, California. They report a vaginal birth rate of 98% in 298 women with a prior cesarean compared with a vaginal birth rate of 99% among a control group of women without prior cesarean matched for age, parity, and gestational age. It is important to note that in this study 84% of the women with prior cesareans also had a history of prior vaginal birth. Women attempting VBAC with no prior vaginal birth were significantly more likely to transfer into hospital care compared to women attempting VBAC having had a prior vaginal birth (25% versus 6%). Among women who were transferred, women with a prior cesarean were more likely to give birth by cesarean (19% versus 6%); however, the difference was not statistically significant due to the low overall number of cesareans. No uterine ruptures were reported (Harrington et al., 1997).

The most comprehensive study of outcomes among women attempting VBAC in U.S. birth centers was published by Lieberman, Ernst, Rooks, Stapleton, and Flamm (2004). Forty-one birth centers offering VBAC services participated in a 10-year data collection effort and provided data for 1,453 women with a prior cesarean who presented to a birth center in labor. Of these women, 7% had more than one prior cesarean and 46% had a prior vaginal birth. The VBAC rate was 87%, with a significantly higher rate of vaginal birth observed in the subgroup of women with a prior vaginal birth (94% versus 81%).

Approximately one quarter of women were transferred into hospital care. Of these women, 7% were transferred immediately upon arrival to the birth center and 11% were otherwise transferred emergently. Women with a prior vaginal birth were significantly less likely to be transferred as compared with women with no prior vaginal birth (11% versus 35%), and the most common reason for intrapartum transfer was lack of progress in labor. Approximately 4% of women were transferred postpartum, with similar proportions transferred for maternal and neonatal indications. The most common maternal indication was laceration repair, and infants were most commonly transferred for respiratory support.

Six women experienced uterine rupture, with five transferring intrapartum for fetal indications and giving birth by cesarean, and one transferring postpartum for hemorrhage. Women with more than one prior cesarean were significantly more likely to experience uterine rupture (3% versus 0.2%). Prior vaginal birth was not protective against uterine rupture, nor was rupture associated with length of labor. Data were collected on the time elapsed from recognition of a complication to arrival at the hospital, and on the time until surgical incision. Four of the five women with intrapartum uterine ruptures arrived at the hospital within 15 minutes. However, only two women had a recognition-to-incision time of 30 minutes or less.

There were seven perinatal deaths, two related to uterine rupture. Women in their 42nd week of pregnancy were more likely to experience infant death as compared with women with a fetal estimated gestational age of less than 42 weeks (4.3% versus 0.4%); however, gestational age and birth weight were not associated with risk of rupture. Overall, 1.7% of women experienced a serious outcome (perinatal death ($n = 7$), Apgar less than 7 at 5 minutes ($n = 15$), uterine rupture ($n = 6$), or hysterectomy ($n = 1$); women in their 42nd week of pregnancy were more likely to experience a serious outcome (6.5% versus 1.6%).

Women who were transferred immediately upon arrival were included in the birth center statistics because presenting to the birth center ultimately delayed initiation of hospital care. However, when these women were excluded from analysis, serious outcomes occurred in 0.9% of births. Furthermore, the authors note that if women who were greater than 42 weeks in pregnancy and women with more than one prior cesarean were excluded from analysis, the rates of both uterine rupture and perinatal death were two per 1,000 births for women in birth center care. Unfortunately, the 10% of women who had either a history of more than one cesarean or a fetus past 42 gestational weeks experienced 50% of the uterine ruptures and 57% of the perinatal deaths observed among the women planning birth center care.

For comparison, 20% of U.S. women with one prior cesarean attempted a trial of labor in 2013, and 70% of these women gave birth vaginally, for an overall VBAC rate of 14% of all women with one prior cesarean (Curtin, Gregory, Korst, & Uddin, 2015). Women attempting VBAC in birth centers have higher rates of vaginal birth; however, they also have high rates of transfer to hospital care, compared with both multiparous and nulliparous women laboring in birth centers. Although absolute rates of uterine rupture are similar among women attempting VBAC in birth centers and in hospitals, there is a delay in accessing surgical resources when uterine rupture occurs in a birth center setting. However, this same delay may also occur in hospitals where surgical or anesthesia staff are not continually in-house.

SYNTHESIS OF NEONATAL OUTCOMES

Neonatal Outcome Data Overview

Although many of the studies described previously in this chapter included information on perinatal and infant outcomes, some focused exclusively on maternal outcomes and were omitted in this section, whereas additional studies on neonatal outcomes were also obtained.

The resulting 24 manuscripts included 19 data sets on neonatal outcomes in birth centers with guidelines consistent with AABC standards. Publication dates ranged from 1986 to 2014. Twelve manuscripts (using 11 data sets) reported on births in the United States (Feldman & Hurst, 1987; Fullerton et al., 1997; Jackson et al., 2003); four studies were set in the United Kingdom, with three analyzing one data set (the Birthplace Study; Brocklehurst et al., 2011; Hollowell et al., 2011; Hundley et al., 1995; Rowe et al., 2013); three studied Australian data (Laws, Tracy, & Sullivan, 2010; Stern et al., 1992; Tracy et al., 2007); three studies analyzed the same Swedish data set (Gottvall et al., 2004; Gottvall, Winbladh, Cnattingius, & Waldenström, 2005; Waldenström & Nilsson, 1993, 1997); and individual studies from Denmark (Overgaard et al., 2011) and Germany (David et al., 1999). Many international studies involved birth centers located within a hospital but adhering to the birth center philosophy of limited technology and intervention, whereas most of the U.S. birth centers studied were freestanding.

Authors used a breadth of study designs, so direct comparisons of data across studies remain difficult. Of the studies included in this review, 12 provided neonatal comparison data from matched or unmatched low-risk women giving birth in hospitals (Brocklehurst et al., 2011; David et al., 1999; Feldman & Hurst, 1987; Gottvall et al., 2004, 2005; Hollowell et al., 2011; Hundley et al., 1995; Jackson et al., 2003; Overgaard et al., 2011, 2012b; Scupholme & Kamons, 1987; Scupholme et al., 1986); six were observational and provided a description of birth center outcomes with no selected comparison group (Fullerton et al., 1997; Roberts & Sward, 2001; Rooks et al., 1992b, 1992c; Stapleton et al., 2013; Stern et al., 1992); one used a randomized controlled design (Waldenström & Nilsson, 1997); and five used birth certificate or other national perinatal tracking data systems (Grünebaum et al., 2013, 2014; Laws et al., 2010; Tracy et al., 2007; Wax et al., 2010). Most of the studies using birth certificate data provided outcomes by location of birth, regardless of where labor was planned or started (e.g., hospital outcome data would include women who transferred from a birth center). All other studies used an intent-to-treat design, and outcomes of newborns of women in the birth center group who transferred to hospital care are included in the birth center statistics. Although most studies limited the birth center sample to women who were admitted in labor, several studies included all women who received antepartum care at the birth center. We did exclude Grünebaum and colleagues' (2013) analysis of Apgar score data as there was a mathematical error in the calculation of the rate of low 5-minute Apgar scores for births with freestanding birth center midwives, and the rate was erroneously elevated by a factor of 100.

Apgar Scores

Thirteen studies reported infant Apgar scores (David et al., 1999; Feldman & Hurst, 1987; Hollowell et al., 2011; Jackson et al., 2003; Laws et al., 2010; Overgaard et al., 2011; Roberts & Sward, 2001; Rooks et al., 1989, 1992c; Scupholme et al., 1986; Stern et al., 1992; Waldenström & Nilsson, 1997; Wax et al., 2010). Although Apgar scores have limited validity as an indicator of long-term outcomes of infants, it is a widely used measure of infant transition to extrauterine life (American Academy of Pediatrics Committee on the Apgar Score, 2015). As these scores are a readily available measure of infant status, researchers have included them within many studies. In particular, it is common to study the percentage of infants who had an Apgar score less than 7 at 5 minutes of life. The incidence of this outcome ranged from 0.4% to 3% among infants born in birth centers, with three quarters of studies reporting the occurrence of low Apgar scores in less than 1% of infants. No study reported a significant difference between infants born in a hospital versus those born to mothers admitted to a birth center in labor. Laws et al. (2010) performed subgroup analysis (population) by parity and found that 1% of primiparas gave birth to infants with low 5-minute Apgar scores, as compared with 0.5% of multiparous women.

Neonatal Transfer

Six studies reported newborn transfer rates ranging from 2% to 5% (Fullerton et al., 1997; Roberts & Sward, 2001; Rooks et al., 1992c; Scupholme & Kamons, 1987; Scupholme et al., 1986; Stapleton et al., 2013). The most common reason for newborn transfer across studies was respiratory distress, which accounted for 60% to 100% of newborn transfers. Additional newborn transfer indications are reported in Table 4.4.

Two studies commented on the urgency of newborn transfer. Roberts and Sward (2001) reported that among the 4% of infants who required transfer after birth (all due to respiratory issues), 75% were transferred by ambulance, which was considered a proxy measure for urgency. The *National Birth Center Study II* (Stapleton et al., 2013) reported that of the 13,030 infants who were born in a birth center, 2.6% required hospital transfer, and 0.7% ($n = 94$) of those transfers were emergent. Rowe et al. (2013)

TABLE 4.4
Common Neonatal Transfer Indications

Common Neonatal Transfer Indications
Respiratory distress*
Hip dislocation
Fractured clavicle/humerus†
Jaundice
Hypoglycemia
Congenital anomaly

*Condition is more common in babies of multiparous women.
†More common in babies of primigravid women.

analyzed the circumstances surrounding transfer in the U.K. Birthplace Study, and noted that all low 5-minute Apgar scores ($n = 6$) were among infants of women transferred for "potentially urgent" indications.

Perinatal and Neonatal Morbidity and Mortality

Respiratory Support

As discussed, the need for some respiratory support is not uncommon at birth and may or may not require hospital transfer. As reported in nine studies, 0% to 5.3% of infants born to mothers in a birth center group required respiratory support. Laws et al. (2010) reported that infants in the birth center group required significantly more "high-level" resuscitation as compared with controls, although the overall numbers were low (0.6% versus 0.4%). This finding was not replicated in other studies. On the contrary, David et al. (1999) noted a higher proportion of newborns in the hospital group required immediate medical care at birth (e.g., mechanical respiration, intubation, or fluid replacement), and Overgaard et al. (2011) reported that a higher number of infants in the hospital group had neonatal asphyxia than those in the birth center group. The need for infant respiratory support may also differ by parity. Laws et al. (2010) reported that infants born to nulliparous women in both settings were approximately twice as likely to require resuscitation at birth.

Admission to NICU

Ten studies reported NICU admission rates among infants whose mothers started labor in a birth center (David et al., 1999; Feldman & Hurst,

1987; Hundley et al., 1995; Jackson et al., 2003; Laws et al., 2010; Overgaard et al., 2011; Scupholme & Kamons, 1987; Stern et al., 1992; Waldenström & Nilsson, 1997; Wax et al., 2010). Admission rates to the NICU ranged from 3% to 10% with the majority of studies reporting admission rates at or below 5%. The majority of studies found no statistically significant differences in the rate of NICU admission of infants born out of versus in the hospital; Wax et al. (2010) and Laws et al. (2010) report that infants born in birth centers were significantly less likely to be admitted to a NICU than those born in a hospital.

Authors of two studies analyzed NICU admission data by maternal parity and found that the infants of nulliparous women were more likely to be admitted to the NICU than the infants of multiparous women receiving birth center care (Laws et al., 2010; Waldenström & Nilsson, 1997). However, Laws et al. (2010) found that NICU admissions among birth center infants were lower than those born in hospitals, whereas Waldenström and Nilsson (1997) found that infants of primiparous women in birth centers were admitted to the NICU more frequently than those of primiparous controls.

Seizures

Three of four studies reported an increased rate of neonatal seizures among infants born in birth centers. Wax et al. (2010) and Grünebaum et al. (2013) used U.S. birth certificate data and noted similar findings: approximately 0.02% of newborns born to low-risk women in a hospital experience temporary seizures compared with 0.04% of infants born in a birth center. In the U.K. Birthplace Study analysis of low-risk women, infants in the birth center group had a rate of 1.5 seizures per 1,000 births, whereas infants born in standard obstetric units had a rate of 1 seizure per 1,000 births (Hollowell et al., 2011). However, Gottvall et al. (2005) found no significant difference in the incidence of seizures between infants born to women receiving birth center versus standard obstetric care. None of these studies provided long-term follow-up information on neonates who experienced seizures. This may be related to the prohibition against continuous electronic fetal monitoring in birth centers using the AABC or similar accreditation guidelines; a Cochrane review meta-analysis found that the only benefit of electronic fetal monitoring was a reduction in neonatal seizures (Alfirevic, Devane, Gyte, & Cuthbert, 2017).

Other Measures of Neonatal Morbidity

Data from the Stockholm birth center study were analyzed for insight into neonatal morbidity within the first month after birth among infants born in an in-hospital birth center (Gottvall et al., 2004). However, it is worth noting that approximately 30% of the women included in the birth center sample actually gave birth in a hospital following antepartum or intrapartum transfer. Authors compared outcomes data from more than 3,000 infants whose mothers received at least some birth center care to the infant morbidity reported by area hospitals throughout Stockholm, and found a statistically lower rate of fractures and hypoglycemia among the infants born to women in the birth center group. Although birth center infants were noted to have a statistically higher incidence of respiratory complications, this finding was not significant when the comparison group was limited to women who gave birth in the same hospital where the birth center was located, and the authors noted this was most likely a difference in documentation practices. There were no other significant differences between the groups in any other measure of morbidity, including brachial plexus injury, seizures, hypoxia or asphyxia, intracranial hemorrhage, infection, and immunization or hyperbilirubinemia (Gottvall et al., 2005).

Perinatal Mortality

Perinatal deaths can be divided in three categories: those occurring after 22 weeks of gestation but before labor begins (antepartum death), those occurring during the process of labor and birth (intrapartum death), and those in the first 28 days of life (neonatal death). Across the studies that provided descriptions of the circumstances surrounding perinatal deaths, most antepartum deaths were due to congenital anomalies, intrauterine fetal demise (often a cord accident), placental abruption, maternal infection, or otherwise unknown causes. Most intrapartum deaths with details available occurred in the hospital after transfer from the birth center for fetal distress, prolonged labor, or placental abruption. Several intrapartum deaths were unexplained stillbirths, where fetal heart tones were lost during labor. Finally, the causes of neonatal death included meconium aspiration, respiratory distress syndrome, isoimmunization, and sepsis.

Twelve studies reported that perinatal deaths occurred among infants born to women planning birth center care (Gottvall et al., 2004; Grünebaum et al., 2014; Hollowell et al., 2011; Hundley et al., 1995; Jackson et al., 2003; Laws et al., 2010; Overgaard et al., 2011; Rooks et al., 1989; Stapleton et al., 2013; Stern et al., 1992; Tracy et al., 2007; Waldenström & Nilsson, 1997). For women admitted to a birth center in labor, the perinatal death rates ranged from 0.59 to 1.5 deaths per 1,000 births. Two studies performed a subgroup analysis and excluded infants with congenital anomalies and reported modified perinatal death rates of 0.4 and 0.7

deaths per 1,000 births (Rooks et al., 1992c; Stapleton et al., 2013). Several studies found slightly higher rates of mortality among the birth center group as compared with controls (Gottvall et al., 2004; Grünebaum et al., 2014; Hollowell et al., 2011; Hundley et al., 1995; Overgaard et al., 2011; Waldenström & Nilsson, 1997), whereas others found lower rates (Jackson et al., 2003; Laws et al., 2010; Tracy et al., 2007). None of the studies that used a low-risk hospital control group reported a statistically significant difference in perinatal mortality rates (Gottvall et al., 2004; Grünebaum et al., 2014; Hollowell et al., 2011; Hundley et al., 1995; Jackson et al., 2003; Laws et al., 2010; Overgaard et al., 2011; Tracy et al., 2007; Waldenström & Nilsson, 1997). Additionally, increased rates of perinatal death experienced by women planning birth center births were observed among primigravidas (Grünebaum et al., 2014; Laws et al., 2010; Tracy et al., 2007; Waldenström & Nilsson, 1997), women past 42 weeks of gestation (Grünebaum et al., 2014; Rooks et al., 1992c; Waldenström & Nilsson, 1997), and women older than 35 years (Tracy et al., 2007).

DISCUSSION

Clinical Outcomes

Clinicians providing care in birth centers have the unique ability to support normal, physiologic birth and routinely provide evidence-based intrapartum care that includes oral nutrition and hydration, intermittent auscultation, ambulation, and continuous support (Hundley et al., 1995; Rooks et al., 1992b). These practices undoubtedly contribute to the high rate of vaginal birth observed in birth centers, more than 90% in the most recent multisite study (Stapleton et al., 2013). Maternal outcomes are excellent, however, there may be a small increase in some poor infant outcomes. While obstetric catastrophes are rare, when they occur, delays in reaching intensive medical and surgical care can affect outcomes. Currently, nearly one third of women giving birth in U.S. hospitals deliver via abdominal incision, which not only increases the maternal morbidity and mortality surrounding that particular birth, but that woman's subsequent pregnancies and births (Curtin et al., 2015). Immediate risks of cesarean include a higher likelihood of blood transfusions, infections, and ICU admissions. Risks in subsequent pregnancies include abnormalities in placental implantation, uterine rupture, and maternal death (Curtin et al., 2015). Women and families need to make their own informed decisions about the location of birth using the best information from the current literature in light of their personal risk factors.

Women who desire out-of-hospital birth should receive informed consent including available data on/about maternal and fetal outcomes. In the past 20 years, priority has been placed on neonatal outcomes as the primary measure of birth safety (American College of Obstetricians and Gynecologists (ACOG) and Society for Maternal-Fetal Medicine, 2015). However, the rising use of cesarean and the subsequent rise in maternal morbidity and mortality have caused practitioners and national organizations to reexamine the focus on neonatal outcomes (ACOG and Society for Maternal-Fetal Medicine, 2015; Curtin et al., 2015). Practitioners can assist women in understanding the maternal and neonatal risks and benefits of out-of-hospital birth in order to make a decision that meets their personal preferences and medical needs. Key aspects that should be addressed in informed consent are included in Box 4.1.

Risks for Poor Clinical Outcomes

Certain populations of women are at higher risk for complications in birth center care. Nulliparous women account for the vast majority of intrapartum transfers and experience almost every obstetric complication at higher rates. This is true of nulliparous women in hospital care as well; a first pregnancy is the initial time that pregnancy-related complications appear, and multiparous women eligible for birth center care likely had uncomplicated prior pregnancies. For example, a woman diagnosed with cephalopelvic disproportion who had a cesarean with her first pregnancy is more appropriate for hospital care with subsequent pregnancies. The evidence is also clear that the risk to infants increases after 42 completed weeks of gestation; therefore, women with postterm pregnancies are not currently eligible for birth center care under CABC guidelines, as well as most other birth centers that publish their exclusion criteria. Finally, although VBAC is acceptable under AABC guidelines for women with one prior low transverse cesarean section, informed consent about the risks of uterine rupture including possible longer time to surgical intervention is required for these women. Discussions about risk status need to be specific to each birth center and include information such as the time required for transfer and the immediate availability of surgical providers at the referring hospital.

BOX 4.1
Information to Include in Informed Consent Discussions

Outcomes in Mothers: Women who are admitted to birth centers in labor have higher rates of vaginal birth and lower rates of cesarean than women who choose hospital birth. The largest and most recent study of women using U.S. birth centers found that only 6% of women admitted to birth centers had a cesarean. Women in birth center care are also less likely to use pain medication during labor and are less likely to need stitches to their perineum. Very few life-threatening maternal problems have been reported among women using birth center services.

Only low-risk women can labor and give birth in accredited birth centers. About 12% of women initially admitted in labor to a birth center will be transferred to a hospital. First-time mothers have a greater risk of needing transfer than women who have already given birth. Most transfers are because of prolonged labor and are not emergencies.

Infant Outcomes: Studies show that babies born in birth centers have Apgar scores similar to those of babies born in the hospital. Although most do very well, 3% to 5% of babies born in birth centers are transferred to a hospital following birth. Difficulty with breathing is the most common reason for infant transfer. Infants born in birth centers may have a slightly increased rate of temporary seizures, but this is very rare; approximately one baby out of 2,500 (0.04%) born in birth centers will have neonatal seizures. The chance that the fetus/newborn of a mother giving birth in a birth center will die in labor or soon after birth is also rare. The largest and most recent study reported that for every 2,000 women admitted to U.S. birth centers in labor, one experienced a fetal or newborn death. This rate of death is slightly higher than in the hospital. A recent study of birth certificates showed a death rate of approximately six per 1,000 babies born in birth centers compared with three per 10,000 in midwife-attended hospital births. This is similar to comparing a lifetime risk of dying due to fire or smoke inhalation (one in 1,666) with the risk of dying from choking (one in 3,333). Infants of first-time mothers may experience problems at a higher rate than babies of multiparous women. Infants of first-time mothers are more likely to need help establishing breathing, more likely to be transferred and receive NICU care, and may have higher rates of infant death.

Birth Center Factors: Characteristics of the birth center may affect outcomes. Birth centers that follow AABC and CABC standards have high standards for safety and quality that include plans for emergencies. The staff of accredited birth centers work within the regional health care system and have ongoing relationships with providers at higher level facilities. The distance to the referring hospital and the quality of collaboration between the birth center providers and their hospital colleagues may affect the speed of transfer during emergencies and influence later maternal and neonatal outcomes.

Health Care System Factors

Most of the non-U.S. birth centers reviewed were located within or adjacent to a hospital, and birth center location plays an important role in the discussion of risk. However, the actual time spent in transport from birth center to hospital is only part of the transfer process. Indeed, Gottvall et al. (2004) identified only one preventable infant death in 10 years of birth center data, and this case involved a mother who was transferred for failure to progress but was then treated as having a low-risk, normal labor, despite having a "very complicated post-dates labor" (p. 76). Thus, positive interprofessional relationships and clear communication between transferring providers are crucial to patient safety. Moreover, it is worth noting that women laboring in many hospitals in the United States do not have instant access to cesarean (ACOG and Society for Maternal-Fetal Medicine, 2015). Without anesthesia and surgical staff in-house, which are uncommon in many small communities, delays can occur even within a hospital.

Up to a third of the birth center sample in these studies actually gave birth in a hospital, meaning that any hospital-associated morbidity or mortality is attributed to the birth center group. Intent-to-treat analysis is important because it keeps all women who intended birth center birth at a given point within the birth center sample, not just those who successfully gave birth in this location. However, much of the mortality and morbidity that was described in these studies occurred in the hospital. Birth centers successfully identified women who were no longer low risk and moved them to a higher level facility. Thus, hospitals and hospital-based providers play an important role in caring for birth center clients who need more specialized obstetric care.

The recent joint guideline from the ACOG and Society for Maternal-Fetal Medicine discussed the expectations for clinical services and systems available in a tiered system of maternity facilities, including birth centers; basic care, specialty care, and subspecialty care facilities; and regional tertiary care centers (ACOG & Society for Maternal-Fetal Medicine, 2015). Birth centers are located within a continuum of care that enables women to receive the appropriate level of care to meet their needs and access to higher level care as needed. Although birth centers are an ideal environment in which to support normal, physiologic birth, midwives continually perform risk assessment with a low tolerance for abnormal findings as evidenced by the relatively high transfer rates across studies.

The guideline advises, "Each facility should have a clear . . . threshold for transferring women to health care facilities that offer a higher level of care. . . . Facilities should collaborate to develop and maintain maternal and neonatal transport plans and cooperative agreements capable of managing the health needs of women who develop complications." The safety of birth center care depends on the level of cooperation between transferring providers and facilities as well as the capabilities of the receiving hospitals. Both women and providers should be aware that transferring women are no longer low risk, and they require some intervention unavailable in the birth center (e.g., Pitocin, continuous monitoring, surgical birth).

It is also important to know that there is great variation in birth center protocols, accreditation status, and provider licensure and certification, all of which potentially impact clinical outcomes. Analyses of birth certificate data do not take into account the heterogeneity of birth centers with regard to adherence to standards. For example, less than 50% of birth centers in the United States are accredited by the CABC, which requires adherence to high standards of patient safety including emergency preparedness, clinical protocols, provider education, and ongoing quality improvement. Nonaccredited birth centers, or those accredited by other organizations such as The Joint Commission, may certainly meet these standards of care. However, in the absence of clear and published guidelines there is no way to compare or evaluate these practices.

DATA COLLECTION: LIMITATIONS AND RECOMMENDATIONS FOR FUTURE RESEARCH

Data Collection in Birth Centers

Nearly all birth centers collect data as part of ongoing quality improvement initiatives. Birth centers accredited by the CABC are required to track their clinical outcomes through the Perinatal Data Registry (PDR), which utilizes a secure web-based portal to allow clinicians to upload and maintain their quality assurance data. Currently, the PDR exists as a robust repository of clearly defined measures for use in quality improvement projects and research studies (Stapleton, 2011). These data collection efforts have been ongoing since 2007. Formerly known as the Uniform Data Set (UDS), the PDR accepts data from diverse practices. A copy of the variables in the PDR can be found on the AABC website. Although individual centers contributing to the PDR may use their own data in outcomes tracking and quality improvement, the use of the registry for research requires institutional review board (IRB) approval and a signed data use agreement. Although birth centers accredited through other mechanisms and those choosing not to pursue accreditation also engage in data collection, these data are not as readily available for aggregation and analysis.

Birth Centers: The Promise and Peril of Data Aggregation

Birth centers are designed to serve the needs of low-risk women and their newborns and provide evidence-based, high-quality, family-centered care to each woman and baby. Ongoing assessment of clinical outcomes is an integral part of quality monitoring and improvement; however, developing clear and meaningful benchmarks for clinical outcomes can be difficult. Severe complications are rare among low-risk women and their infants; therefore, it can often take a large amount of data collected with careful attention to detail to determine a baseline rate for maternal or neonatal complications. Moreover, studies must include even larger samples to accurately detect differences between birth center and hospital groups.

Researchers can obtain large samples by gathering data from multiple locations. Examples include the classic *Birth Center Study* released in 1989 (Rooks et al., 1989), the 2013 *National Birth Center Study II* (Stapleton et al., 2013), and the *U.K. Birthplace Study* (Brocklehurst et al., 2011). Another method of data aggregation is merging results from several studies in a systematic review or meta-analysis. Birth centers are used in many countries and the integration of international data provides additional statistical power to observe the effects of birth center care on maternal and neonatal outcomes. An example of this approach can be found in the Alliman and Phillippi's (2016) study of maternal outcomes in birth centers.

Although multisite studies or systematic aggregation of data allow for greater statistical power, there are pitfalls to merging data from many sites and trials. Maternity care practices have changed over time and vary greatly by country and location. For example, rates of cesarean birth have risen dramatically since studies of birth centers were first published in the 1980s and still vary significantly between countries. In addition, definitions of key outcomes differ between studies; for example, "low-risk," "emergent/nonemergent" transfer, "prolonged labor," or "serious" complications are not consistently defined by researchers. The lack of consistent definitions makes conclusive statistical comparisons difficult. However, careful review of clinical outcomes in birth centers offers valuable information for providers and the women they serve. When multiple studies have similar results, the likelihood of spurious findings is decreased.

There are additional caveats to a systematic analysis of neonatal outcomes in birth centers. The greatest problem is the heterogeneity of measures and the changes in standard care in different locations and over time. For instance, some studies measured fetal morbidity as including everything from a fractured clavicle to neonatal death (Brocklehurst et al., 2011; Waldenström & Nilsson, 1997), whereas other studies include only long-term neonatal injuries as neonatal morbidity and measure mortality separately. In addition, birth centers vary in their clinical guidelines, which can affect the rate of transport and perinatal outcomes.

Differences in clinical practice are especially apparent when examining studies across time. In older studies, ultrasound was not commonly used and congenital anomalies were a more common cause of perinatal morbidity for birth center and hospital-born infants. However, even in recent studies, some women carrying fetuses with a condition known to be incompatible with life are allowed to give birth at centers. Although these infants are sometimes included in mortality statistics, they would not have survived in the hospital. Conversely, hospitals often have a higher risk population than birth centers, so it can be difficult to assess difference in outcomes by setting using large data sets that do not control for risk status at the time of birth. When researchers provide a comparison group, where possible, we note the composition of this sample. The inclusion and exclusion criteria vary greatly among studies and further limit aggregation of studies.

Samples in many older studies include women at 42 weeks or greater fetal gestation (Gottvall et al., 2004; Rooks et al., 1989; Waldenström & Nilsson, 1997), whereas more recent studies exclude women who are postterm (David et al., 1999; Overgaard et al., 2011; Stapleton et al., 2013). Many maternal factors affect neonatal outcomes, most notably age, parity, and obstetric history. Some studies provide more detail on outcomes with these factors as a covariate, whereas other studies only examine outcomes of the entire sample of women or neonates.

Location of the birth center may also affect neonatal outcomes. Birth centers close to the referral hospital may have decreased transport time, which can improve outcomes as treatment delays can increase the likelihood of poor outcomes (Rowe et al., 2013). However even birth centers located in hospitals may experience transfer difficulty. In addition to transport time, delays may also be related to poor communication or collaboration among health care providers or misunderstandings about needs of women who were transferred. Even with these caveats, study of neonatal outcomes in birth centers provides valuable information on the safety of the model and information to facilitate informed consent for women as they decide their location of birth.

Future Research

The PDR is a robust data set for the study of birth center care and outcomes in the United States and has the capacity to be integral to future studies. The growing use of electronic medical records may streamline aggregation of data into registries and enhance statistical power to observe differences among groups. In order to permit large-scale studies, each provider must use identical definitions of outcomes measures. The multidisciplinary reVITALize initiative led by ACOG has a goal of creating standard maternity care definitions for communication, reporting in the medical record, and research (Menard, Main, & Currigan, 2014).

Building on this work, the Clarity in Collaboration process led by ACNM used an interdisciplinary expert panel and a national survey to develop standardized definitions to express the provision of midwifery care (Freytsis, Phillippi, Cox, Romano, & Cragin, 2017). The Clarity in Collaboration Project is a step toward developing measures of the extent of midwifery care received by women to properly attribute outcomes to the provider responsible for the majority of each woman's care. This effort will assist in tracking the outcomes of women who begin care with a midwife in a freestanding birth center.

Researchers should use standardized data definitions across studies to allow for data synthesis and aggregation. Although there is currently not a global data standard for definitions surrounding birth center care, the PDR has well-operationalized definitions that include methods of denoting the timing and type of transfer of care. Ideally, these definitions can be more widely implemented to permit greater data aggregation in the future. In addition, clinicians and researchers should collaborate to create and test new models of interprofessional care utilizing low-intervention birth settings with specialist involvement in individual plans of care. Women and families deserve high-quality, evidence-based care. However, the current literature does not have robust data on effective models of interprofessional collaboration to ensure women receive patient-centered care at the appropriate facility for their immediate and long-term needs.

CONCLUSION

Although there are obvious limitations in aggregating data from multiple countries, birth center locations, and time periods, published literature provides strong evidence that maternal outcomes in birth centers for appropriately selected women are at least equal or improved compared with those in hospitals, whereas infant morbidity and mortality are very rare. However, women and their infants must travel to receive medical interventions when they become needed, which can increase the risk of serious sequelae when emergencies occur. Some groups of women, including nulliparous women and women with a previous cesarean birth, have a slightly increased risk of complications in the birth center setting when compared with the hospital setting. However, overall risk, even for women from these groups, is *very* low. Women and their families can make informed decisions about acceptable levels of risk and priorities of care when determining a location for birth.

The birth center is an important component of a patient-centered maternity care system as developed nations work to decrease cesarean birth and improve maternal health outcomes through promotion of physiologic birth. Individual midwives and other clinicians can contribute to this effort through submission of outcomes data to registries. Continued research is needed to thoroughly study the birth center model of care and its effects on perinatal outcomes, support the safety and continued growth of this model of care, and provide women with information to guide their choices about maternity care.

REFERENCES

Alfirevic, Z., Devane, D., Gyte, G. M. L., & Cuthbert, A. (2017). Continuous cardiotocography (CTG) as a form of electronic fetal monitoring (EFM) for fetal assessment during labour. Cochrane Database of Systematic Reviews, *2012*(2). doi: 10.1002/14651858.CD006066.pub3

Alliman, J., & Phillippi, J. C. (2016). Maternal outcomes in birth centers: An integrative review of the literature. *Journal of Midwifery and Women's Health, 61*(1), 21–51.

American Academy of Pediatrics Committee on the Apgar Score. (2015). The Apgar score. *Pediatrics, 136*(4), 819.

American College of Obstetricians and Gynecologists and Society for Maternal-Fetal Medicine. (2015). Obstetric care consensus no. 2: Levels of maternal care. *Obstetrics and Gynecology, 125*(2), 502–515. doi:10.1097/01.AOG.0000460770.99574.9f

Beckmann, L., Barger, M., Dorin, L., Metzing, S., & Hellmers, C. (2014). Vaginal birth after cesarean in German out-of-hospital settings: Maternal and neonatal outcomes of women with their second child. *Birth, 41*(4), 309–315.

Benatar, S., Garrett, A. B., Howell, E., & Palmer, A. (2013). Midwifery care at a freestanding birth center: A safe and effective alternative to conventional maternity care. *Health Services Research, 48*(5), 1750–1768.

Birthplace in England Collaborative Group. (2011). Perinatal and maternal outcomes by planned place of birth for healthy women with low risk pregnancies: The birthplace in England national prospective cohort study. *British Medical Journal, 343.* doi:10.1136/bmj.d7400

Curtin, S., Gregory, K., Korst, L., & Uddin, S. (2015). Maternal morbidity for vaginal and cesarean deliveries, according to previous cesarean history: New data from the birth certificate, 2013. *National Vital Statistics Reports, 64*(4), 1–14.

David, M., Gross, M. M., Wiemer, A., Pachaly, J., & Vetter, K. (2009). Prior cesarean section—An acceptable risk for vaginal delivery at free-standing midwife-led birth centers? Results of the analysis of vaginal birth after cesarean section (VBAC) in German birth centers. *European Journal of Obstetrics and Gynecology and Reproductive Biology, 142*(2), 106–110.

David, M., von Schwarzenfeld, H. K., Dimer, J., & Kentenich, H. (1999). Perinatal outcome in hospital and birth center obstetric care. *International Journal of Gynaecology and Obstetrics, 65*(2), 149–156.

Feldman, E., & Hurst, M. (1987). Outcomes and procedures in low risk birth: A comparison of hospital and birth center settings. *Birth, 14*(1), 18–24.

Freytsis, M., Phillippi, J. C., Cox, K., Romano, A., & Cragin, L. (2017). ACNM Clarity in Collaboration Project: Defining midwifery care in collaborative care models. *Journal of Midwifery and Women's Health, 62*(1), 101–108.

Fullerton, J. T., Jackson, D., Snell, B., Besser, M., Dickinson, C., & Garite, T. (1997). Transfer rates from freestanding birth centers: A comparison with the National Birth Center Study. *Journal of Nurse-Midwifery, 42*(1), 9–16.

Gottvall, K., Grunewald, C., & Waldenström, U. (2004). Safety of birth centre care: Perinatal mortality over a 10-year period. *British Journal of Obstetrics and Gynaecology: An International Journal of Obstetrics and Gynaecology, 111*(1), 71–78.

Gottvall, K., Winbladh, B., Cnattingius, S., & Waldenström, U. (2005). Birth centre care over a 10-year period: Infant morbidity during the first month after birth. *Acta Paediatrica, 94*(9), 1253–1260.

Grünebaum, A., McCullough, L. B., Sapra, K. J., Brent, R. L., Levene, M. I., Arabin, B., & Chervenak, F. A. (2013). Apgar score of 0 at 5 minutes and neonatal seizures or serious neurologic dysfunction in relation to birth setting. *American Journal of Obstetrics & Gynecology, 209*(4), 321–323.

Grünebaum, A., McCullough, L. B., Sapra, K. J., Brent, R. L., Levene, M. I., Arabin, B., & Chervenak, F. A. (2014). Early and total neonatal mortality in relation to birth setting in the United States, 2006–2009. *American Journal of Obstetrics & Gynecology, 211*(4), 390.e1–390.e7.

Harrington, L. C., Miller, D. A., McClain, C. J., & Paul, R. H. (1997). Vaginal birth after cesarean in a hospital-based birth center staffed by certified nurse-midwives. *Journal of Nurse-Midwifery, 42*(4), 304–307.

Hollowell, J., Puddicombe, D., Rowe, R., Linsell, L., Hardy, P., Stewart, M., . . . Macfarlane, A. (2011). The birthplace national prospective cohort study: Perinatal and maternal outcomes by planned place of birth. Birthplace in England research programme. Final report part 4. NIHR Service Delivery and Organisation Programme.

Hundley, V. A., Cruickshank, F. M., Milne, J. M., Glazener, C. M. A., Lang, G. D., Turner, M., . . . Mollison, J. (1995). Satisfaction and continuity of care: Staff views of care in a midwife-managed delivery unit. *Midwifery, 11*(4), 163–173.

Jackson, D. J., Lang, J. M., Swartz, W. H., Ganiats, T. G., Fullerton, J., Ecker, J., & Nguyen, U. (2003). Outcomes, safety, and resource utilization in a collaborative care birth center program compared with traditional physician-based perinatal care. *American Journal of Public Health, 93*(6), 999–1006.

Laws, P. J., Tracy, S. K., & Sullivan, E. A. (2010). Perinatal outcomes of women intending to give birth in birth centers in Australia. *Birth, 37*(1), 28–36.

Lieberman, E., Ernst, E. K., Rooks, J. P., Stapleton, S., & Flamm, B. (2004). Results of the national study of vaginal birth after cesarean in birth centers. *Obstetrics and Gynecology, 104*(5 Part 1), 933–942.

MacVicar, J., Dobbie, G., Owen-Johnstone, L., Jagger, C., Hopkins, M., & Kennedy, J. (1993). Simulated home delivery in hospital: A randomised controlled trial. *British Journal of*

Obstetrics and Gynaecology: An International Journal of Obstetrics and Gynaecology, 100(4), 316–323.

Menard, M. K., Main, E. K., & Currigan, S. M. (2014). Executive summary of the reVITALize initiative: Standardizing obstetric data definitions. *Obstetrics and Gynecology, 124*(1), 150–153. doi:10.1097/AOG.0000000000000322

Nguyen, U. S. D., Rothman, K. J., Demissie, S., Jackson, D. J., Lang, J. M., & Ecker, J. L. (2009). Transfers among women intending a birth center delivery in the San Diego birth center study. *Journal of Midwifery and Women's Health, 54*(2), 104–110.

Overgaard, C., Fenger-Grøn, M., & Sandall, J. (2012a). Freestanding midwifery units versus obstetric units: Does the effect of place of birth differ with level of social disadvantage? *BMC Public Health, 12*(1), 478.

Overgaard, C., Fenger-Grøn, M., & Sandall, J. (2012b). The impact of birthplace on women's birth experiences and perceptions of care. *Social Science and Medicine, 74*(7), 973–981.

Overgaard, C., Møller, A. M., Fenger-Grøn, M., Knudsen, L. B., & Sandall, J. (2011). Freestanding midwifery unit versus obstetric unit: A matched cohort study of outcomes in low-risk women. *BMJ Open, 1*(2). doi:10.1136/bmjopen-2011-000262

Roberts, L., & Sward, K. (2001). Birth center outcomes reported through automated technology. *Journal of Obstetric, Gynecologic, and Neonatal Nursing, 30*(1), 110–120.

Rooks, J. P., Weatherby, N. L., & Ernst, E. K. M. (1992a). The National Birth Center Study. Part I—Methodology and prenatal care and referrals. *Journal of Nurse-Midwifery, 37*(4), 222–253.

Rooks, J. P., Weatherby, N. L., & Ernst, E. K. M. (1992b). The National Birth Center Study. Part II—Intrapartum and immediate postpartum and neonatal care. *Journal of Nurse-Midwifery, 37*(5), 301–330.

Rooks, J. P., Weatherby, N. L., & Ernst, E. K. M. (1992c). The National Birth Center Study. Part III: Intrapartum and immediate postpartum and neonatal complications and transfers, postpartum and neonatal care, outcomes, and client satisfaction. *Journal of Nurse-Midwifery, 37*(6), 361–397.

Rooks, J. P., Weatherby, N. L., Ernst, E. K. M., Stapleton, S., Rosen, D., & Rosenfield, A. (1989). Outcomes of care in birth centers: The National Birth Center Study. *New England Journal of Medicine, 321*(26), 1804–1811.

Rowe, R. E., Townend, J., Brocklehurst, P., Knight, M., Macfarlane, A., McCourt, C., . . . Silverton, L. (2013). Duration and urgency of transfer in births planned at home and in freestanding midwifery units in England: Secondary analysis of the birthplace national prospective cohort study. *BMC Pregnancy and Childbirth, 13*(1), 224.

Scupholme, A., & Kamons, A. S. (1987). Are outcomes compromised when mothers are assigned to birth centers for care? *Journal of Nurse-Midwifery, 32*(4), 211–215.

Scupholme, A., McLeod, A. G., & Robertson, E. G. (1986). A birth center affiliated with the tertiary care center: Comparison of outcome. *Obstetrics and Gynecology, 67*(4), 598–603.

Stapleton, S. R. (2011). Validation of an online data registry for midwifery practices: A pilot project. *Journal of Midwifery and Women's Health, 56*(5), 452–460.

Stapleton, S. R., Osborne, C., & Illuzzi, J. (2013). Outcomes of care in birth centers: Demonstration of a durable model. *Journal of Midwifery and Women's Health, 58*(1), 3–14. doi:10.1111/jmwh.12003

Stern, C., Permezel, M., Petterson, C., Lawson, J., Eggers, T., & Kloss, M. (1992). The Royal Women's Hospital Family Birth Centre: The first 10 years reviewed. *Australian and New Zealand Journal of Obstetrics and Gynaecology, 32*(4), 291–296.

Tracy, S. K., Dahlen, H., Caplice, S., Laws, P., Wang, Y. A., Tracy, M. B., & Sullivan, E. (2007). Birth centers in Australia: A national population-based study of perinatal mortality associated with giving birth in a birth center. *Birth, 34*(3), 194–201.

Waldenström, U., & Nilsson, C.-A. (1993). Women's satisfaction with birth center care: A randomized, controlled study. *Birth, 20*(1), 3–13.

Waldenström, U., & Nilsson, C.-A. (1994). Experience of childbirth in birth center care. *Acta Obstetricia et Gynecologica Scandinavica, 73*(7), 547–554.

Waldenström, U., & Nilsson, C.-A. (1997). A randomized controlled study of birth center care versus standard maternity care: Effects on women's health. *Birth, 24*(1), 17–26.

Wax, J. R., Pinette, M. G., Cartin, A., & Blackstone, J. (2010). Maternal and newborn morbidity by birth facility among selected United States 2006 low-risk births. *American Journal of Obstetrics & Gynecology, 202*(2), 152.e1–152.e5.

CHAPTER 5

A Profile of Birth Center Use in the United States and the Potential Demand for Birth Center Use in the Future

EUGENE R. DECLERCQ AND ERIKA R. CHENG

LEARNING OBJECTIVES

Upon completion of this chapter, the reader will be able to:

1. Describe the recent trends in birth center births in the United States
2. Identify the characteristics of mothers who give birth in birth centers in the United States
3. Describe the characteristics of mothers who gave birth in a hospital but express an interest in using birth centers for their future births

This chapter focuses on the "who" and "where" of birth centers in the United States—examining trends in birth center use in the United States over time, the distribution of birth center births by state, the characteristics of mothers who choose a birth center birth, and some unique data from women who recently gave birth in a hospital on their attitudes toward birth center births. Our goal is to provide the most recent data available on birth center births. Given normal delays in the production of a book, we also have a website (www.birthbythenumbers.org) where updates to the figures presented here are posted as new data become available.

THE GROWING DEMAND FOR BIRTH CENTER BIRTHS

Relatively systematic data on the use of birth centers in the United States only begins to appear after the 1989 revision to the U.S. Standard Certificate of Live Birth (an agreement among states that specifies what variables all states agree to collect data on), which refined an earlier measure that simply defined births as occurring either in or out of a hospital. The 1989 revision added a category of "freestanding birth center" as a possible place of delivery (National Center for Health Statistics [NCHS], 2013). Figure 5.1 is drawn from that birth certificate item and presents the overall trend of nonhospital births from 1989 to 2015 (NCHS, 1991, 2017). The pattern of home births and births in freestanding birth centers roughly parallel each other with a very gradual decline from 1989 to 2004 followed by a more rapid increase to the point where, by 2015, about one in every 70 births (1.4%) in the United States occurred at home or in a birth center.

Figure 5.2 presents the data specifically for birth centers. In 1989, there were 14,273 births recorded as occurring at freestanding birth centers in the United States, representing 0.36% of all U.S. births. That total declined slowly such that by 2004 fewer than one in 400 U.S. births (0.23%) were in birth centers. The total increased slightly in 2005 (from 9,620 in 2004 to 10,217 in 2005), then remained relatively steady until 2008 when another

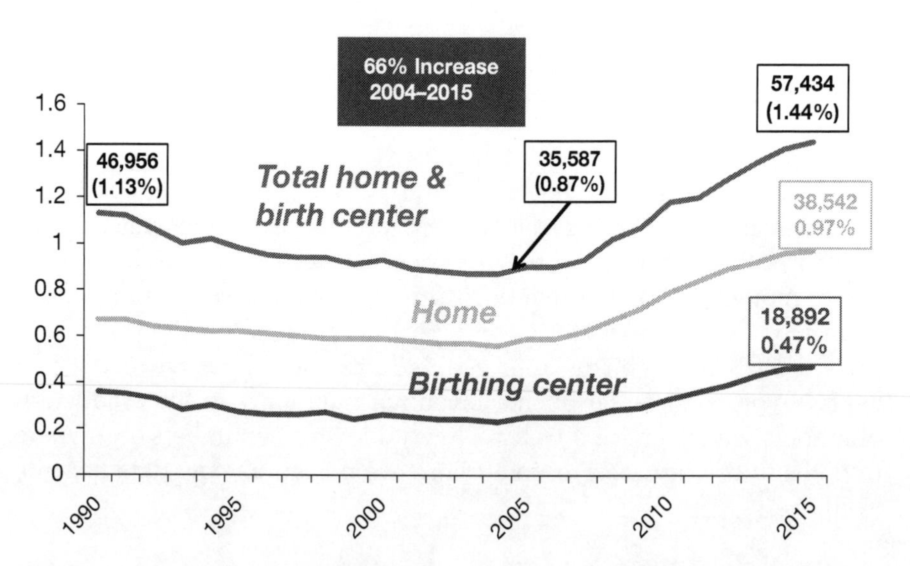

FIGURE 5.1 Percentage of all births at home or in a birthing center, United States, 1990–2015.
Adapted from CDC (2015) and Hamilton, Martin, Osterman, Curtin, and Matthews (2015).

significant increase occurred (12,014 or 0.28% of all births). Since 2008, the number of birth center births has increased rapidly with 18,219 occurring by 2014. Between 2004 and 2014, the proportion of all U.S. births occurring in freestanding birth centers has doubled, from 0.23% to 0.46%. Although starting from a very small base, this represents a notable increase and is consistent with the overall trend toward an increasing reliance on out-of-hospital births.

Where Are Birth Center Births Occurring?

Figure 5.3 presents the rate of birth center births by state and notable differences that emerge. Although there is a regional pattern to home births (MacDorman & Declercq, 2016; MacDorman, Declercq, & Mathews, 2013), the potential for state differences in birth center births is even more pronounced, since the establishment and operations of birth centers are typically regulated by a state agency, with some states having no birth centers and others having many (see American Association of Birth Centers' (AABC) website: www.birthcenters.org). As a result, we see both some regional clustering with five states in the Pacific Northwest all having more than 1% of their births occurring in birth centers, and also some adjoining states (North Dakota and Nevada) reporting fewer than 10

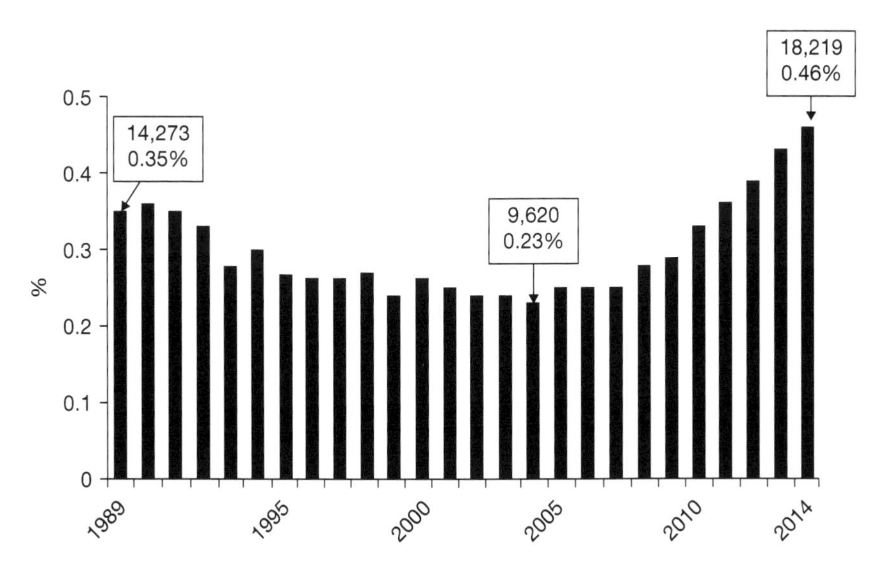

FIGURE 5.2 Trend in numbers of births at a birthing center in the United States, 1989–2014. Adapted from CDC (2015) and Hamilton et al. (2015).

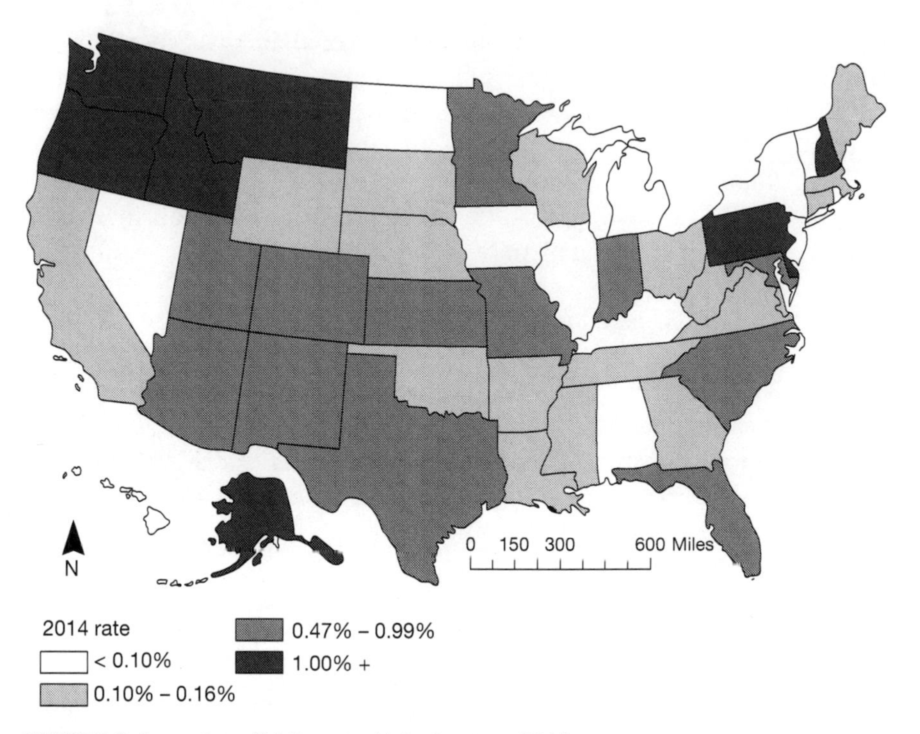

FIGURE 5.3 Proportion of birth center births by state, 2014.

Source: Birth By the Numbers, www.birthbythenumbers.org. Data presented in the map were provided by Dr. Eugene Declercq. Map created by Dr. Veronica Vieira, December 2015. Data adapted from CDC (2015) and Hamilton et al. (2015).

mothers in the entire state who gave birth in a birthing center. Birth center births are also more common in the Southwest and less common in the Deep South and, with the exception of New Hampshire, the Northeast.

Two notes of caution should be mentioned when interpreting birth center data by state. First, state figures are based on residence of the mother, not the location of the delivery. Hence, states with recorded birth center births may not actually have any birth centers located within their borders; rather, resident mothers may have travelled to an adjoining state to utilize a birth center. Second, when the data are broken down by state, we are dealing with relatively small numbers. For example, in 2014, 16 states reported fewer than 40 total birth center births. Therefore, when looking at such data over time a small absolute difference can seem proportionally large.

Table 5.1 presents specific data for the states with the 20 highest rates of birth center births in 2004 and in 2014. Alaska leads all states by a large margin in both years, with a larger proportion of birth center births than

TABLE 5.1
Top 20 States for Birth Center Births, 2004 and 2014

2004			2014		
State	Total Birth Center Births	% Birth Center Births	State	Total Birth Center Births	% Birth Center Births
Alaska	296	2.86	Alaska	590	5.18
Idaho	230	1.02	Montana	212	1.71
Arizona	671	0.72	Oregon	673	1.48
District of Columbia	56	0.71	Washington	1,304	1.47
Washington	565	0.69	Delaware	153	1.39
Pennsylvania	997	0.69	Pennsylvania	1,759	1.24
Delaware	78	0.69	Idaho	275	1.20
Maryland	444	0.59	New Hampshire	128	1.04
Indiana	502	0.58	Kansas	356	0.91
Utah	246	0.49	Utah	459	0.90
Ohio	640	0.43	Florida	1,747	0.79
Florida	894	0.41	South Carolina	443	0.77
Oregon	185	0.41	Texas	3,001	0.75
Maine	53	0.38	New Mexico	183	0.70
Massachusetts	298	0.38	Indiana	555	0.66
Tennessee	288	0.36	Arizona	511	0.59
New Mexico	99	0.35	Colorado	337	0.51
Texas	1,276	0.33	Missouri	382	0.51
Kansas	128	0.32	Maryland	374	0.51
Montana	37	0.32	Minnesota	351	0.50

Data adapted from CDC (2015) and Hamilton et al. (2015).

the next three highest states combined. The consistency of these trends over time—nine of the top 10 states in 2004 were on the list again in 2014 (the District of Columbia was the only exception)—reflects the long-term potential impact of establishing a sustainable birth center in a state with a favorable policy climate. The rapid growth in birth center use is evidenced by several factors. Although only two states reported more than 1% of their births being in birth centers in 2004, eight did in 2014. Also, states that maintained roughly the same (e.g., Maryland) or even increased (e.g., Idaho) the proportion of birth center births between 2004 and 2014 dropped substantially in the rankings as birth center births increased across U.S. states. Overall, 35 states reported an increase in birth center births between 2004 and 2014, whereas 16 reported decreases or no change.

Table 5.2 presents data from states with the largest increases in birth center births between 2004 and 2014. Although the increase in birth center

TABLE 5.2
States With the Largest Increase in Birth Center Births, 2004–2014

State	2004–2014 Increase in Absolute Numbers	2004–2014 % Increase
U.S. (total)	8,599	96
Texas	1,725	124
Florida	853	94
Pennsylvania	762	80
Washington	739	113
California	561	155
Oregon	488	265
South Carolina	423	2,076
North Carolina	369	177
Minnesota	351	35,362
Missouri	341	861
Colorado	337	—*

*Colorado reported zero birth center births in 2004.
Data adapted from CDC (2015) and Hamilton et al. (2015).

births occurred in a majority of states, there was a notable increase in the 10 states listed, which, between them, accounted for three fourths (77%) of the total national increase in the past decade. Texas and Florida alone account for 30% of the national increase in absolute terms. The impact of the movement toward birth centers can also be seen in two states that went from fewer than five recorded birth center births in 2004 to more than 300 in 2014, specifically Minnesota (351 births) and Colorado (337 births).

Who Is Having Birth Center Births?

Table 5.3 compares the characteristics of mothers who gave birth in a free-standing birth center in 2014 with mothers who gave birth in a hospital and shows several notable differences that emerge. Mothers giving birth in a birth center are distinct demographically from mothers giving birth in

TABLE 5.3
Characteristics of Mothers Giving Birth in Hospitals and Birth Centers in United States, 2014

	Birth Center (%)	Hospital (%)
White non-Hispanic	83.4	53.9
Age 30+	48.1	42.7
Parity 3+	32.2	28.8
Foreign born	9.3	22.1
Gestation 37+ weeks	98.3	88.6
County with less than 100,000 population	20.8	20.1
No reported prenatal care	0.1	1.5
Nonsmoker	98.7	91.5
College graduate	46.5	30.0
Prepregnancy BMI 25+	33.7	50.6
Self-pay for birth	31.9	3.4

BMI, body mass index.
Source: CDC (2015) and Hamilton et al. (2015).

a hospital, being much more likely to be non-Hispanic White, U.S. born, college graduates and less likely to be obese when they begin pregnancy and slightly more likely to be parity 3 or above. Behaviorally, birth center mothers virtually all report having prenatal care, and rarely report smoking. They are also much less likely to give birth prematurely, though that distinction is likely related to the tendency for mothers who go into premature labor to be transferred from birth centers to hospitals. Finally, mothers giving birth in birth centers are almost 10 times more likely to report having to pay for their birth out of pocket, reflecting continuing limitations of insurance coverage for birth center births.

Who Attends Birth Center Births?

Figure 5.4 presents the data on reported birth attendants at birth center births. Although a handful of birth center births are attended by physicians, they are primarily the domain of midwives in the United States. A majority (54%) of birth center births are attended by certified nurse-midwives (CNMs), whereas almost two in five (39%) are attended by "other" midwives, typically certified professional midwives (CPMs; Declercq, 2015). There is a similar pattern in home births with midwives attending the vast majority; however, in the case of home births, it is CPMs who attend a larger share (MacDorman & Declercq, 2016).

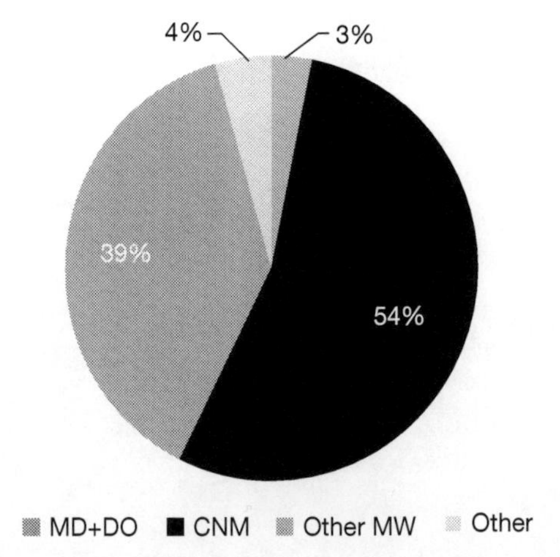

FIGURE 5.4 Birth center births by attendant in United States, 2014.

CNM, certified nurse-midwife; MW, midwife.

Adapted from CDC (2015) and Hamilton et al. (2015).

INTEREST IN BIRTH CENTER BIRTHS AMONG MOTHERS WHO GAVE BIRTH IN A HOSPITAL

Although there are no national survey data yet collected from mothers who gave birth in birth centers, a 2011–2012 national survey of mothers who had recently given birth in a hospital entitled *Listening to Mothers III* (Declercq, Sakala, Corry, Applebaum, & Herrlich, 2013) included the question, "For any future births, how open would you be to giving birth at a birth center that is separate from a hospital?" The results from this survey are presented in Figure 5.5 and show considerable interest in future birth center births among mothers who had just experienced a hospital birth. More than one quarter of mothers said they would "definitely" want a birth center birth in the future, whereas 39% responded that they "would consider" the option. In essence, almost two thirds of mothers who had recently experienced a hospital birth were open to a freestanding birth center birth in the future.

We examined mothers' responses to this question by a variety of maternal characteristics to identify from our data that mothers were most open to a birth center birth in the future. The results are presented in Tables 5.4 and 5.5. Table 5.4 presents maternal characteristics for all women who responded to the question about birth centers, excluding those who did not take a position (i.e., responded "not sure" or "don't want to have any more biological children") resulting in slightly different totals than seen in Figure 5.5. There was little variation across most of the categories with only parity and payer source showing statistically significant differences. Multiparous mothers were more favorable than first-time mothers

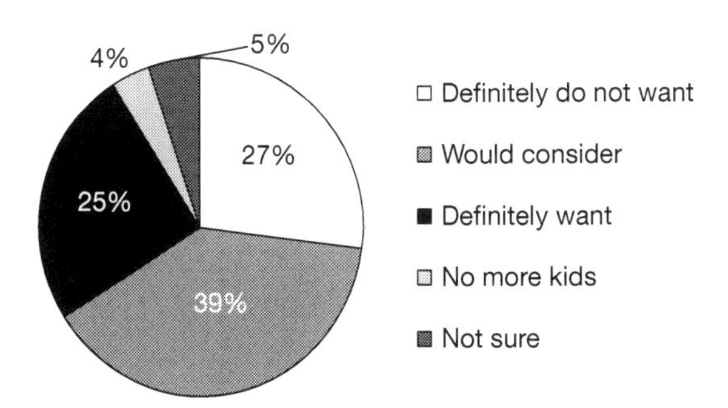

FIGURE 5.5 For any future births, how open would you be to giving birth at a birth center that is separate from a hospital?

Source: Declercq et al. (2013).

TABLE 5.4
Variations in Interest in Birth Center Birth by Maternal Characteristics*

	Total *n* (%)	Definitely Would Not Want	Would Consider	Definitely Would Want	*p*-value
	651 (100)	219 (30.1)	299 (42.4)	133 (27.6)	
Maternal Characteristic					
Age, Years					0.346
18–24	139 (34.5)	27.1	45.5	**27.4**	
25–29	198 (31.9)	27.1	37.0	**35.8**	
30–34	211 (23.8)	35.1	44.2	**20.7**	
35–39	80 (8.7)	38.6	42.1	**19.3**	
40 and older	23 (1.1)	33.4	60.0	**6.6**	
Education Status					0.308
High school or less	93 (43.4)	28.9	39.2	**31.9**	
Some college or associate's	228 (28.0)	27.3	44.1	**28.6**	
College graduate	247 (20.4)	37.4	41.0	**21.7**	
Graduate degree	83 (8.2)	27.6	56.8	**15.6**	
Race/Ethnicity					0.571
Non-Hispanic White	426 (56.7)	31.0	43.8	**25.1**	
Non-Hispanic Black	66 (14.1)	33.0	42.3	**24.7**	
Other race, Non-Hispanic	43 (7.5)	15.5	53.5	**30.9**	
Hispanic or Latina	112 (21.8)	30.7	34.5	**34.8**	

(continued)

TABLE 5.4
Variations in Interest in Birth Center Birth by Maternal Characteristics *(continued)*

	Total *n* (%)	Definitely Would Not Want	Would Consider	Definitely Would Want	*p*-value
Parity					0.048
Primiparous	359 (47.6)	29.5	49.1	**21.5**	
Multiparous	292 (52.4)	30.6	36.3	**33.1**	
Prepregnancy BMI					0.876
Underweight (less than 18.5)	56 (11.5)	25.6	44.3	**30.1**	
Normal (18.5–24.9)	349 (49.1)	27.1	43.8	**29.0**	
Overweight (25.0–29.9)	138 (20.9)	35.3	42.5	**22.1**	
Obese (30 or higher)	108 (18.6)	34.8	37.1	**28.1**	
Self-Reported Insurance Type					0.001
Public	399 (49.8)	34.9	47.7	**17.4**	
Private	203 (45.4)	28.6	37.2	**34.2**	
Self-Pay	28 (4.8)	25.9	18.8	**55.2**	
Prenatal Care Provider					0.226
OB/GYN	508 (75.7)	34.2	40.0	**25.8**	
Family practitioner	53 (10.2)	13.8	52.3	**33.9**	
Midwife	56 (8.1)	24.4	48.8	**26.7**	
Other	34 (6.0)	24.4	48.8	**26.7**	

(continued)

TABLE 5.4
Variations in Interest in Birth Center Birth by Maternal Characteristics *(continued)*

	Total *n* (%)	Definitely Would Not Want	Would Consider	Definitely Would Want	*p*-value
Birth Characteristics					
Type of Birth					0.645
Vaginal	484 (70.5)	29.6	44.1	**26.3**	
Cesarean	167 (29.5)	31.3	38.1	**30.6**	
Birth Attendant					0.822
OB/GYN	466 (67.9)	31.7	40.2	**28.2**	
Family practitioner	79 (14.6)	25.8	49.9	**24.4**	
Midwife	64 (10.2)	20.2	51.0	**28.8**	
Other	42 (7.2)	37.7	35.6	**26.7**	
Ever Took Childbirth Education Classes					0.233
Yes	423 (57.3)	27.3	46.9	**25.9**	
No	228 (42.7)	33.9	36.3	**29.8**	

BMI, body mass index.

*The figures in the rows of this table do not always total 100% because of rounding.

toward future birth center births, and most notably, mothers who had to self-pay for their hospital birth were much more favorable toward future birth center births, with a majority of these women (55%) definitely wanting this option. Factors that were not related to the desire for a future birth center birth included whether or not a mother had a midwife as a prenatal care provider or birth attendant, had taken childbirth education classes, or gave birth vaginally or by cesarean. Table 5.5 examines some additional variables from the *Listening to Mothers III* survey that assessed women's attitudes toward their recent maternity care experience. Perhaps not surprisingly, mothers who reported they had been treated poorly in the hospital were more likely to be interested in a future birth center birth. Once again, some nonsignificant relationships are of some interest.

TABLE 5.5
Variations in Interest in Birth Center Birth by Attitudinal Factors*

Maternal Factors	Total *n* (%)	Definitely Would Not Want	Would Consider	Definitely Would Want	*p*-value
Mother considered whether or not provider was a "good match" a "major" factor when choosing a maternity care provider					0.104
Yes	441 (67.3)	26.1	43.6	**30.3**	
No	210 (32.7)	38.2	39.9	**21.9**	
Mother felt provider was "not at all," "somewhat," or "moderately" trustworthy					0.113
Yes	528 (75.2)	33.7	39.4	**26.9**	
No	123 (24.8)	19.0	51.5	**29.5**	
Mother reported being treated poorly in hospital because of					
Race, ethnicity, or cultural background	28 (5.3)	17.4	24.2	**58.4**	0.005
Insurance status	30 (7.8)	11.4	39.0	**49.7**	0.064
A difference of opinion with caregivers about the right care for herself or baby	39 (9.6)	9.2	44.1	**46.7**	0.027

(continued)

TABLE 5.5
Variations in Interest in Birth Center Birth by Attitudinal Factors *(continued)*

Maternal Factors	Total *n* (%)	Definitely Would Not Want	Would Consider	Definitely Would Want	*p*-value
Mother believes birth is a process that should not be interfered with (strongly agree or agree)					0.640
Yes	380 (56.7)	30.9	39.8	**29.2**	
No	271 (43.3)	29.0	45.7	**25.4**	
Rated quality of the maternity care system as excellent					0.126
Yes	554 (82.7)	31.9	39.6	**28.5**	
No	97 (17.3)	21.5	55.6	**22.8**	

* The figures in the rows of this table do not always total 100% because of rounding.

Mothers' general attitude toward intervention in birth was statistically unrelated to their interest in delivering at a birth center as was their overall rating of the maternity care system.

DISCUSSION

In the United States, both home births and birth center births have been increasing rapidly in the past decade from a very small base to the point where more than 56,000 births occurred outside of hospitals in the United States in 2014. In the case of birth center births, the proportion of all births in birth centers has doubled (0.23%–0.46%) in the past decade, although the absolute numbers remain relatively small (18,219 in 2014) in a country that reports almost 4 million births every year. The data presented here suggest some reasons for both future growth in birth center births and the limitations on that growth.

The survey data from mothers who had recently given birth in a hospital showed widespread interest (64%) in a future birth center birth. The fact that these responses were related to mothers' reported experience in the hospital suggests that at least for some mothers, their treatment in a hospital during labor and delivery may have been an impetus for their response. For example, it seems plausible that women who reported being treated poorly in the hospital would consider seeking alternative sources of care for future obstetric events. Finances may also play a role, as mothers who had to self-pay for their hospital birth were more interested in a birth center option. Furthermore, the map presenting the wide variation of birth center births by state suggests a major reason birth center births have not increased more rapidly in recent years. State context, both in terms of the laws that govern birth centers and in the maternity care financing systems that can be crucial to sustaining them, can play a major role in any potential future growth in birth center births.

The limited past research on mothers' satisfaction with birth centers suggests that they may be seen as an alternative to hospital births among women. This is an area ripe for future studies since the published studies on mothers' experiences with birth centers in the past have had limited relevance to the U.S. context described here for several reasons. First, most have been from other countries, including Germany (David, Gross, Wiemer, Pachaly, & Vetter, 2009), Australia (Coyle, 1998), Denmark (Overgaard, Fenger-Grøn, & Sandall, 2012), England (Walsh, 2006), and Sweden (Waldenström & Nilsson, 1993). The studies may also involve hospital-based (Waldenström & Nilsson, 1993) rather than freestanding centers. Third, studies have often focused more on mothers' descriptive reports of their experience in the center (Coyle, Hauck, Percival, & Kristjanson, 2001; Walsh, 2006) rather than overall satisfaction with that experience. Nonetheless, when asked, mothers responded positively to their experiences in birthing centers, as in the case of the Australian study, which found, "Women wanted carers who viewed birth as a natural process rather than as an illness, and who engaged in a sharing, rather than a controlling, relationship" (Coyle, 1998, p. ii). A small qualitative study in the United States also found the theme of maternal empowerment to be central to mothers' satisfaction in using birthing centers (Pewitt, 2008).

CONCLUSION

What do these data suggest for future trends in the use of birth centers in the United States? Analysts are inevitably better at explaining the past than predicting the future, but the combination of three factors will likely dictate the level of future expansion. First, there appears to be continued interest among mothers in birth centers. The parallel and much larger growth in home births in the past decade was driven by consumer demand, and although birth centers face more regulatory obstacles than home births, a much larger proportion of mothers reported an interest in future birth center births than in home births (Declercq et al., 2013). One substantial and largely untapped area of possible growth is among mothers of color who currently account for almost half of all U.S. births, but only one in six birth center births. Notably, in our national survey, Hispanic mothers reported the highest level of interest in a future birth center birth. That deals with the demand side, whereas a second issue concerns supply. The political, regulatory, and financing systems will dictate how challenging it will be to establish and sustain birth centers. Birth centers do not happen organically—regulations vary widely by state and can be an inducement or barrier to future growth, leading to the third factor.

A final key element going forward will be building on a foundation of clinical excellence and compassionate care to cultivate business and political sophistication among birth center leaders. Changing the state context for birth center development and maintenance happens only through ensuring that advocates understand the political and regulatory climate in their state. This requires regular communication with policy makers to ensure their voices are heard, having a sound business plan that will attract foundations and investors, and working with the medical community to minimize miscommunication concerning clinical and financing issues in sensitive areas such as transfers. This combination of continued excellence in care and savvy business and political leadership will ensure that the growth in birth center births documented in this chapter will continue going forward.

REFERENCES

Centers for Disease Control. (2015). National Vital Statistics System. Retrieved from https://www.cdc.gov/nchs/nvss.births.htm

Coyle, K. (1998). *Women's perception of birth centre care: A qualitative approach.* Joondalup, Western Australia: Edith Cowan University.

Coyle, K. L., Hauck, Y., Percival, P., & Kristjanson, L. J. (2001). Normality and collaboration: Mothers' perceptions of birth centre versus hospital care. *Midwifery, 17,* 182–193.

David, M., Gross, M. M., Wiemer, A., Pachaly, J., & Vetter, K. (2009). Prior cesarean section: An acceptable risk for vaginal delivery at free-standing midwife-led birth centers? Results of the analysis of vaginal birth after cesarean section (VBAC) in German birth centers. *European Journal of Obstetrics and Gynecology and Reproductive Biology, 142,* 106–110.

Declercq, E. (2015). Midwife-attended births in the United States, 1990–2012: Results from revised birth certificate data. *Journal of Midwifery and Women's Health, 60,* 10–15.

Declercq, E. R., Sakala, C., Corry, M. P., Applebaum, S., & Herrlich, A. (2013). *Listening to Mothers III: Pregnancy and birth.* New York, NY: Childbirth Connection.

Hamilton, B. E., Martin, J. A., Osterman, M. J., Curtin, S. C., & Matthews, T. J. (2015). Births: Final data for 2014. *National Vital Statistics Reports, 64*(12), 1–64.

MacDorman, M. F., & Declercq, E. (2016). Trends and characteristics of United States out-of-hospital births 2004–2014: New information on risk status and access to care. *Birth, 43*(2), 116–124.

MacDorman, M. F., Declercq, E., & Mathews, T. J. (2013). Recent trends in out-of-hospital births in the United States. *Journal of Midwifery and Women's Health, 58,* 494–501.

Martin, J. A., Hamilton, B. E., Osterman, M. J., Driscoll, A. K., Matthews, T. J. (2017). Births: Final data for 2015. *National Vital Statistics Report, 66*(1). Hyattsville, MD: National Center for Health Statistics.

National Center for Health Statistics. (1991). *Advance report of final natality statistics, 1989.* Hyattsville, MD: Public Health Service.

Overgaard, C., Fenger-Grøn, M., & Sandall, J. (2012). The impact of birthplace on women's birth experiences and perceptions of care. *Social Science and Medicine, 74,* 973–981.

Pewitt, A. T. (2008). The experience of perinatal care at a birthing center: A qualitative pilot study. *Journal of Perinatal Education, 17,* 42–50.

Waldenström, U., & Nilsson, C-A. (1993). Women's satisfaction with birth center care: A randomized, controlled study. *Birth, 20,* 3–13.

Walsh, D. J. (2006). "Nesting" and "Matrescence" as distinctive features of a free-standing birth centre in the UK. *Midwifery, 22,* 228–239.

CHAPTER 6

Cost Outcomes and Finances of Freestanding Birth Centers

VICTORIA G. WOO AND NEEL T. SHAH

LEARNING OBJECTIVES

Upon completion of this chapter, the reader will be able to:

1. List elements of birth center care that contribute to lower cost care for low-risk women
2. Describe challenges birth centers and birth center clients face with insurance coverage and negotiations
3. Discuss long-term cost savings due to improved health measures and reduced societal costs associated with birth center care

Approximately 98% of the nearly 4 million births a year (Martin, Hamilton, Osterman, Driscoll, & Matthews, 2017) occur in the hospital (MacDorman, Declercq, & Matthews, 2013). In fact, childbirth is among the most common reasons for hospitalization in the United States (Moore, Witt, & Elixhauser, 2014). Hospitalization is costly. One night in the hospital can cost more than an entire week at a luxury hotel. As a result, health care delivery reform efforts have focused on ensuring that healthy patients have access to health care services in alternative settings. For childbirth, birth centers can provide a high-quality and affordable solution for well-selected patients.

Although the cumulative cost of hospital birth is very hard to quantify, Truven Health Analytics Marketscan Survey (2013) examined average payment for a maternal and neonatal birth episode for both Medicaid and commercial payers. For an uncomplicated, normal vaginal delivery, the average payment covering facility and professional fees for a commercially insured mother was $18,329, whereas the average payment for a Medicaid-insured mother was $9,131 (Truven Health Analytics Marketscan Survey, 2013). The facility fee, or hospital fee, comprised almost 60% of payments.

Hospital facility fees tend to be high due to the high overhead that hospitals carry, and can range from $1,189 to $11,986 (Xu et al., 2015). This overhead may include the cost of maintaining expensive imaging equipment, operating rooms, and blood banks, all of which are often passed on to the patient or payer whether they use these services or not. For childbirth, high staffing ratios (often approaching similar nurse-to-patient ratios as the intensive care unit) lead to even greater costs.

In many parts of the country, expensive facility fees may present a barrier to accessing care. Because hospital labor and delivery units are so costly to operate, many rural hospitals have stopped offering maternity services (Andrews, 2016). In broad swaths of the United States, it is not uncommon for pregnant women to travel for several hours to receive care. In fact, 50% of U.S. counties currently do not even have a qualified provider (including obstetricians, midwives, and family practice physicians who attend births; Salamon, 2012).

At the time of this writing, the United States spends more than $3 trillion on health care annually, which amounts to nearly one out of every five dollars spent in the economy (California HealthCare Foundation, 2014). Despite spending considerably more than other peer countries, we rank last in the Organization for Economic Cooperation and Development on key health indicators, including maternal mortality. The goal of improving our health care system can be summarized by the "triple aim": (a) improving the individual experience of care, (b) improving the health of populations, and (c) reducing the per capita costs of care for populations (Berwick, Nolan, & Whittington, 2008). Many believe that birth centers may provide a unique opportunity to achieve the triple aim in maternity care.

BIRTH CENTERS AS A LOWER COST ALTERNATIVE

Freestanding birth centers are an attractive solution for delivering care to the plurality of low-risk mothers at a substantially lower cost. These potential savings can be attributed to four factors: (a) difference in facility costs (leading to differences in payments per birth episode); (b) difference in staffing; (c) differences in intervention rates, especially in the case of cesarean births; and (d) differences in patient population.

Lower Cost for Birth Episode

Approximately 45% of births in the United States are paid for by Medicaid. Due to higher facility costs, Medicaid reimbursement for a normal spontaneous vaginal delivery in a hospital is almost twice the rate reimbursed to a birth center ($3,998 versus $1,907 on average in 2009; Rohde & Machlin, 2012; Stapleton, Osborne, & Illuzzi, 2013). One prospective cohort study examined births in 79 midwifery-led birth centers and calculated a savings to state Medicaid programs of $27.25 million in facility fee payments for their 13,030 cumulative births compared with hospital births (Stapleton, Osborne, & Illuzzi, 2013). Others have more conservatively calculated that birth centers are able to achieve at least a 16% reduction in costs for every woman cared for at a birth center when compared with "usual care" (Howell, Palmer, Benatar, & Garrett, 2014). This translates to a potential savings of $11.64 million for every 10,000 births for women insured by Medicaid. When private payments are taken into account, the differences remain equally stark. Even with transfer rates of up to 62% from birth centers to hospitals, planned hospital births were still more costly (Stone & Walker, 1995). A formal cost-effectiveness analysis that took hospital transfers and potential complications into account validated the claim that birth centers may provide both higher quality and more affordable care for low-risk women (Henderson & Petrou, 2008).

Difference in Staffing

Birth centers and hospital labor and delivery units are staffed very differently. Staff on labor and delivery units care for a much broader range of women than those at birth centers. Birth centers are an option for healthy low-risk women, whereas labor and delivery units must accommodate all comers. Labor and delivery units also maintain the capacity to perform emergency surgery, and, in some cases, manage multiple obstetric emergencies simultaneously. Although all labor and delivery units are required to have anesthesiologists either in the hospital or within close range of the hospital, birth centers are not (the average salary of an anesthesiologist was $258,100 in May 2015 according to the U.S. Bureau of Labor Statistics [2016a]; see Table 6.1).

Nursing requirements also differ between the two facilities as a result of their differences in scope and capacity. On the hospital labor and delivery suite, nurses staff the unit 24 hours a day, and most hospitals require a minimum number of nurses to be present, regardless of volume, to be able to assist in case of an emergency. Many birth centers, on the other hand,

TABLE 6.1
Average Salary of Maternity Care Providers

Maternity Care Provider	Average Salary
Certified nurse-midwife	$93,610
Obstetrician and gynecologist	$222,400
Anesthesiologist	$258,100
Registered nurse	$71,000

*U.S. Bureau of Labor Statistics (2016a, 2016b, 2016c, 2016d).

call in staff when a woman is in labor and being admitted to the center. A prevalent model at many birth centers is to have a midwife present through most of labor, and then, once delivery is close, the nurse is called to come in from home to assist. The nurse is then responsible for postpartum care until the woman is ready to be discharged, typically 6 to 8 hours after the birth. Because of the smaller patient volumes, and difference in minimum number of nurses required to be on the unit at all times, birth centers have a smaller nursing staff compared with hospital units (the national salary for a registered nurse in 2015, according to the U.S. Bureau of Labor Statistics [2016b], is $71,000; see Table 6.1).

The vast majority of women in the United States receive their prenatal care from an obstetrician, and give birth with an obstetrician in a hospital. In 2013, medical doctors attended 85.4% of all hospital births (Curtin, Gregory, Korst, & Uddin, 2015). Birth centers are primarily midwife led. The average salary of an obstetrician in the United States in 2015 was $222,400 (U.S. Bureau of Labor Statistics, 2016c), whereas the average salary of a nurse-midwife in 2015 was $93,610 (U.S. Bureau of Labor Statistics, 2016d; see Table 6.1). Thus, birth centers that only employ midwives and nurses as medical staff have a significant savings in cost in provider salaries.

The role of obstetricians in birth centers tends to vary by state. Some states require birth centers to have a medical director with a medical license; others do not require an MD to be involved. A birth center may even be fully staffed by obstetricians, although this is largely uncommon. For example, the University of Kansas at Wichita offers a birth center that is a physically separate building from labor and delivery, but is staffed by physicians onsite. The birth center building is connected to the hospital via an underground tunnel. The physicians include obstetric and gynecology residents at the university, family medicine residents, university-employed attending obstetricians and gynecologists, and private practice obstetricians (O'Hara et al., 2013). This birth center is considered a unit of the hospital, therefore the providers that are employees of the hospital are paid through their agreements with the hospital.

Differences in Cesarean Rate

The average cesarean rate in the United States was 32% in 2015, with a 25.8% cesarean rate for low risk first-time mothers (nulliparous, term, singleton, vertex; Martin et al., 2017) and a 21.8% primary cesarean rate (National Center for Health Statistics, 2015). Women who initiate care at birth centers are less likely to undergo a cesarean compared with women who initiate care at hospitals; one study of almost 50,000 women showed that women who delivered in the birth center were significantly less likely to deliver via cesarean compared with women who delivered at the hospital (OR = 0.59; $p < .01$; Benatar, Garrett, Howell, & Palmer, 2013). One reason for this is that only very low-risk women who are committed to achieving a vaginal birth deliver in birth centers. Patients who require cesareans or are at an increased risk for having a cesarean typically have planned deliveries in the hospital. Additional research could help further elucidate the reasons women choosing birth center care have fewer cesareans. The care model, the care providers, and the environment may have an effect.

A number of observational studies have demonstrated twofold to threefold lower cesarean rates for low-risk women who intend to deliver at birth centers (O'Hara et al., 2013). These differences persist even when the type of provider is taken into account. A study from Canada found that midwives in out-of-hospital settings have lower cesarean rates (7.2%) compared with midwives in the hospital (10.5%) when taking care of similar low-risk populations (Janssen et al., 2009).

These differences in rates of surgery have significant implications for the costs of birth centers. A 2013 study on behalf of the American Association of Birth Centers (AABC) looked at the potential cost savings birth centers could offer, taking into account the effect of intervention rates. The authors reported that, given the increased payments for facility services for cesarean birth compared with vaginal birth in the hospital, the lower cesarean birth rate potentially saved an additional $4.49 million (several others have arrived at similar estimates; Dekker, 2013). A study by Howell et al. (2014) specifically examined cost savings within the Medicaid population. They found that for a matched group of similar patients, the difference in cesarean rates in birth centers compared with hospitals saved Medicaid about $244 per patient, or $2.44 million per 10,000 Medicaid births (Howell et al., 2014).

In addition to a lower cesarean rate, birth centers tend to use other costly interventions less frequently, particularly with regard to anesthesia and analgesia. Use of epidurals and narcotic analgesia in birth centers is uncommon. Instead, nonpharmacological forms of pain control such as walking, massage, water immersion, and using birthing balls are more typical. Some birth centers do offer nitrous oxide (N_2O), which is a self-administered blend of 50% N_2O and 50% oxygen, a tasteless and odorless gas, which is more commonly used as a labor analgesic in other countries (Collins, Starr, Bishop, & Baysinger, 2012). A basic Nitronox nitrous oxide system costs about $5,000 (Boschert, 2013) for the equipment to the facility and lasts about 15 years. N_2O and oxygen are purchased separately from a local medical gas supplier, relatively inexpensively. Although each patient uses the gas differently (e.g., different durations of use, or different size inhalations), it is estimated that the cost is about $5 to $10 per patient. Additional consumables such as breathing circuits or masks could add another $15 to $20 to the total cost of care for the patient. Finally, the use of N_2O within birth centers tends to depend on the scope of practice in the state or municipality. Some areas require an order from an MD to administer the gas, whereas others do not have that requirement, influencing the feasibility of using N_2O in this setting (Mike Civitello, Sales Manager, Porter Instruments, personal communication, March 31, 2016).

Difference in Patient Population

Birth centers serve low-risk clients, whose need for specialists and specialist services are minimal. As a result, birth centers strive to provide care for women who will deliver term, normal weight infants. Among women who obtain prenatal care at birth centers, preterm birth is less common (11% in usual care, compared with 7.9% in birth centers; Howell et al., 2014). Average birth weight also tends to be higher at birth centers, although this contributes a small portion of the cost difference when viewed independently from staffing and intervention rates.

LONG-TERM COST SAVINGS AND HEALTH IMPROVEMENTS PROMOTED BY BIRTH CENTERS

By promoting normal vaginal birth for low-risk women, birth centers may also present long-term cost savings. Vaginal births are associated with decreased maternal risks in subsequent pregnancies compared with cesareans. Women are more likely to have subsequent vaginal births after an initial vaginal birth. This fact contrasts sharply with the fact that almost 90% of women who have an initial cesarean go on to have a subsequent cesarean in a later pregnancy in the United States (Curtin et al., 2015). Furthermore, subsequent cesareans are associated with a higher likelihood of serious, morbid, and costly medical complications, including placenta accreta, hysterectomy, and uterine rupture (Curtin et al., 2015).

Shorter recovery periods after low-intervention vaginal birth may also have an impact on economic productivity. Compared with normal vaginal births, women who have cesareans report more exhaustion, lack of sleep, and bowel problems; in addition, they are more likely to be readmitted to the hospital within 8 weeks of the birth (Thompson, Roberts, Currie, & Ellwood, 2002). Savings are realized by the health care system when there are lower readmission rates and fewer visits for postsurgery problems or complications. Additional savings are realized by society because the faster recovery time allows women to be able to care for themselves and their children sooner following vaginal births. A vaginal birth may also allow either the women themselves or their family members to take less time off of work.

High intervention or cesarean births may also have cost implications for the neonate. Even in full-term infants, cesareans may pose risks of increased likelihood of respiratory distress and breastfeeding complications (Neu & Rushing, 2011). There is also some association between mode of delivery and development of childhood disease, particularly asthma, allergic rhinitis, celiac disease, diabetes mellitus, and gastroenteritis (Neu & Rushing, 2011). The hypothesis is that there could be some sort of causal relationship between cesarean delivery, shift of microbiota in the neonate, and childhood disease state, although it is not yet well understood. Nonetheless, childhood asthma is one of the top five most costly children's diseases in the United States each year (Soni, 2014).

Birth centers also place a high emphasis on breastfeeding, which has been shown to have numerous benefits for mother and baby. A report assessing breastfeeding practices in the United States was published in June 2008 by the Centers for Disease Control and Prevention (CDC). Researchers sent surveys to both birth centers and hospitals asking about breastfeeding practices. The response rate was high for both parties (greater than 80% for both), and researchers assigned each facility a score from 0 to 100, with 100 representing the most favorable practices toward breastfeeding. When researchers compared mean total score, birth centers scored 86, whereas hospitals scored a 62, indicating that birth centers appeared to be doing a much better job at promoting breastfeeding (National Center for Chronic Disease Prevention and Health Promotion, 2014).

The higher breastfeeding rate that birth centers support may also have long-term cost implications. Using breast milk substitutes has been associated with higher rates of childhood diseases, including gastrointestinal infection, lower respiratory tract infections, acute otitis media in infants, and necrotizing enterocolitis in preterm infants (Pokhrel et al., 2015). Nonetheless, it is unclear whether increased breastfeeding in low-risk women would reduce the burden of disease, and any potential savings are challenging to quantify. An economic analysis from the United Kingdom suggests that programs that support exclusive breastfeeding may result in net savings by reducing the incidence of associated childhood diseases (Pokhrel et al., 2015).

FINANCIAL BARRIERS AND CHALLENGES AT BIRTH CENTERS

Despite their empirically demonstrated value, new birth centers face significant initial hurdles in surmounting the initial start-up costs. Initial start-up costs can be thought of in three broad categories: (a) physical/structural costs (fixed costs); (b) accreditation and licensing costs; and (c) staffing costs, which have been discussed in more detail in the previous paragraphs (see Chapter 13).

The physical/structural costs for birth centers range widely depending on the birth center. Some owners choose to build their own structure, whereas others renovate an already existing building. Additional fixed costs include large equipment (showers, beds, and so forth). These numbers differ vastly across the country, and can be challenging to obtain. For this chapter, we spoke to the founder of the Minnesota Birth Center (MBC), Steve Calvin, MD, and his administrative director, Tricia Balazovic, who estimated that it costs them about $500,000 per room in terms of physical start-up costs. Typical start-up costs for birth centers from the group of birth center owners we spoke to appeared to range from slightly under $1 million to almost $2 million, depending on the size and location of the birth center.

Another start-up cost is incurred with the decision to seek accreditation. The Commission for the Accreditation of Birth Centers (CABC) is a national accreditation body specifically focused on birth centers (see Chapter 8). It sets forth a set of specific safety and practice requirements that must be met in order to achieve accreditation. Birth centers apply for accreditation every 3 years, after initial accreditation. The cost is approximately $4,000 in fees for every accreditation cycle, and the operational costs of compliance are challenging to quantify. There is also the option to receive accreditation through The Joint Commission or the Accreditation Association for Ambulatory Health Care. Accreditation under these bodies is for accreditation as an ambulatory center, and is not specific to being a freestanding birth center. Some states offer licensure as well through the Department of Public Health, which certifies that the birth center is meeting a certain standard of safety codes. The California Department of Public Health offers licensure to birth centers, deemed "alternative birthing centers." Their fee per year in 2014 was listed as $2,380.19 (California Department of Public Health, 2016). Accreditation and licensure requirements vary by state. Some states require both, some require just one, and some require neither. In Minnesota, for example, birth centers are required to be accredited in order to be licensed.

After initial start-up costs are paid for, birth centers must also turn their attention to volume, which plays an important role in whether birth centers are able to create an operating margin, and ultimately provide societal cost savings. A study by Stone, Zwanziger, Hinton-Walker, and Buenting (2000) examined the importance of economies of scale and found that volume played a significant role in whether birth centers were cost-effective in delivering full prenatal care to low-risk pregnant women, compared with prenatal care provided by a traditional medical model. Sixty-nine subjects were enrolled in a freestanding birth center group and 77 subjects were in the traditional medical center group. In the freestanding birth center group, prenatal costs were higher (mean difference $751; $p < .001$), whereas the costs for the birth itself were less expensive ($1,472; $p < .01$). When costs for the entire maternity care episode were totaled, there were no significant differences between groups ($6,087 versus $6,803). Sensitivity analysis demonstrated that the freestanding birth center group could be more cost effective than the traditional medical center group if it increased its volume (Stone et al., 2000). Birth center providers spent notably more time with each patient than the providers in the traditional medical care model, and thus saw substantially fewer women in a given time period.

Once operating at scale, birth centers are often challenged by the need to coordinate with higher acuity facilities. Birth centers plan for a certain number of women to be transferred to the hospital, which is an anticipated and expected part of the business (Stapleton et al., 2013). Birth is not predictable. According to Dr. Calvin, his center plans for about 15% of patients to require some kind of hospital-based intervention to give birth and require transfer. First-time mothers are much more likely to require transfer than mothers who have had previous successful vaginal births. In a study from the United Kingdom comparing outcomes for women who delivered in the hospital compared with women who planned out-of-hospital births, 45% of British first-time mothers who intended to give birth at home ultimately were transferred to a hospital obstetrical unit during the course of labor (Birthplace in England Collaborative Group, 2011). If the transfer rate is high, the result is lost revenue for birth centers and can be costly. As Dr. Calvin explains, there are multiple scenarios for billing and insurance reimbursement in this model. The providers are reimbursed for their professional fees via a "maternity global fee," or a lump payment from insurance companies that provides payment for prenatal care, delivery care, and postpartum care. When a birth takes place at the birth center, there is also a facility fee. Newborn charges are also billed for both professional and facility fees.

If clients risk out of a birth center birth during the antepartum period, they will be directly admitted to the hospital for labor; if the nurse-midwife attends the birth, the "maternity global fee" is still applicable; however, the birth center is no longer able to bill for the facility and newborn fees. If patients are transferred from the birth center to the hospital during the intrapartum period, a reduced facility fee rate is assessed. In the event that the nurse-midwife transfers care to an obstetrician in either the antepartum or intrapartum period, the "maternity global fee" is broken. The birth center then receives some reimbursement for the prenatal care provided, but the fee for delivery goes to the provider that attends the birth. Thus, both parties end up making less money than if one of them had covered the whole pregnancy experience for that patient (the birth center may receive a fraction of the facility fee for the portion of time the patient labored there). Like all childbirth facilities, birth centers may face financial disincentives to transfer. Birth centers that are integrated within a hospital delivery system may not face this disincentive.

HOW BIRTH CENTERS ARE CURRENTLY FINANCED

Given the substantial cost of having a baby, the majority of patients prefer to deliver in a venue where their insurance is accepted. Thus, in order for birth centers to attract customers, they need to negotiate with insurers for reimbursements. Currently, these negotiations end up occurring on a center-by-center basis with rates differing by insurance plan, state, and birth center. Actual rates of reimbursement are considered proprietary information and therefore challenging to obtain. However, negotiating a rate that allows for financial solvency is key for freestanding birth centers to be able to remain in business, and many birth centers have successfully negotiated with private payers. Cara Osborne, SD, CNM, the founder of the birth center chain, Baby + Co, believes that this necessitates negotiating with the leadership of the insurance company to help them see the overall value of birth centers as potential cost savers as opposed to negotiating with the individual sales representatives, whose goal is to negotiate the lowest possible rate. Dr. Calvin of the MBC also reported that these negotiations are supported by making a strong clinical case as to why freestanding birth center births actually save insurance companies money. He shares evidence that birth centers maximize the likelihood of a normal spontaneous vaginal birth for the patient using a low intervention approach, resulting in cost savings for insurance companies. If insurance companies can see birth centers as an asset to their business to help decrease overall expenses associated with birth, he believes they can be convinced to reimburse at a rate that allows the birth center to be sustainable.

Medicaid

Almost 50% of births in the United States are covered by Medicaid (Howell et al., 2014). Negotiating reimbursement rates with Medicaid to cover births in birth centers expands access for women interested in delivering in birth centers. Prior to the introduction of the Affordable Care Act (ACA) in 2010, there was not a unified approach to reimbursing freestanding birth centers. Section 2301 of the ACA provided a definition for a freestanding birth center and required states to provide separate payments to providers who provide prenatal care, labor and delivery, and postpartum care in these centers. The law allowed a grace period for states needing to enact legislation to implement the requirements, but was in effect immediately. Because the reimbursement rate is at the state level, funding differs widely by state. It is uncertain how possible changes to the ACA will affect birth centers. Some states pay a facility fee for services rendered in the birth centers; others only pay for professional services provided. Certified professional midwives (CPMs) are reimbursed as birth attendants in some states; others only pay for births attended by certified nurse-midwives (CNMs). Differences also exist in whether prenatal care provided at the centers is reimbursed, or if payment is limited to labor and birth care. Reimbursement policy varies as well. The Kaiser Family Foundation has a comprehensive website, which summarizes benefits, coverage, and reimbursement methodology by state for freestanding birth centers, and demonstrates the wide variation across states (see their website: http://kff.org/other/state-indicator/medicaid-benefits-freestanding-birth-center-services/?currentTimeframe=0&sortModel=%7B%22colId%22:%22Location%22,%22sort%22:%22asc%22%7D). As the website notes, some states establish global payment rates for services or a fee schedule and pay on a fee-for-service basis; other states pay based on a percentage of the rate for the same service in a hospital setting.

The wide range in reimbursement rates by state has impacted birth centers' ability to accept Medicaid-reimbursed patients. For many centers, their state reimbursement rate is so low that accepting women insured under Medicaid is not economically feasible, thereby limiting access to many women who might otherwise be eligible for birth center care. However, some states (such as Minnesota) have a higher reimbursement rate, allowing centers to more feasibly accept patients insured by Medicaid. At the MBC, the vast gap between commercial and public program reimbursement rates led staff to initially limit the Medicaid-to-private patient ratio in the first 18 months of operations. Once the center became profitable, it was able to expand the number of patients who were insured under Medicaid.

The Midwife Center for Birth and Women's Health in Pittsburgh, Pennsylvania, had a slightly different approach. Christine Haas, CNM, the executive director of the center, explained:

> When women are first approved for Medicaid from state, they can pick a Medicaid MCO [managed care organization]. We encourage women to sign up for one of the MCO's because they have a much better reimbursement rate than "straight Medicaid" and some offer incentives, such as free car seats and doulas. Some of the Medicaid MCO reimbursements are even better than some of the national commercial carriers, making it more financially feasible to care for patients insured by these plans.

Birth centers that are not able to receive adequate payments from straight or managed Medicaid plans are sometimes able to use the tax-exempt status to seek donations or apply for grants. Through fund raising, they are able to supplement the costs of patients who are insured by straight Medicaid, allowing women covered by any insurance the option of delivering at the birth center.

Expanded Services Offered

In addition to routine prenatal care and vaginal deliveries, many birth centers have expanded into other services that also provide a source of revenue (see Chapter 10). Baby + Co offers a small retail section selling pregnancy-related products such as lactation cookies and breastfeeding pillows. Because as many as half of pregnancies are unplanned, many birth centers offer some basic well-woman exams and basic contraceptive services. The Strong Start Initiative, an effort by the U.S. Department of Health and Human Services to reduce preterm birth and improve outcomes for newborns and pregnant mothers, has helped to fund several initiatives including enhanced prenatal care at birth centers. This includes intensive case management, counseling, and psychosocial support (Centers for Medicare and Medicaid Services, 2017). The Santa Rosa Birth Center is one of the recipients of this grant and so offers these expanded services. Linda Cole, DNP, CNM, director of the Lisa Ross Birth and Women's Center in Tennessee from 2000 to 2010, noted that another service their birth center offered was a comprehensive breastfeeding clinic. Even women who had not delivered at the birth center were welcome to come to the breastfeeding clinic and learn from lactation consultants. The Tennessee birth center also ran a pediatric clinic for children aged 0 through 12 years, staffed by a pediatric nurse practitioner (PNP). As Dr. Cole explains, as birth centers explore their role in the community, they can expand to offer services and fill niches that are otherwise missing in the medical community. This allows them to become more financially viable and secure additional business.

Private Individual Payments and Venture Investment

Although the majority of funding comes from insurance reimbursement for specific patient services, some birth centers receive funding from other sources. Self-pay is an option for some patients who do not have insurance, or prefer not to use their insurance. With the increasing rise in high deductible plans as a result of the ACA, more women may be exploring birth centers as an attractive option to receive personalized maternity care services for less than the cost of their high deductible plan. Charges for birth centers average around $6,400 according to the AABC. Those who self-pay remain a small percentage of the clientele; the MBC estimates this percentage at about 0.5%, and this rate appears to be consistent across other birth centers. Funding can also come in the form of investment capital. More recently, the birth center company, Baby + Co, has set about to show that birth centers can overcome start-up costs by seeking venture capital funding and attracting equity.

CASE STUDY: Baby + Co

Cara Osborne, a CNM and SD in maternal and child health, has spent her career closely affiliated with birth centers. After spending some time working on the *National Birth Center Study II*, a study describing outcomes for approximately 15,000 women planning to give birth in birth centers across the United States, she became interested in the idea of creating "a real brick and mortar demonstration of what a feasible birth center could look like." She opened her first birth center in Arkansas in 2013. She was then approached by a private investor, who was interested in seeing if they could create a chain of birth centers that could be funded by investment firms and attract equity. They created a business plan, and Baby + Co was formed in January 2014. From there, they pitched to investors, and were able to gain enough funding to replicate their model in four additional locations. Although the model has not yet made a return on investment, at this point they are meeting projections and are on track to make a return on investment, with the breakeven point estimated at around 2 years from initial start-up. Dr. Osborne believes that their success is based around three major points. First is negotiating with payers to obtain "reasonable" rates. For example, in North Carolina, where two of the Baby + Co centers are located, they found a willing partner in Blue Cross Blue Shield (BCBS), and were able to negotiate rates that allowed sustainability. Second, she partnered closely with hospital systems that were interested in fostering a relationship between the birth center and the hospital. This relationship ensured buy-in from the local community and that collaboration mechanisms were in place. Lastly, she took the business aspect of the company very seriously. A chief executive officer (CEO) who previously ran a chain of ambulatory surgery centers has been brought in to become the new CEO and help to market the brand.

Not-for-Profit and Grant Funding From Private and Public Sectors

Some birth centers are not-for-profit and so can engage in grant writing and regular fund raising to help offset costs. Although the majority of the center's revenue comes from reimbursement from services provided, the Midwife Center for Birth and Women's Health in Pittsburgh, Pennsylvania, also receives grants, mostly from local private foundations and individual donors. These grants help to fund additional services that the birth center offers, such as postpartum follow-up calls and class scholarships. The members of the 15- to 17-member board tend to be professionals with expertise that assist the center with many functions, including fund-raising activities. Fund-raising campaigns have also proved successful to help fund specific projects, like their current project to expand the size of the birth center. In addition, birth centers may receive additional funding from their local government. The Lisa Ross Birth and Women's Center in Tennessee began receiving county funding when the county health department stopped providing direct patient care services for pregnant women.

ECONOMIC CHALLENGES CAN LEAD TO BIRTH CENTER FAILURE

Like any other business, birth centers around the country have failed for various reasons. From an economic standpoint, they have primarily been challenged due to reimbursement rates. Elizabeth Smith, CNM and owner of the Santa Rosa Birth Center, explains the problem in this way: "Freestanding birth centers often struggle to stay open because their reimbursement rates have historically been too low to stay in business. The paradox is that they save the system money, but they're not powerful enough to negotiate a reimbursement high enough to be sustainable. Of further concern, individual consumers (families that choose to birth at the center) are not able to utilize their health care benefits to the fullest. They are forced to pay either the out-of-network rates or self-pay in full. This makes the cost of birth center care to the consumer significantly greater than more traditional care. That the less expensive option ends up costing the individual the most is the truest irony of all!"

Jonathan Bush, the founder of Athena Health, an electronic medical record company, further describes the problem. Prior to starting Athena Health, Mr. Bush and some colleagues had initially tried to open a birth center chain. However, the chain ultimately went out of business due to problems with reimbursement. As Jonathan Bush states in an interview on Athena Health and Birth, "It was clear that the reason we weren't succeeding was that we were dying the death of a thousand paper cuts. . . . It was this numbing exhausting sort of bureaucratic paper chase" (Bush, 2013).

COST INNOVATIONS IN BIRTH CENTERS

Although birth centers present an attractive solution for delivering care at a substantially lower cost, there are also opportunities for further innovation. In April 2009, Childbirth Connection hosted a national policy symposium, entitled "Transforming Maternity Care: A High Value Proposition" in Washington, DC. A white paper was published by Angood et al. (2010) the following year, listing some interesting ideas for cost innovation, which are discussed here.

The first idea that emerged from the paper was to identify birth centers that have strong relationships with tertiary hospitals and disseminate a white paper discussing what has been going well. The goal is to help existing birth centers and those interested in starting birth centers understand the key concepts needed to build a strong relationship with a tertiary hospital. These relationships are important on many levels, and can be seen as a good financial investment. Strong relationships allow for mutual trust and the ability to work together to maximize efforts to provide great patient care. They also allow for smoother and easier transfer of patients from the birth center to the hospital, often resulting in better outcomes. Sometimes birth center providers can also obtain privileges at the associated hospital and thus continue caring for their patients following transfer, which is good for both patient continuity and reimbursement. Furthermore, if hospital systems have a strong relationship with a birth center, they will refer their low-risk patients, increasing volume for the birth center. In fact, their strong partnership can attract patients to utilize the system as a whole, which increases clientele for both parties. As more partnerships are developed, or as more health care systems consider adding birth centers to their delivery units, we hope that more rigorous methodologies will be applied to understand how to successfully implement these centers within a health care system. Results can then be disseminated, allowing other birth centers to learn from these experiences.

Another idea that emerged was to campaign for reimbursement rates to birth centers to be equivalent to the reimbursement rate that a hospital receives. This is likely to prove challenging, however, because, as discussed in this chapter, the cost of a birth at the two settings is drastically different. There is also a concern that if birth centers receive equivalent payments to hospitals, they might lose the ability to negotiate with insurance companies, demonstrating that they offer great care for low-risk women for less cost. This could even lead to lost contracts if insurance companies no longer see a financial gain by paying for a birth center birth.

A third, controversial, proposed idea was to only reimburse birth centers with accreditation. This would effectively prevent birth centers without accreditation from opening, and ensure a certain level of standards among birth centers. One could argue that this could lead to better outcomes and improved safety, which could attract more patients and lead to better negotiating power for birth centers with insurance companies and health care systems.

Lastly, the paper suggested providing financial incentives to education programs that creatively incorporate birth centers with education. One specific idea that was proposed is to have obstetric residents work at birth centers. The University of Kansas at Wichita has a freestanding birth center as part of its health care system, known as the Wesley Birth Care Center. This center has 21 large labor and delivery units, and is managed by a second year resident (University of Kansas School of Medicine-Wichita, 2017). The advantages of having residents work in birth centers is that they become comfortable with this environment and are more accepting and open to birth centers. This allows them to build better relationships with birth centers in their future career, actively refer appropriate candidates, and even encourage more birth centers to be built as a viable model for providing care to mothers.

CONCLUSION

Birth centers are widely used in maternity care systems throughout the world but are seldom used in the United States. There has been a recent increase in the number of birth centers available, although the absolute number is still small. Abundant evidence documents that expanded use of birth centers may lead to better quality of care at lower cost for the majority of healthy low-risk mothers. Nonetheless, birth centers currently face numerous financial barriers ranging from steep start-up costs to limited leverage to negotiate reimbursements.

In the era of value-based health care, health care delivery systems are increasingly taking ownership of the need to ensure that each patient receives the right care at the right time in the right place from the right provider. It is not clear that every pregnant patient requires or even benefits from the hospital, and some evidence indicates that for low-risk women hospital birth may even increase the risk of avoidable interventions. Currently, innovators in disparate pockets of the country are finding ways to build sustainable birth centers through creative business models. Ultimately, for birth centers to move from the fringe to the mainstream of maternity care, patients, purchasers, payers, and other stakeholders will need to increase the economic demand for birth center services.

REFERENCES

Andrews, M. (2016, February 24). More rural hospitals are closing their maternity units. *National Public Radio*. Retrieved from http://www.npr.org/sections/health-shots/2016/02/24/467848568/more-rural-hospitals-are-closing-their-maternity-units

Angood, P. B., Armstrong, E. M., Ashton, D., Burstin, H., Corry, M. P., Delbanco, S. F., . . . Salganicoff, A. (2010). Blueprint for action: Steps toward a high-quality, high-value maternity care system. *Womens Health Issues, 20*(Suppl. 1), S18–S49. Retrieved from http://www.whijournal.com/article/S1049386709001406/fulltext

Benatar, S., Garrett, A. B., Howell, E., & Palmer, A. (2013). Midwifery care at a freestanding birth center: A safe and effective alternative to conventional maternity care. *Health Services Research, 48*(5), 1750–1768. Retrieved from http://www.pubmedcentral.nih.gov/articlerender.fcgi?artid=3796112&tool=pmcentrez&rendertype=abstract

Berwick, D. M., Nolan, T. W., & Whittington, J. (2008). The Triple Aim: Care, health, and cost. *Health Affairs, 27*(3), 759–769. doi:10.1377/hlthaff.27.3.759

Birthplace in England Collaborative Group. (2011). Perinatal and maternal outcomes by planned place of birth for healthy women with low risk pregnancies: The Birthplace in England national prospective cohort study. *British Medical Journal, 343*. Retrieved from http://www.bmj.com/content/343/bmj.d7400

Boschert, S. (2013). Nitrous oxide returns for labor pain management. Retrieved from http://www.mdedge.com/obgynnews/article/59258/obstetrics/nitrous-oxide-returns-labor-pain-management

Bush, J. (2013, April 10). Plenty to say: Behind the scenes with Jonathan Bush, part III [web log post]. Retrieved from http://www.athenahealth.com/blog/2013/04/10/plenty-to-say-behind-the-scenes-with-jonathan-bush-part-iii

California Department of Public Health. (2014). Center for Health Care Quality Licensing & Certification Program. Annual fee report for 2014–2015. Appendix A. Retrieved from https://www.cdph.ca.gov/pubsforms/forms/Documents/LicCertFeeListing15.pdf

California HealthCare Foundation. (2014). U.S. health care spending: California Health Care Almanac Quick Reference Guide. Retrieved from http://www.chcf.org/~/media/MEDIA LIBRARY Files/PDF/PDF H/PDF HealthCareCostsQRG14.pdf

Centers for Medicare and Medicaid Services. (2017). Strong Start for Mothers and Newborns Initiative: General information. Retrieved from https://innovation.cms.gov/initiatives/strong-start/

Collins, M. R., Starr, S. A., Bishop, J. T., & Baysinger, C. L. (2012). Nitrous oxide for labor analgesia: Expanding analgesic options for women in the United States. *Reviews in Obstetrics and Gynecology, 5*(3–4), e126–e131. Retrieved from http://www.pubmedcentral.nih.gov/articlerender.fcgi?artid=3594866&tool=pmcentrez&rendertype=abstract

Curtin, S. C., Gregory, K. D., Korst, L. M., & Uddin, S. F. G. (2015). Maternal morbidity for vaginal and cesarean deliveries, according to previous cesarean history: New data from the birth certificate, 2013. *National Vital Statistics Reports, 64*(4). Retrieved from http://www.cdc.gov/nchs/data/nvsr/nvsr64/nvsr64_04.pdf

Dekker, R. (2013). National Birth Center Study II. Retrieved from http://www.birthcenters.org/?page=NBCSII#16

Henderson, J., & Petrou, S. (2008). Economic implications of home births and birth centers: A structured review. *Birth, 35*(2), 136–146. doi:10.1111/j.1523-536X.2008.00227.x

Howell, E., Palmer, A., Benatar, S., & Garrett, B. (2014). Potential Medicaid cost savings from maternity care based at a freestanding birth center. *Medicare and Medicaid Research Review, 4*(3). doi:10.5600/mmrr.004.03.a06

Janssen, P. A., Saxell, L., Page, L. A., Klein, M. C., Liston, R. M., & Lee, S. K. (2009). Outcomes of planned home birth with registered midwife versus planned hospital birth with midwife or physician. *Canadian Medical Association Journal, 181*(6 7), 377–383. Retrieved from http://www.pubmedcentral.nih.gov/articlerender.fcgi?artid=2742137&tool=pmcentrez&rendertype=abstract

MacDorman, M. F., Declercq, E., & Mathews, T. J. (2013). Recent trends in out-of-hospital births in the United States. *Journal of Midwifery and Women's Health, 58*(5), 494–501. doi:10.1111/jmwh.12092

Martin, J. A., Hamilton, B. E., Osterman, M. J., Driscoll, A. K., & Matthews, T. J. (2017). Births: Final data for 2015. *National Vital Statistics Report, 66*(1). Hyattsville, MD: National Center for Health Statistics.

Moore, J. E., Witt, W. P., &. Elixhauser, A. (2014). Complicating conditions associated with childbirth, by delivery method and payer, 2011. HCUP statistical brief #173. Rockville, MD: Agency for Healthcare Research & Quality. Retrieved from http://www.hcup-us.ahrq.gov/reports/statbriefs/sb173-Childbirth-Delivery-Complications.pdf

National Center for Chronic Disease Prevention and Health Promotion. (2014). Breastfeeding report card: United States, 2014. Retrieved from http://www.cdc.gov/breastfeeding/pdf/2014breastfeedingreportcard.pdf

National Center for Health Statistics. (2015). The public use natality file—2015 update. Retrieved from http://www.cdc.gov/nchs/data_access/Vitalstatsonline.htm

Neu, J., & Rushing, J. (2011). Cesarean versus vaginal delivery: Long-term infant outcomes and the hygiene hypothesis. *Clinics in Perinatology, 38*(2), 321–331. Retrieved from http://www.pubmedcentral.nih.gov/articlerender.fcgi?artid=3110651&tool=pmcentrez&rendertype=abstract

O'Hara, M. H., Frazier, L. M., Stembridge, T. W., Mckay, R. S., Mohr, S. N., & Shalat, S. L. (2013). Physician-led, hospital-linked, birth care centers can decrease cesarean section rates without increasing rates of adverse events. *Birth, 40*(3), 155–163. doi:10.1111/birt.12051

Pokhrel, S., Quigley, M. A., Fox-Rushby, J., McCormick, F., Williams, A., Trueman, P., . . . Renfrew, M. J. (2015). Potential economic impacts from improving breastfeeding rates in the UK. *Archives of Disease in Childhood, 100*(4), 334–340. Retrieved from http://www.ncbi.nlm.nih.gov/pubmed/25477310

Rohde, F., & Machlin, S. (2012). Health care expenditures for uncomplicated pregnancies 2009. Research Findings No. 32. Rockville, MD: Agency for Healthcare Research and Quality. Retrieved from http://meps.ahrq.gov/data_files/publications/rf32/rf32.pdf

Salamon, M. (2012, May 8). Half of U.S. counties have no OB-GYN. *US News and World Report.* Retrieved from http://health.usnews.com/health-news/news/articles/2012/05/08/half-of-us-counties-have-no-ob-gyn-study

Soni, A. (2014). STATISTICAL BRIEF #434: The Five Most Costly Children's Conditions, 2011: Estimates for U.S. Civilian Noninstitutionalized Children, Ages 0–17. Retrieved from http://meps.ahrq.gov/data_files/st434/stat434.shtml

Stapleton, S. R., Osborne, C., & Illuzzi, J. (2013). Outcomes of care in birth centers: Demonstration of a durable model. *Journal of Midwifery and Women's Health, 58*(1), 3–14. Retrieved from http://www.ncbi.nlm.nih.gov/pubmed/23363029

Stone, P. W., & Walker, P. (1995). Cost-effectiveness analysis: Birth center vs. hospital care. *Nursing Economics, 13*(5), 299–308.

Stone, P. W., Zwanziger, J., Hinton-Walker, P., & Buenting, J. (2000). Economic analysis of two models of low-risk maternity care: A freestanding birth center compared to traditional care. *Research in Nursing and Health, 23*(4), 279–289.

Thompson, J. F., Roberts, C. L., Currie, M., & Ellwood, D. A. (2002). Prevalence and persistence of health problems after childbirth: Associations with parity and method of birth. *Birth, 29*(2), 83–94. Retrieved from http://www.ncbi.nlm.nih.gov/pubmed/12051189

Truven Health Analytics Marketscan Survey. (2013). *The cost of having a baby in the United States.* Ann Arbor, MI: Truven Health Analytics.

U.S. Bureau of Labor Statistics. (2016a). Occupational wages and employment, 2015: Anesthesiologists. Retrieved from http://www.bls.gov/oes/current/oes291061.htm

U.S. Bureau of Labor Statistics. (2016b). Occupational wages and employment, 2015: Registered nurses. Retrieved from http://www.bls.gov/oes/2011/may/oes291111.htm

U.S. Bureau of Labor Statistics. (2016c). Occupational wages and employment, 2015: Obstetricians and gynecologists. Retrieved from http://www.bls.gov/oes/current/oes291064.htm

U.S. Bureau of Labor Statistics. (2016d). Occupational wages and employment, 2015: Nurse midwives. Retrieved from http://www.bls.gov/oes/current/oes291161.htm

University of Kansas School of Medicine-Wichita. (2017). Obstetrics and gynecology. Retrieved from http://wichita.kumc.edu/obgyn/birthcare-center.html

Xu, X., Gariepy, A., Lundsberg, L. S., Sheth, S. S., Pettker, C. M., Krumholz, H. M., & Illuzzi, J. L. (2015). Wide variation found in hospital facility costs for maternity stays involving low-risk childbirth. *Health Affairs, 34*(7), 1212–1219. doi:10.1377/hlthaff.2014.1088

SECTION III

Political and Regulatory Landscape

CHAPTER 7

Care Providers in Freestanding Birth Centers

AUTUMN VERSACE VERGO AND KAYE KANNE

LEARNING OBJECTIVES

Upon completion of this chapter, the reader will be able to:

1. Describe the providers who most commonly work in freestanding birth centers
2. Describe the typical scope of practice and skills unique to birth center providers
3. Review national trends currently shaping provider practice in the birth center setting

HISTORY OF PROVIDERS IN COMMUNITY SETTINGS

The foremothers of today's birth center providers were caring for childbearing women in community settings long before the Maternity Center Association (MCA) opened the first modern birth center in New York City in 1975. Although many of these early midwives' stories are lost to history, we can surmise that they served their communities as helpers, companions, and experts. Native American midwives gave advice on healthy eating, herbal medicine, positioning, and ritual to guide women through pregnancy and labor. Midwives in the American colonies not only attended women in labor but also nursed their sick neighbors throughout the life span. Some had training in nursing and British herbal medicine. The capture and forced relocation of West African women to the colonies brought community midwives versed in traditional healing practices and herbalism who primarily attended women enslaved on southern plantations. All of these early community midwives had some important qualities in common. Although they occasionally traveled short distances to attend those in need, they rose from and lived as members of the communities they served. Some had formal training in an apprenticeship model, but most relied on experience, intuition, and their deep knowledge of the values, challenges, and hopes of women in their home communities to guide their practice (Borst, 1995; Maxwell, 2009; Rooks, 1997; Ulrich, 1990).

During the next 100 years, the role of community midwife evolved from women with homegrown expertise and apprentice training to midwives formally educated in professional nursing and/or midwifery programs. The goals of community midwifery care also shifted, from the necessary attendance of family, friends, and neighbors to public health efforts to improve outcomes for mothers and babies. The 1900s brought an influx of immigrants with training from rigorous programs in Italy and France, and apprentice-trained midwives from other parts of Europe (Rooks, 1997). In New York City, public health nurses were sent out into communities and pregnant and postpartum women's homes to teach nutrition, self-care, and hygiene. The Boston Female Medical College created the first formal midwifery program in the United States, graduating a class of 12 women in 1850 (Boston University School of Medicine [BUSM], 2014). The Frontier Nursing Service, founded by Mary Breckenridge in 1925 to reduce maternal and infant mortality in rural Kentucky, brought midwives trained in the British model of nurses dually educated in midwifery to Appalachia (Breckinridge, 1981). In the 1940s, apprentice-trained "granny" midwives attended two thirds of births in Mississippi, South Carolina, Arkansas, Georgia, Florida, Alabama, and Louisiana. They were joined by graduates of the Tuskegee School of Nurse-Midwifery, which opened in 1941 and graduated 31 Black nurse-midwives before its closure in 1946 (Dawley, 2003; Kenney, 1942).

THE MODERN BIRTH CENTER: ENVIRONMENT-SHAPING PRACTICE

The early professionalization of providers of childbirth care in the United States saw a dramatic shift in place of birth from homes to hospitals; however, community midwives were largely prevented from following their patients into this new setting (Smith, 2008). Early hospital birth brought access to advances such as antibiotic therapy and anesthesia but also focused on the use of sophisticated and sometimes proprietary technology, the enforcement of institution-defined processes and standards of care, and pregnancy itself, often viewed as a disease process. Expansion of midwifery practice into the hospital setting was hampered by restrictive licensing and supervision laws and physician's concerns over shared and vicarious liability (Rooks et al., 1989). The closure of many early midwifery training programs and the inability of trainees to secure midwifery preceptorships in hospitals further limited practice. Health care consumers, meanwhile, became increasingly disillusioned with the loss of autonomy experienced during institutionalized birth; in an effort to maintain safety and satisfaction, some families sought to avoid hospital birth altogether (Turkel, 1995). Hospitals had become the physician's place for birth. Midwives needed to create a new place for birth outside of the hospital system, in order to protect their professional autonomy and model of care (Rothman in Turkel, 1995).

In 1975, the MCA opened Manhattan's Childbearing Center (CbC) as a demonstration project, developed in response to rising rates of home birth unattended by a skilled provider (Rooks, 1997). The MCA considered other strategies to meet the needs of childbearing couples, including efforts to humanize the hospital setting, a return to home birth, and opening an independent hospital, but settled on opening a freestanding birth center (Turkel, 1995). The founders of the MCA CbC recognized the need to test a model of care that provided midwives with autonomy in their practice and women the safety and expert guidance of trained caregivers whose practice was integrated with the larger health care system. MCA Director Ruth Watson Lubic, EdD, CNM, spent 2 years preparing to open the center, extensively reviewing data pertaining to the safety of out-of-hospital birth. The CbC participated in the wider health care system by creating protocols for consultation, transport, and follow-up care. Outcome data were examined by multiple agencies in 1978 and demonstrated that the CbC operated safely while providing care that was much less expensive than hospital birth (Canoodt, 1982). The MCA CbC demonstrated the importance of providing care based on evidence, full integration into the health care system, and quality improvement through the examination of outcome data.

PROVIDERS OF BIRTH CENTER CARE

The American Association of Birth Centers (AABC) recognizes several types of providers able to care for women delivering in birth centers. Most are midwives; in the United States, birth centers are owned or operated by certified professional midwives (CPMs) or certified nurse-midwives/certified midwives (CNMs/CMs), or both CNM/CMs and CPMs. The standards for birth centers specify that providers in birth centers must be licensed according to state guidelines; the Commission for the Accreditation of Birth Centers (CABC) indicators for compliance with the standards specify that professional staff be licensed to practice in accordance with state and local laws (AABC, 2016; CABC, 2015; see Chapters 8 and 9). Therefore, the types of providers practicing in birth centers vary from state to state. CNMs are licensed providers in all states, CPMs are licensed providers in 28 states, and CMs are licensed providers in five states with a sixth anticipated soon. Physicians, including obstetrician/gynecologists and family practice physicians, also attend a small percentage of birth center births. According to 2004 to 2014 birth certificate data from 47 states and Washington, DC, 53.6% of birth center births were attended by CNMs/CMs; 39.0% by "other" midwives including CPMs, licensed midwives (LMs), and direct-entry midwives; 3.1% by physicians; and 4.3% by "other" (MacDorman & Declercq, 2016).

Certified Professional Midwives: Definition, History, Education, and Practice Model

CPMs are a rapidly growing segment of the midwifery profession in the United States. The number of CPMs increased from 500 in early 2000 to more than 1,400 in 2008, and more than 2,000 as of July 2016 (Ida Darragh, personal communication, August 6, 2016). A new generation of direct-entry (non-nurse) midwives emerged in the 1970s to serve women who were rejecting the medical model of care, rediscovering physiologic birth, and choosing to give birth at home. The CPM credential includes multiple routes of entry to the profession including accredited direct-entry programs and an apprenticeship model, which is currently evolving to meet international standards for midwifery education (U.S. Midwifery Education, Regulation, & Association [USMERA], 2015; International Confederation of Midwives, 2013). All CPMs meet the standards for certification set by the North American Registry of Midwives (NARM, 2016). Today approximately half of new CPMs are graduates of programs of study accredited by the Midwifery Education Accreditation Council (MEAC, 2016; Ida Darragh, personal communication, August 2016), a national accrediting agency recognized by the U.S. Department of Education (2016). CPM training occurs exclusively in out-of-hospital community settings focusing on supporting physiologic birth. Most CPMs attend birth in homes; however, more are moving to birth center practice as opportunities for legal practice expand, and health care consumers increasingly recognize that birth center care is associated with lower rates of unnecessary intervention, lower risk of cesarean birth, and excellent outcomes for mothers and babies (Dekker, 2013).

Certified Nurse-Midwives/Certified Midwives: Definition, History, Education, and Practice Model

Nurse-midwives are primary health care providers for women and newborns, focusing on health promotion and disease prevention for women of all ages. Nurse-midwives are dually educated; as nurses, they gain a solid grounding in the provision of skilled care inclusive of patients' physical, emotional, and spiritual wellness (American College of Nurse-Midwives [ACNM], 2012a). To become a CNM, candidates complete a graduate program accredited by the Accreditation Commission for Midwifery Education (ACME) and pass the American Midwifery Certification Board (AMCB) national certification exam (AMCB, 2013). The Core Competencies for Basic Midwifery practice (ACNM, 2012b; Walker, Lannen, & Rossie, 2014) include ongoing, comprehensive assessment and treatment, prescribing, oversight and interpretation of appropriate laboratory testing, and individualized counseling about wellness (Walker, Lannen, & Rossie, 2014). Nurse-midwifery originated in the 1920s through the efforts of public health nurses and other advocates who believed nurse-midwives could play an important role in meeting the needs of underserved populations. Nurse-midwifery grew gradually until the 1970s when national standards for education and certification were established by the American College of Nurse-Midwives (ACNM, 2011), and federal funding was provided for nurse-midwifery education. Approximately 95% of all births attended by CNMs occur in hospitals; however, more CNMs are entering birth center practice as the number of birth centers in the United States increases.

The CM credential was created in 1994 as a direct-entry equivalent to the CNM. CMs are not nurses, and may hold other health care-related degrees or certifications. Like CNMs, they pass the same AMCB certification exam following completion of a graduate program accredited by ACME. CMs are licensed in New Jersey, New York, and Rhode Island. They are authorized by permit to practice in Delaware, and authorized to practice in Missouri (AMCB, 2013). Maine recently passed legislation that will award licensure to CMs as of January 1, 2020 (Whittle, 2016).

Other Midwives

Midwifery is an ancient profession whose origin predates formal education and government-granted regulation and licensure. There remains in the United States a small number of midwives who do not hold certification or license, practicing in states where licensure and/or certification is not required. The education of these individuals varies and may include apprenticeship, international education, and both degree-granting and non–degree-granting formal education. In addition, some individuals from specific communities, religious groups, or indigenous cultures may refer to themselves as midwives. These midwives are unlikely to practice in accredited freestanding birth centers, as both the standards for accreditation and state-level statute regarding outpatient medical facilities require all employed care providers to be licensed in accordance with state and local laws.

Additional Providers of Birth Center Care

Midwife leaders of birth centers function locally as health care entrepreneurs and often design care models and service offerings around needs specific to their home communities. Family practice physicians; pediatricians; family practice, pediatric, and mental health nurse practitioners (NPs); and physician assistants may provide services at freestanding birth centers. National data on extended services is limited (see Chapter 10).

In addition to the providers attending births and supervising prenatal and other women's and infant health care, birth centers employ a variety of ancillary health professionals to further help integrate care delivery into the pregnant patient's home community. These clinicians and others include birth assistants, registered nurses, doulas, nurse or peer home visitors, childbirth and health educators, and community health workers. Birth doulas may be hired by birth centers or by birthing mothers and provide skilled labor support. Birth assistants are most often employed by the midwife or birth center, and assist with providing care and monitoring the mother and baby. Perinatal community health workers are trained to provide support and education to women during the perinatal period by focusing on comfort measures, relaxation techniques, nutrition for pregnancy and breastfeeding, basic lactation management, and assessment for perinatal mood disorders in ways that are culturally appropriate (Mamatoto Village, 2013). Providers of lactation support including certified lactation consultants may also work in birth centers.

QUALITIES OF BIRTH CENTER PROVIDERS

Although midwives and others who work in birth centers come from different educational, practice model, and cultural backgrounds, they share several qualities in common. First, they all develop expertise in promoting physiologic labor and birth. Care delivery in community settings requires providers to be flexible and adapt their practice to the patient's needs and often, as with home visiting, his or her physical environment as well. Birth center providers must develop clear, respectful, professional communication skills to be used in consultation, collaboration, and transfer or transport. To support the goal of remaining eligible for birth center birth, prenatal care must focus on keeping women in excellent health and low risk by promoting good nutrition, physical activity, and thorough preparation for unmedicated labor. Birth center providers deliver immediate postpartum and newborn care as part of their practice. And finally, birth center providers and staff often participate in the management of the birth center, necessitating a working knowledge of billing and coding, the business plan of the birth center, the quality assurance and improvement program, and marketing and community outreach (see Chapter 13). Facility tasks such as cleaning, ordering and stocking supplies, and maintaining equipment are sometimes carried out by providers as well.

NATIONAL TRENDS SHAPING PROVIDER PRACTICE IN BIRTH CENTERS

The number of pregnant women choosing to deliver in community settings is increasing. Birth rates in nonhospital settings have been rising since 1990; the Centers for Disease Control and Prevention (CDC) reported that 0.87% of births occurred outside the hospital setting in 2004 and has increased to 1.5% in 2014 (MacDorman & Declercq, 2016). In response to this increased demand, new systems are evolving to integrate community-based care with the larger health care system. For example, the Home Birth Summit meetings and resulting collaborative statements recognize women's right to autonomous choice of birth setting, and Summit workgroups have developed guidelines for safe and respectful intrapartum transfer of care to hospitals from out-of-hospital settings (Home Birth Summit, 2016).

The American College of Obstetricians and Gynecologists and Society for Maternal-Fetal Medicine consensus statement "Levels of Maternal Care" (Menard et al., 2015) defined birth centers as providing care to low-risk women with uncomplicated singleton term pregnancies with vertex presentations who are expected to have uncomplicated births. This statement marked the first time these organizations included birth centers in the conceptual continuum of maternity care in the United States. Over the past several years, new, collaborative guidance on interprofessional communication and transport has been published by several organizations, including ACNM, American College of Obstetricians and Gynecologists (ACOG), and Society for Maternal-Fetal Medicine's (SMFM) Transforming Communication and Safety Culture in Intrapartum Care: A Multi-Organization Blueprint (Lyndon et al., 2015). Others include Washington State's Smooth Transitions program (Washington State Perinatal Collaborative, 2015), the Maine CDC Transport Guidelines (Maine Center for Disease Control and Prevention, 2014), and the Northern New England Perinatal Quality Improvement Network's (NNEPQIN) Out of Hospital to In Hospital Perinatal Transfer Form (NNEPQIN, 2011).

CONCLUSION

"The birth center is the place for the practice of midwifery," stated Kitty Ernst, Mary Breckenridge Chair of Midwifery at Frontier Nursing University (Ernst, 2012). Birth centers today are the exemplar of midwifery-led care and a haven for undisturbed, physiologic birth. The model of care continues to evolve, and further information is needed about the providers in birth centers, the range of services they offer, and how best to prepare new midwives and providers to work in this unique setting. As the national health care system shifts toward value-based payment models, supporting population health, and delivering care designed around patients' needs, midwifery practice is gaining notice as a powerful tool to improve outcomes and patient satisfaction. From the beginning, birth center practice was directly shaped by the needs of women: safety, autonomy, and access to care within their own communities. The forces that gave rise to the birth center's unique practice environment produced a care delivery model well equipped to meet the Institute of Healthcare Improvement's Triple Aim of improved patient experience, improved population health, and lower health care cost. Assuring a full complement of birth center providers and staff will be important as the model continues to grow.

EXEMPLAR

Birth Center: Flagstaff Birth and Women's Center, Flagstaff, Arizona

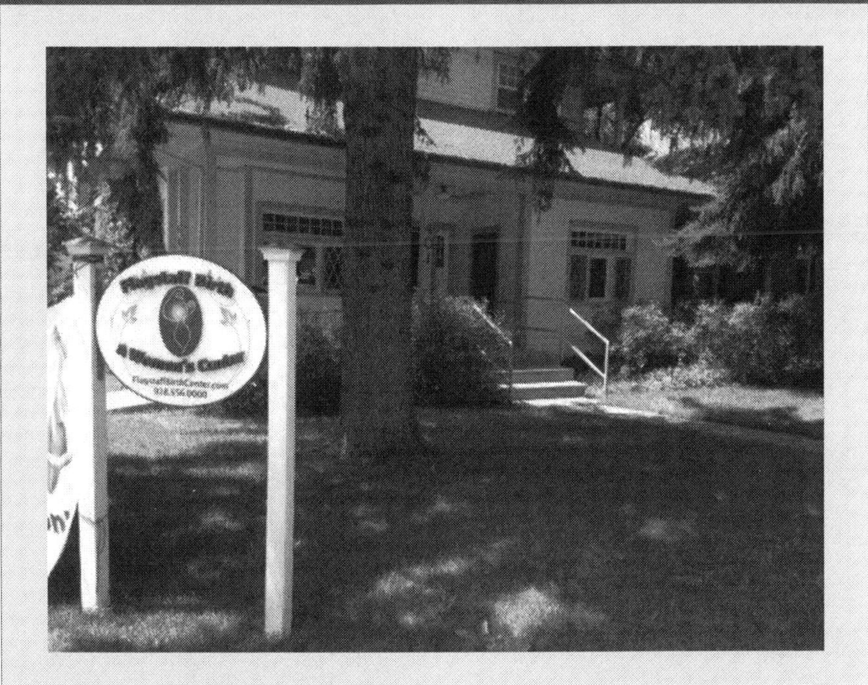

Year established: 2013

Type of building/square feet/architectural features: Older, 1908 home converted to business in mid-1980s, historical features, outdoor space, classroom space, offices and birth suites, built in approximately 3,100 square feet

Location: Urban

Business structure: For-profit

Ownership: Jointly LM, CPM, and CNM-owned

Licensed as: Outpatient treatment facility

Accredited by: Commission for the Accreditation of Birth Centers

Number of births to date/births per year: 191 births thus far, average 65 births per year

Services/enhanced services: IBCLC/lactation services

(continued)

EXEMPLAR *(continued)*

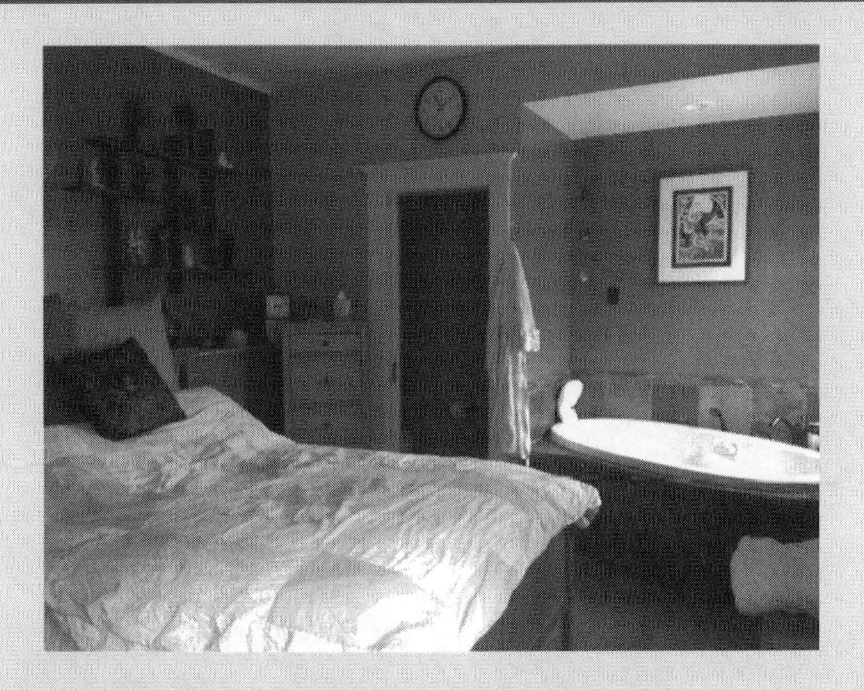

Providers: Two CNMs, one LM, CPM, and one ND, CPM

Client mix: Insurance, Medicaid, and cash-pay. Demographic: mostly White with small percentage of Hispanic, Black, and Native American

The Flagstaff Birth and Women's Center (FBWC) is Northern Arizona's first and only accredited birth center, located in the historic district of Flagstaff, Arizona, providing compassionate midwifery services and well-woman care. Our clients receive personal attention and exceptional care in an intimate, safe, home-like setting with a family- and community-centered approach to care.

FBWC is a unique birth center utilizing a variety of professional credentials for the care of women and their families during pregnancy, birth, and beyond. The owners are an LM, CPM, and CNM partnership with two other CNMs and an ND, CPM on staff. In addition, we have an acupuncturist, massage therapist, nutritionist, and lactation consultant also providing care here. The multidisciplinary group provides a well-rounded team of support for women and their families in Flagstaff.

(continued)

EXEMPLAR *(continued)*

FBWC is more than just a place to give birth or to receive quality health care; it is a place where community is welcomed and supported no matter the birth location. We are a culturally sensitive resource center that collaborates with other health care professionals when necessary to assure that all of the client's needs are met. It is our personal and professional mission to make midwifery services available and affordable to all women who desire our care. FBWC is a participating provider for most insurance companies including Medicaid.

Dar a Luz Exemplar, Abigail Eaves. Flagstaff Birth and Women's Center, Flagstaff, AZ.

REFERENCES

American Association of Birth Centers. (2016). Standards for birth centers (Revised). Retrieved from https://aabc.site-ym.com/?page=Standards

American College of Nurse-Midwives. (2011). Standards for the practice of midwifery. Retrieved from http://www.midwife.org/ACNM/files/ACNMLibraryData/UPLOADFILENAME/000000000051/Standards_for_Practice_of_Midwifery_Sept_2011.pdf

American College of Nurse-Midwives. (2012a). Definition of midwifery and scope of practice of certified nurse-midwives and certified midwives. Retrieved from http://www.midwife.org/ACNM/files/ACNMLibraryData/UPLOADFILENAME/000000000266/Definition%20of%20Midwifery%20and%20Scope%20of%20Practice%20of%20CNMs%20and%20CMs%20Feb%202012.pdf

American College of Nurse-Midwives. (2012b). Core competencies for basic midwifery practice. Retrieved from http://www.midwife.org/ACNM/files/ACNMLibraryData/UPLOADFILENAME/000000000050/Core%20Comptencies%20Dec%202012.pdf

American Midwifery Certification Board. (2013). Why AMCB certification. Retrieved from http://www.amcbmidwife.org/amcb-certification/why-amcb-certification-

Borst, C. G. (1995). *Catching babies: The professionalization of childbirth, 1870-1920*. Cambridge, MA: Harvard University Press.

Boston University School of Medicine. (2014). Boston University School of Medicine historical timeline: Boston Female Medical College. Retrieved from http://medlib.bu.edu/generic/timeline.php

Breckinridge, M. (1981). *Wide neighborhoods: A story of the Frontier Nursing Service*. Lexington: University Press of Kentucky.

Canoodt, L. J. (1982). *Utilization and economic analysis of the Maternity Center Association's Childbearing Center*. New York, NY: Blue Cross/Blue Shield of Greater New York, Health Affairs Research Department.

Commission for the Accreditation of Birth Centers. (2015). Indicators of compliance with the standards for birth centers. Retrieved from https://www.birthcenteraccreditation.org/go/get-cabc-indicators

Dawley, K. (2003). Origins of nurse-midwifery in the United States and its expansion in the 1940s. *Journal of Midwifery and Women's Health, 48*(2), 86–95.

Dekker, R. (2013). Evidence confirms birth centers provide top-notch care. Retrieved from http://www.birthcenters.org/?page=NBCSII

Ernst, E. (2012). Interview with Eunice (Kitty) Ernst, RN, CNM, MPH, DSc (hon)—Mary Breckinridge Chair of Midwifery. Retrieved from http://seattleschools.com/resources/interview-with-eunice-kitty-ernst-rn-cnm-mph-dsc-hon-mary-breckinridge-chair-of-midwifery

Home Birth Summit. (2016). Best practice guidelines: Transfer from planned home birth to hospital. Retrieved from http://www.homebirthsummit.org/best-practice-transfer-guidelines/transfer-guidelines-model-forms

International Confederation of Midwives. (2013). Global standards for midwifery education. Retrieved from http://www.internationalmidwives.org/assets/uploads/documents/CoreDocuments/ICM%20Standards%20Guidelines_ammended2013.pdf

Kenney, J. A. (1942). The first graduating class of the Tuskegee School of Midwifery. *Journal of the National Medical Association, 34*(3), 107–109.

Lyndon, A., Johnson, M. C., Bingham, D., Napolitano, P. G., Joseph, G., Maxfield, D. G., & O'Keefe, D. F. (2015). Transforming communication and safety culture in intrapartum care: A multi-organization blueprint. *Journal of Obstetric, Gynecologic and Neonatal Nursing, 44*(3), 341–349.

MacDorman, M. F., & Declercq, E. (2016). Trends and characteristics of United States out-of-hospital births 2004–2014: New information on risk status and access to care. *Birth, 43*(2), 116–124. doi:10.1111/birt.12228

Maine Center for Disease Control and Prevention. (2014). *Best practice recommendations for handoff communication during transport from a home or freestanding birth center to a hospital setting.* Augusta, ME: Author.

Mamatoto Village. (2013). Perinatal community health workers. Retrieved from http://www.mamatotovillage.org/#!pchw-training/cbzf

Maxwell, K. R. (2009). Birth behind the veil: African American midwives and mothers in the rural south, 1921–1962. Retrieved from https://ictcmidwives.org/wp-content/uploads/2015/04/Birth-Behind-the-Veil.pdf

Menard, M. K., Kilpatrick, S., Saade, G., Hollier, L., Joseph, G. F., Barfield, W., . . . Conry, J. (2015). Levels of maternal care. *American Journal of Obstetrics & Gynecology, 125*, 259–271. doi:10.1016/j.ajog.2014.12.030

Midwifery Education Accreditation Council. (2016). About us. Retrieved from http://meacschools.org

North American Registry of Midwives. (2016). Candidate information bulletin. Retrieved from http://narm.org/pdffiles/CIB.pdf

Northern New England Perinatal Quality Improvement Network. (2011). Out of Hospital to In Hospital Perinatal Transfer Form. Retrieved from http://www.nnepqin.org/Guidelines.asp#tabs-7

Rooks, J. P. (1997). *Midwifery and childbirth in America.* Philadelphia, PA: Temple University Press.

Rooks, J. P., Weatherby, N. L., Ernst, E. K. M., Stapleton, S., Rosen, D., & Rosenfield, A. (1989). Outcomes of care in birth centers: The National Birth Center Study. *New England Journal of Medicine, 321*(26), 1804–1811.

Smith, B. (2008). Midwifery. In *The Oxford encyclopedia of women in world history* (pp. 221–226). New York, NY: Oxford University Press. doi:10.1093/acref/9780195148909.001.0001

Turkel, K. D. (1995). *Women, power, and childbirth: A case study of a free-standing birth center.* Westport, CT: Greenwood Publishing Group.

Ulrich, L. T. (1990). *A midwife's tale: The life of Martha Ballard based on her diary, 1785–1812.* New York, NY: Alfred A. Knopf.

U.S. Department of Education. (2016). Specialized accrediting agencies database. Retrieved from http://www2.ed.gov/admins/finaid/accred/accreditation_pg7.html#health

U.S. Midwifery Education, Regulation, & Association Professional Regulation Committee. (2015). Statement on the licensure of certified professional midwives (CPM). Retrieved from http://www.usmera.org/index.php/2015/07/01/statement-on-the-licensure-of-certified-professional-midwives-cpm

Walker, D., Lannen, B., & Rossie, D. (2014). Midwifery practice and education: Current challenges and opportunities. *Online Journal of Issues in Nursing, 19*(2), Manuscript 4.

Washington State Perinatal Collaborative. (2015). Smooth transitions: Enhancing the safety of planned out-of-hospital birth transfers. Retrieved from http://www.washingtonmidwives.org/documents/Smooth-Transitions-Hospital-Transport-QI-Project.pdf

Whittle, P. (2016). New Maine midwifery rules reflect licensure drive around US. Retrieved from https://www.boston.com/news/health/2016/05/29/maine-midwives-license

CHAPTER 8

Reaching for Excellence: Birth Center Standards and Accreditation

SUSAN RUTLEDGE STAPLETON AND
ROSEMARY SENJEM

LEARNING OBJECTIVES

Upon completion of this chapter, the reader will be able to:

1. Describe the history of the development of the national *Standards for Birth Centers* and birth center accreditation
2. Understand the difference between accreditation and regulation
3. Discuss perceived barriers to accreditation and opportunities for wider adoption of birth center accreditation

HISTORY OF THE DEVELOPMENT OF BIRTH CENTER STANDARDS AND ACCREDITATION

Focus on quality and safety has been a key aspect of the birth center movement from its inception. The foundation for quality and safety is the triad of evidence-based standards, state licensure, and national accreditation. Pioneering experts in maternity care have worked collaboratively for decades to assure this strong foundation for today's birth centers. This story of foresight and vision describes the process of establishing national birth center standards based on the best available evidence, development of an accreditation mechanism that includes peer review,

---

This history has been edited and updated with permission from its original author, Eunice "Kitty" Ernst. The original text was published in 2015 in a birth center trade association newsletter (Ernst, 2015).

and the impact of these pioneering achievements on contemporary birth centers.

In 1975, after 5 years as the director of Maternity Center Association (MCA), nurse-midwife/anthropologist Ruth Watson Lubic opened the first demonstration of a *licensed, accredited, freestanding* birth center with reimbursement for services from the largest health care insurer at the time, Blue Cross and Blue Shield (BCBS) of Greater New York. Since there were no birth center-specific standards for accreditation, regulations for licensure, or contracts for payment of services in place, MCA worked with existing agencies. This set the precedent for the future development of the essential foundation for birth centers. The MCA's Childbearing Center (CbC) was given a temporary license under the New York Ambulatory Surgery Center Regulations and was accredited by the combined American Public Health Association (APHA) and National League for Nursing's Accreditation of Community-Based Health Care.

The negotiation of a contract with BCBS included permission to monitor and evaluate the safety, satisfaction, and savings of the demonstration birth center. The payer found that the birth center provided safe care based on evaluation of basic perinatal outcomes; women reported high levels of satisfaction with their care, and the birth center achieved a cost savings of up to 40% over hospital confinement (Canoodt, 1982). This study set a precedent for the rigorous and objective evaluation of the birth center that continues today. Meanwhile, there was vigorous and often contentious debate opposing out-of-hospital birth (Lubic, 1979). Opponents ultimately accepted that women were seeking an alternative to the medical routines of hospital-based maternity care, and there was agreement that development of systems to assure safety and quality care was critical.

In 1979, MCA brought together directors of 14 early birth centers to identify their needs and discuss how best to meet them. The major issues identified were the need for national standards, licensure regulations, reimbursement for services, and evaluation of the birth center model of care. In May 1981, MCA received a grant from the John A. Hartford Foundation to convene a group of maternity care experts to explore:

- Promoting a wider public understanding of the birth center concept
- Supporting the development of a birth center trade association
- Developing and publishing national standards
- Making recommendations for regulations to guide public health officials, policy planners, and payers

Standards and regulations for licensure as an ambulatory surgical center were not appropriate; thus, it was critical to develop standards specific to the birth center midwifery model of care. Information collected from existing birth centers was used to define the birth center, and Recommendations for Establishing Standards or Regulations for Freestanding Birth Centers was published in the February 1982 issue of the newsletter of the Cooperative Birth Center Network (CBCN; American Association of Birth Centers [AABC], 1982). CBCN became the trade association for birth centers and is now called the AABC (see Chapter 1). In 1982, the APHA published its Guidelines for Licensing and Regulating Birth Centers (APHA, 1982). These guidelines have served as the basis for birth center regulations across the United States, and continue to be used as the foundation for new state regulations. Table 8.1 summarizes the APHA guidelines.

As the debate about safety of out-of-hospital birth intensified, the Institute of Medicine (IOM) appointed a research committee to review all of the scientific literature on all birth settings. The IOM and National Research Council report, *Research Issues in the Assessment of Birth Settings* (1982), essentially found no reliable evidence about the safety of *any* birth setting and offered recommendations for conducting future research on

TABLE 8.1
American Public Health Association Guidelines for Licensing and Regulating Birth Centers (APHA, 1983)

Guideline	Areas Addressed
Definitions	Birth center; low risk and licensed birth attendants
Staffing	Administration; clinical, staff; volunteers and personnel providing patient and other services; advisory council
Facility	Design; fire and safety; equipment
Services	Selection of clients; orientation and education; prenatal care; surgical services; intrapartum care; analgesia and anesthesia; postpartum and newborn care; food service; referral to other community services
Policies and procedures	Organization; consultation; transfer and transportation; health records; program evaluation; quality assurance; accreditation

Source: APHA (1983).

all birth settings (IOM and National Research Council (NRC) Committee on Assessing Alternative Birth Settings, 1982).

Exploratory meetings with both the Joint Commission on Accreditation of Hospitals (JCAH), now The Joint Commission (TJC), and the Association for the Accreditation of Ambulatory Health Care (AAAHC) occurred in 1984 and participants determined that accreditation within their organizations was not feasible. Consequently, in December 1984 MCA obtained funding from the Pew Charitable Trusts and brought together representatives of birth centers, consumer organizations, and maternity care professionals from the private and public sectors in Philadelphia to discuss writing national standards for birth centers and establishing a mechanism for accreditation. This meeting was called the Forum on Health Policy Issues of the Freestanding Birth Center and the trade association published essays by some participants in its newsletter. The issues were identified, with a particular focus on safety, and debated before arriving at the general consensus that the standards should reflect midwifery care, and be flexible enough to allow continued development of an evidence-based model of care to be evaluated by an accreditation process. AABC board member Charles Mahan, MD, FACOG, volunteered to chair the trade association's new standards committee; Eunice Cole, RN, immediate past president of the American Nurses Association, volunteered to chair the new Commission for the Accreditation of Birth Centers (CABC), which was yet to be formed under the AABC; and birth center midwives and administrators volunteered to train and serve as CABC site visitors (Ernst, 2015).

In March 1985, AABC published the first national *Standards for Birth Centers* after the standards were unanimously adopted by the trade association members. Here is an excerpt from the introduction section of this landmark document:

> Quality assurance is an evaluation function that is both external and internal to the birth center. Licensure and accreditation constitute two arms of external quality assurance. Licensing agencies are officially charged by the federal, state or local governments to protect the public and monitor safety through codes, ordinances and a variety of regulations. This first level of external quality control requires that the birth center meet defined criteria for licensure in order to operate as a business or health care facility. But the level of quality required for licensure may vary from one locality to another. Some states and municipalities are non-specific or uneven in their requirements

for regulations while other states may be very specific and uniform in the level of requirements for safe operation.

A second level of external quality assurance is a national program of accreditation. Standards and attributes for accreditation are uniformly applied in all localities, thereby eliminating state and local inconsistency. It is a voluntary program that places the level of quality desired above that which the state may require.

Internal quality assurance begins at the earliest stages of planning of the birth center and comprises a systems approach to evaluation of operation and services. Like all new health care facilities, the birth center has the opportunity to build evaluation mechanisms into all facets of the organization and operation. If attention is given to establishing a strong program of quality assurance in planning the freestanding birth center, application for licensure and accreditation are simply a form of external review—an opportunity to be evaluated or measured by established yardsticks for required and desired levels of excellence. (Standards for Birth Centers, American Association of Birth Centers. [1985–2013]. Reprinted with permission.)

This achievement was the result of the culmination of nationwide efforts by birth center founders and stakeholders since 1975, including the demonstration CbC by MCA of New York. MCA's demonstration project included (Ernst, 2015):

- Identification of criteria for low-risk pregnancy and birth
- Development of policies and procedures for operation of a birth center as a place for the midwifery model of care, and connected to the existing system of health care
- Design of record forms including an extensive informed consent
- A health record that reflects the care provided and the instruction of clients on health relating to pregnancy, birth, and early parenting
- Evaluation mechanisms for all aspects of the program offered

At this same first annual meeting of the trade association, their board voted to "establish a separate association to be called tentatively, the Association for Accreditation of Birth Centers." This would become the

CABC and was ultimately founded under the trade association to (Ernst, 2015):

- Evaluate the quality of birth center services
- Promote the development of national guidelines for licensure
- Review state regulations for birth centers
- Explore and evaluate the programs of other accrediting agencies
- Support the expensive process of accreditation with resources from the trade association

In the fall 1985 newsletter, the trade association announced that "Additional funds have been secured to continue the Pilot Program on Accreditation of Freestanding Birth Centers" (AABC, 1985b). MCA funded this program to develop and conduct an accreditation process for 12 birth centers, which led to the establishment of the CABC.

Then, a landmark meeting was held in Philadelphia of the newly formed CABC and newly recruited advisory council to the CABC to evaluate the work of establishing the national standards and applying them in the pilot program for accreditation. The advisory council to CABC, led by H. Robert Cathcart, who was president of Pennsylvania Hospital and a commissioner for JCAH, included representatives from a broad group of stakeholders and experts, including midwifery, obstetrics, neonatology, nursing, public health, birth center parents, birth centers, vice president of the Health Insurance Association of America (HIAA), vice president of Pennsylvania Hospital in charge of hospital accreditation, and federal policy maker.

After one and a half days of deliberation, the consensus for how best to reach for excellence through *National Standards and Accreditation for Freestanding Birth Centers* was that "in this time of rapid change, the CABC had the best prospects of developing a high quality program of accreditation for birth centers and should continue to pursue it, cooperating with other agencies as the opportunities arise" (Ernst, 2015). The following are excerpts from papers presented by advisory council members and later published in the trade association's newsletter:

- "The Health Insurance Association of America (HIAA) supports the development of quality care review programs by member companies as well as by other entities within the private and public sectors. . . .

HIAA recognizes that birth centers address the desires and demands of many childbearing families. However, the birth center holds the same potential for being abused or corrupted as nursing homes, hospices or any other care facility that may emerge outside of established mechanisms for measuring the quality of care provided. The established mechanisms are state licensure and national accreditation." —Stanley B. Peck, MBA, vice president, HIAA (Peck, 1987)

- "Quality assurance mechanisms must be expanded into non-traditional settings. . . . It is important for birth centers to give attention to accreditation if they want to retain responsibility for development of the birth center concept." —Eunice Cole, chair, Commission for Accreditation of Freestanding Birth Centers (Cole, 1987)
- "The importance of accreditation to 'emerging' organizations like freestanding birthing centers is critical. Accreditation of birth centers like the accreditation of hospitals will become a franchise to do business. Loss of accreditation for hospitals in Philadelphia means loss of reimbursement. Accreditation for birth centers will, in all probability, also become a preclusion of entry into 'the market' for those who cannot meet select standards. It provides a legitimacy and will be valued in the face of skepticism from childbearing women or from physicians who have been trained to view the hospital labor floor as the only safe and responsible location for childbirth. Hospitals that dare to associate with such iconoclasm as the birthing center will dare more readily if a center is 'accredited' by a reputable body. . . . Hospitals will be eager to see that birthing centers have in place systematic and comprehensive Quality Assurance mechanisms that parallel the licensure, accreditation, quality assurance and insurance data systems that affect hospitals. There must be assurance that birthing centers have been deliberate in their self-evaluation, that they will not admit or hold women unwisely and that providers' practice patterns are reviewed periodically. These practices, in my opinion, will contribute significantly to acceptance and trust of birthing centers by hospitals providing back-up services to birth centers."—Bruce Herdmon, PhD, vice president, Pennsylvania Hospital, responsible for hospital accreditation (Herdmon, 1987)

The first CABC board of commissioners, led by Eunice Cole, also included nurse-midwives, obstetricians, a pediatrician, and a representative of the public. The advisory council to CABC remained in place through 1988. CABC accreditation was designed as a peer review process and birth center midwives and administrators volunteered to train and serve as CABC site visitors and continued to do so up to the end of September 2014, when CABC hired staff to fulfill this role.

CABC separated from AABC in 2002 as planned from its founding, and incorporated as a separate not-for-profit entity. CABC continued to conduct accreditation activities with a volunteer corps of commissioners and site visitors until October 2014. With the support of accredited birth centers, CABC was able to raise its fees substantially and adopted a different business model with all staff site visitors to meet the demands of growth. In March 2015, CABC added a board of governors to allow for fund raising to retool for growth and further develop the organization's outreach.

In September 2015, CABC published its first reference edition of the Indicators of Compliance With the Standards for Birth Centers, which revealed CABC requirements for accreditation, listed unacceptable practices, and included a glossary of terms, linked index, and reference citations. In January 2016, after more than 30 years, CABC reached the milestone of 100 currently accredited birth centers.

ACCREDITATION: WHAT IS IT? WHY DOES IT MATTER?

Accreditation is a nongovernmental process in which certification of competency, authority, or credibility is presented. A wide and growing array of fields use accreditation, including health care, veterinary medicine, engineering and manufacturing, education, language translation and interpretation, and public relations.

It is common for standards and accreditation to originate in a trade association or professional organization, for example, TJC was created jointly by the American College of Surgeons, American College of Physicians, American Hospital Association, and American Medical Association (TJC, 2016). When the accreditor's scope is confined to the review of a small or finite number of organizations, the accreditor typically remains under the originating organization for support. For example, Accreditation Commission for Midwifery Education (ACME) is a commission of the American College of Nurse-Midwives (ACNM), which provides some funding for this function (ACNM, n.d.). When an accrediting organization has enough volume to spread out the costs, it can achieve financial independence as seen with larger accrediting organizations, such as TJC and the Commission on Collegiate Nursing Education (CCNE).

The purposes of birth center accreditation are to:

- Hold the accredited birth centers accountable to the community of interest—childbearing families, collaborative health care professionals, payers, other birth centers
- Assess the extent to which a birth center meets national accreditation standards
- Inform the public of the purposes and values of accreditation and identify birth centers that meet accreditation standards
- Foster continuing improvement in birth centers—and, thus, in professional practice and maternity care in general

To achieve these purposes, an accrediting organization does more than conduct periodic site visits (or surveys) and decision processes. Accreditors of birth centers must do all of the following:

- Continuously review relevant current research, best practices, and national guidelines
- Publish periodic updates to standards and indicators
- Disseminate alerts and communications regarding accreditation
- Implement a public complaint mechanism and review process
- Provide a birth center appeal mechanism and review process
- Provide a mechanism for sentinel event reporting and review, including dissemination of knowledge garnered from these reviews for quality improvement
- Provide ongoing verification of the credential
- Represent the credential at professional meetings
- Inform the public regarding the value of the credential and the need to look for accreditation when selecting a maternity care provider and facility
- Educate policy makers and payers on the value of accreditation for their constituents and subscribers
- Provide ongoing training for staff and board members
- Offer education and training to assist the organizations seeking accreditation

ACCREDITATION AND REGULATION: WHAT IS THE DIFFERENCE?

In general, regardless of the field of expertise, regulations are obligatory and seeking accreditation is voluntary, although the latter is changing in the field of health care. Birth centers are obliged to abide by the laws and regulations that govern them in order to maintain a current license. Birth centers choose to become accredited to demonstrate their accountability and dedication to best practices. Regulations represent a minimum level of performance, whereas accreditation represents excellence.

As of 2015, Minnesota and Illinois required CABC accreditation for licensure; others were considering it. In Montana, birth centers can choose either CABC accreditation or going through the state licensing process with state inspections in order to be licensed. CABC-accredited birth centers in Florida may defer the annual inspection by the Agency for Health Care Administration in the year in which they have a CABC site visit. A growing number of health care insurers, such as some Medicaid plans (Louisiana and North Carolina), Anthem Blue Cross and Highmark Blue Shield (Pennsylvania), and Regence Blue Cross Blue Shield (Washington), wanting evidence for safety and quality, require CABC accreditation for contracting with and reimbursing birth centers.

As of September 2015, approximately one third of U.S. birth centers known to AABC were CABC accredited or in the process. According to CABC's 2014 annual report, that represents a significant increase over prior years and the number of birth centers seeking accreditation is expected to continue to rise as both consumers and payers demand that birth centers demonstrate they are providing high-quality care (CABC, 2015a).

Regulations currently refer to birth center accreditation in one of two ways. In some states, accreditation is granted by deeming status for licensure, for example, Montana and Florida; the credential is used by the regulatory body in lieu of all, or part, of the process for granting the license. In other states—for example, Minnesota and Illinois—a birth center must attain accreditation from an approved accrediting body, either CABC or TJC in order to be eligible for the license. In this case, this credential may also be used in lieu of part, or all, of the regulator's process for granting the license. In either case, the birth center is responsible to first obtain the CABC accreditation credential and provide it to the regulatory agency. Some regulatory agencies request a copy of the CABC decision letter as part of this step in their process. The regulatory agency can then contact CABC to verify the credentials provided or accreditation can be verified on the CABC website (CABC, 2015d). If the birth center has provided the regulator with a copy of the accreditation decision letter, CABC will verify the letter and its contents for the regulatory body upon request. The CABC has a direct relationship and legal agreement with the birth center. The CABC has an indirect relationship with the regulatory body.

The CABC is currently the only accreditor that uses the national *Standards for Birth Centers* and accredits facilities as birth centers. TJC reviews birth centers as ambulatory care centers, thus side-stepping the midwifery model of care that is the hallmark of CABC accreditation and the *Standards for Birth Centers*. Some birth centers are accredited both by CABC as a birth center and by TJC as an ambulatory care center.

CABC accreditation can be verified at this website (www.VerifyMyBirthCenter.org), allowing stakeholders to rely on the national Standards for Birth Centers and informing their decision making. Table 8.2 shows the benefits of birth center accreditation to stakeholders.

NATIONAL STANDARDS FOR BIRTH CENTERS: THE BASIS FOR ACCREDITATION

In the field of accreditation, the accreditor is usually the publisher of the standards used for accreditation and, as part of the accreditor's own quality assurance program, seeks stakeholder input periodically. However, the birth center model is a disruptive innovation in maternal and newborn care. As a disruptive innovation, its definition is fragile until well established; the members of the trade association did not release the standards to the CABC in 2001, when CABC separated from the trade association. This was due to fears of potential for eventual corruption of the standards of this new model away from the midwifery model of care toward the medical model of care. Instead, the two organizations set out to collaborate, as described later in this chapter. Despite this anomaly in the field of accreditation, the *Standards for Birth Centers*, published by the AABC, have withstood the test of time, and much of what we know about the safety and good outcomes in birth centers is based upon the model of care reflected in these standards (AABC, 1985–2016).

Figure 8.1 shows the process used by the trade association for reviewing and revising the *Standards for Birth Centers* (CABC, 2015c). The AABC Standards Committee is chaired by an AABC board member and made up of three AABC members and three CABC commissioners. All members of the AABC Standards Committee must be members of AABC. Thus, AABC membership retains control of the standards, but provides

TABLE 8.2
Benefits of CABC Accreditation to Stakeholders

Stakeholder	Benefits
Childbearing families	Know that this birth center and its care providers are dedicated to national standards for safe, evidence-based maternity care and avoid inappropriate use of technology.
Local employers	Rely on this credential as a verifiable measure of quality when negotiating health insurance contracts to cover the care their employees prefer.
Birth centers and midwives	Learn from experienced experts in birth center operations and be verifiably accountable to the community and maternity care colleagues.
Hospitals and physicians receiving transfers	Count on complete records and communications for consultation or transfer of care, as well as participate in interviews during the CABC accreditation site visit.
Health care insurance companies	Use this credential to support payment for CABC-accredited birth centers, as well as in-network status. (Some birth centers initially seek CABC accreditation because it is required by a major health insurance payer in their region.)
Liability insurance companies	Use this credential as one measure of risk in evaluating rates as an underwriter. (Two liability insurance companies offer up to a 10% discount for CABC-accredited birth centers.)
Funders of not-for-profit birth centers	In addition to rigorous evaluation of clinical practices, an important part of the CABC's accreditation is looking at the long-term viability of each birth center. Three of the nine national Standards for Birth Centers are devoted to organization governance, planning, and administration, including financial practices. Birth centers that are ready to open are eligible to seek 1-year accreditation, making it easier for funders to verify a not-for-profit start-up.

CABC, Commission for the Accreditation of Birth Centers.

Reprinted with permission from Commission for the Accreditation of Birth Centers.

CABC with the opportunity to contribute based on its experiences with implementing the standards in its accreditation process.

The impetus for proposed changes in the *Standards for Birth Centers* may arise from the AABC Standards Committee itself, AABC board or members, CABC, or other stakeholders. In 2015, AABC conducted an

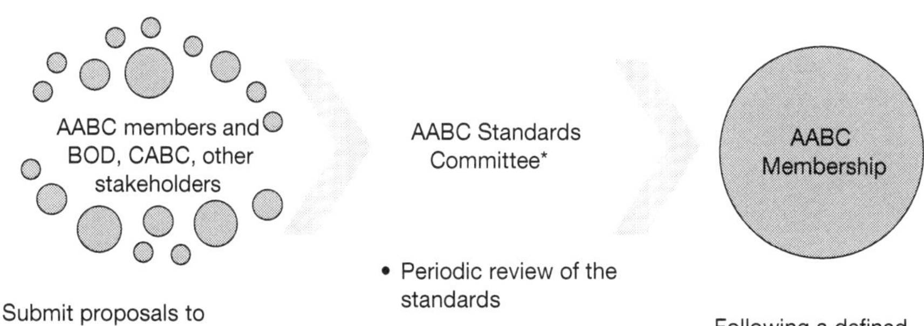

FIGURE 8.1 Revision process for the *Standards for Birth Centers*, published by the AABC.

AABC, American Association of Birth Centers; BOD, Board of Directors; CABC, Commission for the Accreditation of Birth Centers.

*The Standards Committee is chaired by an AABC board member and composed of representatives of AABC (6) and CABC (maximum 3). All members of the AABC Standards Committee must be members of AABC.

Reprinted with permission from American Association of Birth Centers (AABC).

extensive review of the standards that included literature review, inviting comments from AABC members and convening an expert panel of consumer advocates and representatives from professional organizations of maternity care providers. Recommendations for revisions were approved by AABC membership, and include updates to reflect current evidence-based practices in perinatal care and enhanced elucidation of the birth center model of care.

CABC uses the *Standards for Birth Centers*, published by the trade association, as the basis for its accreditation process because these standards are nationally recognized as the gold standard for birth center practice and operations. No other standards specific to birth centers currently exist in the United States, although the *Standards for Birth Centers* incorporate many endorsed and evidence-based national guidelines and standards for maternity and neonatal care.

INDICATORS OF COMPLIANCE WITH THE STANDARDS FOR BIRTH CENTERS: MEASURES OF EXCELLENCE

Standards are, intentionally, very broad guidelines, and, thus, are not sufficient for use as measures in evaluating quality in a facility. Consequently, accrediting organizations also develop detailed performance indicators for measuring whether the standards are being met. The CABC's (2015) Indicators of Compliance with the Standards for Birth Centers are used to determine the degree to which each birth center is adhering to the *Standards for Birth Centers,* and to develop requirements and recommendations for improvement for a birth center when indicated.

The CABC's *Indicators of Compliance with the Standards for Birth Centers* are available to the public on the CABC website, where registration allows one to receive both the current indicators and alerts regarding updates as they occur. Indicators or measures are based on the best available evidence and accepted professional guidelines. Indicators are revised much more frequently than standards as they are designed to provide specific guidance for the accreditation process. An example of the need for such flexibility in indicators is the dissemination in 2015 of revisions in its Guidelines for Cardiopulmonary Resuscitation and Emergency Cardiovascular Care of the Neonate to be published in its release of the Neonatal Resuscitation Program (NRP) 7th edition (AHA & AAP, 2015). Although the *Standards for Birth Centers* simply state that birth centers should adhere to current NRP guidelines, CABC indicators specify specific measures, including equipment and medications available; staff competency maintenance and drills; and content of clinical practice guidelines for neonatal resuscitation. Consequently, changes in the NRP guidelines usually require revision of the CABC indicators in order to assure that birth centers remain in compliance with the new guidelines and thus the *Standards for Birth Centers.* The development and revision process for the CABC indicators also helps to inform the work of the AABC Standards Committee in identifying aspects of the *Standards for Birth Centers* needing revision for greater clarity or to align with updated evidence and guidelines.

Figure 8.2 illustrates the process for maintaining and revising the CABC indicators. The CABC Indicators and Research Committee (IRC) is responsible for maintaining the indicators and conducting a full review periodically. Suggestions for review or revision are also initiated by other stakeholders, including CABC-accredited birth centers and their clients; CABC commissioners, site visitors, and staff; and collaborating professional organizations. Publication or endorsement of national guidelines and standards in perinatal care and other relevant fields often trigger review of the indicators as well. Specific revisions are approved by the board of commissioners in response to recommendations from the IRC, with final approval by the Joint Assembly of Boards. CABC then communicates the revisions to CABC-accredited birth centers, publishes the

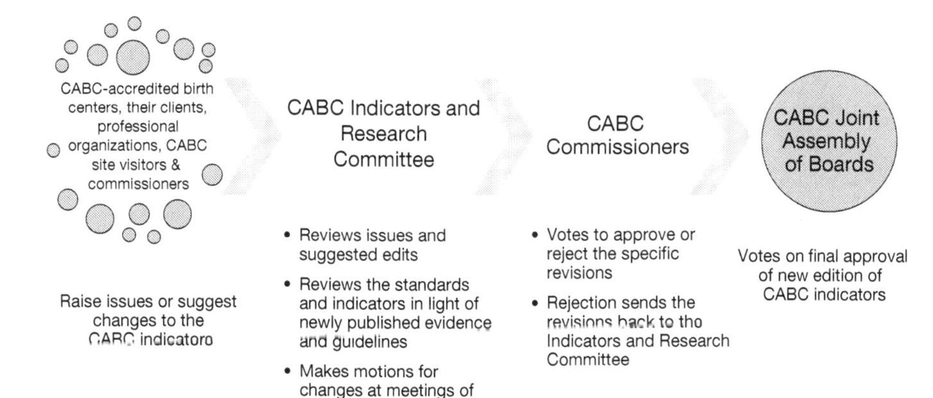

FIGURE 8.2 Revision process for the CABC indicators.

CABC, Commission for the Accreditation of Birth Centers.

Reprinted with permission from Commission for the Accreditation of Birth Centers.

new edition of the CABC indicators on the website, and notifies registered subscribers.

CABC ORGANIZATIONAL STRUCTURE

The Commission for the Accreditation of Birth Centers, Inc. is a 501(c)3 not-for-profit organization, with a three-board structure (commissioners, governors, and together they are the CABC Joint Assembly of Boards). This allows CABC to manage conflicts of interest and ethical and legal responsibilities of the peer review accreditation process, as well as raise funds to provide support for the organization beyond accreditation fees. Figure 8.3 shows the current organizational structure of the CABC.

The commissioners are birth center experts who have either owned, been employed by, or been a client at a CABC-accredited birth center. They develop and approve CABC indicators, serve as panelists for review of accreditation documents, and make decisions as to whether a birth center meets the requirements for CABC accreditation. The consumer representatives on the board of commissioners play a special role that is both ombudsman and watchdog for the process. The governors are advocates for CABC accreditation and are not involved in accreditation decisions. CABC staff are responsible for day-to-day operations, and conduct

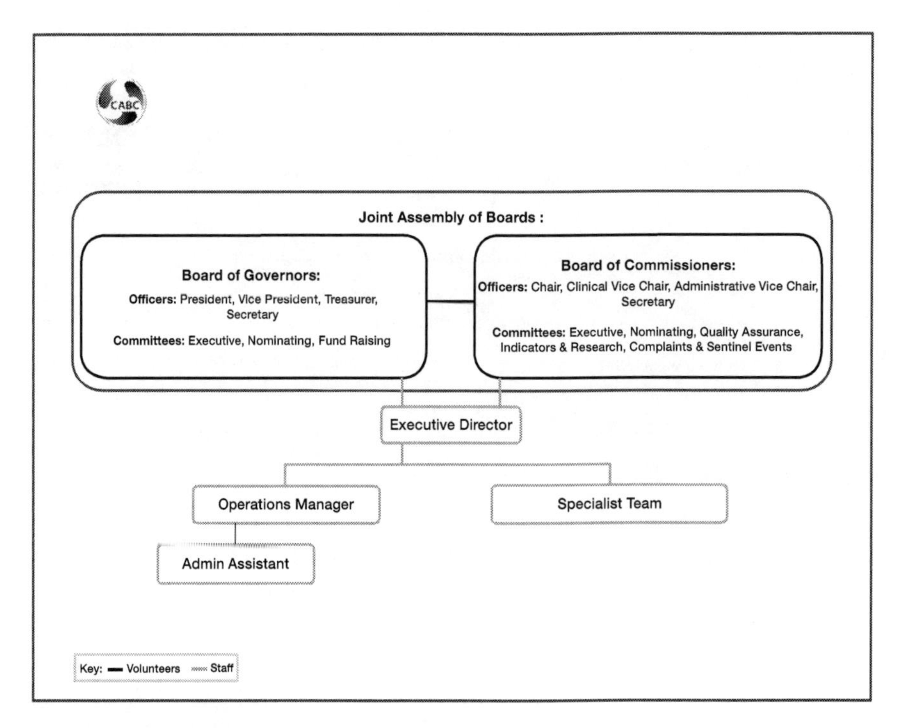

FIGURE 8.3 Organizational chart for the Commission for the Accreditation of Birth Centers.
Reprinted with permission from Commission for the Accreditation of Birth Centers.

site visits to collect data for accreditation panel reviews and to educate birth center staff.

ROLE OF EDUCATION IN CABC ACCREDITATION

CABC's organizational approach is always educative, whether during a phone call with a birth center, a site visit at the birth center, or the decision letter and progress report correspondence. The entire organization works to create buy-in from a birth center so the birth center's staff will become champions of the standards and accreditation. The goal is to assist birth centers to identify and implement best clinical and business practices and evaluate their own performance in achieving excellence. In 2016, CABC launched online tutorials for birth centers seeking accreditation.

CABC accreditation requires that the birth center enter data in a national data registry and track its own statistics to drive best practices, as well as implement a continuous quality improvement program, including quality assurance policies and procedures, review of clinical management, and root cause analysis for sentinel events, unusual incidents, and adverse outcomes. Aggregate data regarding sentinel events is used by CABC as one basis for birth center education, as well as to help inform maintenance of the CABC indicators.

CABC ACCREDITATION PROCESS

The process for CABC accreditation is dynamic and changes in response to CABC internal quality improvement activities, including analysis of feedback data from all involved in the process. Learn the steps of the current accreditation process at the CABC website (www.birthcenteraccreditation.org).

RECOGNITION OF THE CABC ACCREDITATION CREDENTIAL

The certification mark of the CABC Seal of Accreditation is displayed by each CABC-accredited birth center along with a current certificate of accreditation in public view. Parents seeking birth center care, their health insurance companies, state regulatory bodies, graduate education programs for health professionals, liability insurance companies, and health professional organizations recognize the CABC accreditation credential.

The American College of Obstetricians and Gynecologists (ACOG) in its 2015 Obstetric Care Consensus on the Levels of Maternal Care document acknowledged birth centers and CABC accreditation (ACOG, 2015). This document was endorsed or supported by AABC, ACNM, Association of Women's Health, Obstetric and Neonatal Nurses, CABC, the American Academy of Pediatrics leadership, the American Society of Anesthesiologists leadership, and the Society for Obstetric Anesthesia and Perinatology leadership. Endorsement represents a growing recognition of the role of birth centers in the maternity care system, and of the value of CABC accreditation in assuring high-quality birth center care.

PERCEIVED BARRIERS TO ACCREDITATION

The perceived barriers to accreditation fall into two main categories: financial burdens (staff time and cost) and disagreements with the requirements for CABC accreditation. The AABC conducted a 2016 survey of

307 known birth centers, including nonmembers, with 164 (53.42%) responding to questions regarding accreditation status. Of these, 117 (71.34%) were AABC members (AABC, 2017).

Eighty-five (53.46%) of the 159 U.S. birth centers responding reported they are accredited by the CABC as a birth center; eight (4.88%) are accredited by TJC as an ambulatory care facility or a department of a larger facility; and five (3.05%) of these are accredited by both the CABC and TJC. Five others are located outside the United States, where no accreditation mechanism is available. The CABC reports that it is the only known accreditor of birth center facilities in the world and currently only reviews birth centers in the United States.

Seventy-three (45.91%) of the 159 U.S. birth centers responding reported they are not accredited, with 15 of the unaccredited U.S. birth centers (20.55%) reporting a plan to seek accreditation within the next year. Twenty-two (30.14%) of the 73 nonaccredited U.S. birth centers report two or more barriers to becoming accredited, including seven of those indicating that they would seek accreditation within the next year. The most common barrier to seeking accreditation for these birth centers was time and fitting preparing for accreditation into a busy staff schedule. All except two of the birth centers planning to seek accreditation in the next year have been open for 5 years or less, with four open for less than 1 year with fewer than 100 births, and thus ineligible for CABC accreditation.

Fifty-eight (79.45%) of the 73 nonaccredited U.S. birth centers responding reported they are not in the process, nor plan to seek accreditation in the next year. These birth centers have been open anywhere from 1 year to 36 years, with 23 (41.07%) founded in the past 5 years. The most common reasons for not seeking accreditation in these birth centers were cost and a perception of insufficient value for their circumstances (see Table 8.3).

Financial burdens are perceived differently around the United States, and are dependent upon the market forces in that community. For example, in a state where CABC accreditation is required or is granted deemed status for the birth center's license, the birth center owner is more likely to consider accreditation a normal cost of doing business. Likewise, in regions in which major payers mandate accreditation, birth centers desiring payer contracts perceive accreditation as a necessary business expense. However, in a state where accreditation is not yet recognized and the public and the health insurance companies in that region are underinformed, the birth center owner will find little to no financial incentive and tend to see the cost of accreditation as an unnecessary burden. In this case, the barriers include lobbying legislators or regulators to

TABLE 8.3
2016 AABC Birth Center Survey: Perceived Barriers to Accreditation

Perceived Barriers to Accreditation Among Unaccredited U.S. Birth Centers ($n = 73$)	Cost ($n = 30$)		Insufficient Value ($n = 26$)		Time & Scheduling ($n = 23$)		Disagree With Requirements of Accreditation ($n = 7$)	
Planning to seek accreditation within the next year ($n = 15$)	6	8.22%	1	1.37%	8	10.96%	2	2.74%
Not planning to seek accreditation in the next year ($n = 58$)	24	32.88%	25	34.25%	15	20.55%	5	6.85%

AABC, American Association of Birth Centers.

Source: AABC (2017)

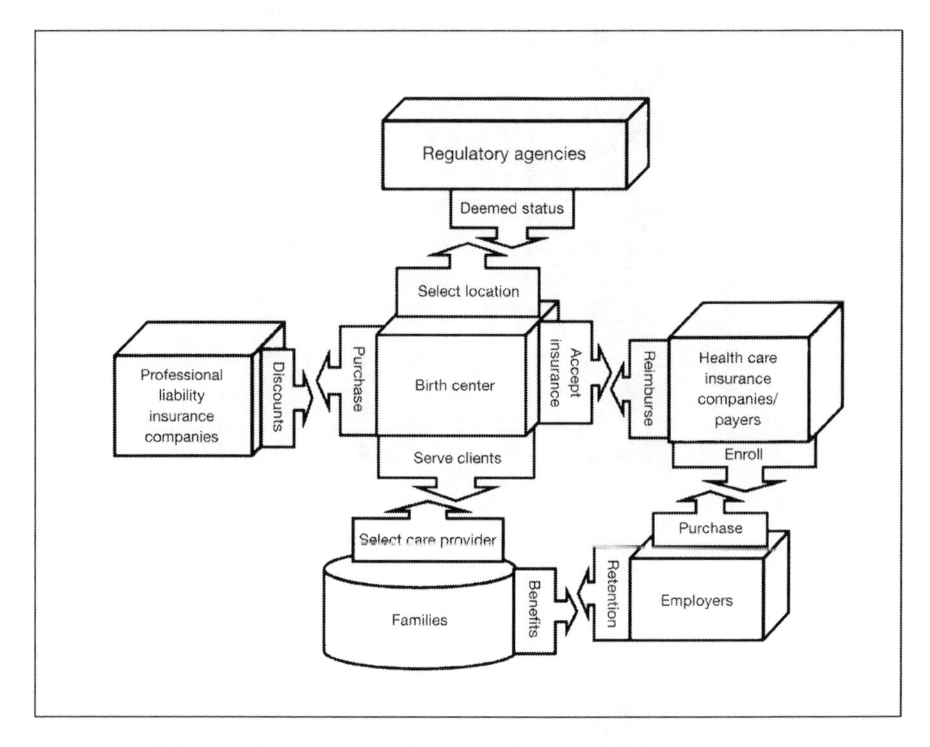

FIGURE 8.4 Marketplace relationships affected by CABC accreditation.

CABC, Commission for the Accreditation of Birth Centers.

Reprinted with permission from Commission for the Accreditation of Birth Center.

mandate accreditation, significant public relations efforts to raise awareness with the community and employers, and relationship building and negotiations to educate insurance companies.

In Figure 8.4, consider the various players and their choices that can be affected by CABC accreditation in the birth center's marketplace. Incentives for CABC accreditation can occur in these relationships like this (AABC, 2017):

- **Families ask the birth center,** "Is this birth center using best practices and CABC accredited?" If so, they select that birth center.
- **Families ask their employers,** "Do health care benefits include birth centers and midwives?" If so, they use and find value in the benefits.
- **Employers ask employees,** "Are you interested in a health care plan that includes CABC-accredited birth centers?" If so, employers hope to

boost staff retention with plans that include CABC-accredited birth centers.

- **Employers ask health insurance companies,** "Do you have a plan that includes CABC-accredited birth centers?" If so, the employer purchases it for the employees.
- **Health insurance companies ask employers,** "Are you interested in our plans that include CABC-accredited birth centers?" If so, the insurance company enrolls these employers.
- **Health insurance companies ask birth centers,** "Is this birth center CABC accredited?" If so, the insurance company provides reimbursement for care and the facility, as well as includes this birth center in-network.
- **Professional liability insurance companies ask birth centers,** "Is this birth center CABC accredited?" If so, the insurance company offers discounts on liability insurance.
- **Regulatory agencies ask birth centers,** "Is this birth center CABC accredited?" If so, the regulatory agency grants deemed status for the birth center license or site inspections.
- **Birth centers ask regulatory agencies,** "Do you offer deemed status for CABC accreditation?" If so, the birth center chooses this jurisdiction to locate the facility.
- **Birth centers ask professional liability insurance companies,** "Do you offer discounts for CABC accreditation?" If so, the birth center selects this liability insurance.
- **Birth centers ask health insurance companies,** "Do you reimburse CABC-accredited birth centers at full rates?" If so, the birth center chooses to accept this health insurance for payment.
- **Birth centers ask families,** "Are you seeking care in alignment with CABC accreditation?" If so, the birth center knows they are marketing successfully to their target clients.

For a more detailed diagram, download marketplace incentives for CABC accreditation: www.birthcenteraccreditation.org/wp-content/uploads/2016/07/Incentives-for-Accreditation.pdf

Disagreements with the requirements for CABC accreditation can be a more challenging barrier to accreditation. To overcome this barrier, birth center owners may need to experience uninvited challenges from stakeholders and peers, which eventually bring about cognitive dissonance and then a change in opinion. Conversely, birth center owners who want the benefits of CABC accreditation may need to present a winning argument and evidence to CABC for changing Indicators of Compliance with the Standards for Birth Centers.

CONCLUSION

Birth center accreditation is a valuable tool for establishing the birth center as a quality model in the health care system for the benefit of mothers, babies, and their families. This change in the system is expected to transform the birth center from a disruptive innovation into a widely accepted facility and model of care. Much work has been done to establish birth center accreditation, and there is more yet to be done in order to realize the full value of birth center accreditation for all of its stakeholders. The challenges ahead include increasing the number of birth centers in the United States, increasing the marketplace incentives for birth centers to become accredited, and sustaining birth center accreditation until there is enough growth to support this valuable credential.

REFERENCES

American Association of Birth Centers. (1982). Recommendations for establishing standards or regulations for freestanding birth centers. *AABC News, 1*(2–3). Perkionmenville, PA: Author. Retrieved from http://www.birthcenters.org

American Association of Birth Centers. (1985–2013). Standards for birth centers (revised). Retrieved from http://www.birthcenters.org/resource/resmgr/AABC_STANDARDS-RV2016.pdf

American Association of Birth Centers. (2015). Birth center regulations map. Retrieved from http://www.birthcenters.org/?page=bc_regulations

American Association of Birth Centers. (2017). *The state of birth centers: Report on the 2016 AABC Birth Center Survey*. Perkiomenville, PA: Author. Submitted for publication.

American College of Nurse-Midwives. (n.d). Accreditation Commission for Midwifery Education. Retrieved from http://www.midwife.org/Accreditation

American College of Obstetricians and Gynecologists. (2015). Obstetric care consensus on the levels of maternal care. Retrieved from http://www.acog.org/Resources-And-Publications/Obstetric-Care-Consensus-Series/Levels-of-Maternal-Care

American Heart Association and American Academy of Pediatrics. (2015). 2015 guidelines for cardiopulmonary resuscitation and emergency cardiovascular care of the neonate. Retrieved from https://www2.aap.org/nrp/docs/15535_NRP%20Guidelines%20Flyer_English_FINAL.pdf

American Public Health Association. (1982). Guidelines for licensing and regulating birth centers. Retrieved from https://www.apha.org/policies-and-advocacy/public-health-policy-statements/policy-database/2014/07/10/13/29/guidelines-for-licensing-and-regulating-birth-centers

Canoodt, L. J. (1982). *Utilization and economic analysis of the Maternity Center Association's Childbearing Center.* New York, NY: Blue Cross Blue Shield of Greater New York, Health Affairs Research Department.

Cole, E. (1987). The role of accreditation. *AABC News, 4*(All), 25–26. Retrieved from http://www.birthcenters.org/global_engine/download.asp?fileid=A59499B6-63CB-4439-8186-C5A0DB21F010&ext=pdf

Commission for the Accreditation of Birth Centers. (2015a). Annual report 2014. Retrieved from https://www.birthcenteraccreditation.org/wp-content/uploads/2015/04/2CABCAnnualReport2014.pdf

Commission for the Accreditation of Birth Centers. (2015b). Indicators of compliance with the standards for birth centers. Retrieved from https://www.birthcenteraccreditation.org/go/get-cabc-indicators

Commission for the Accreditation of Birth Centers. (2015c). *AABC and CABC – Two Distinct Organizations*, p. 3. Retrieved from https://www.birthcenteraccreditation.org/wp-content/uploads/2014/07/AABC-CABC-Relationship-2017.pdf

Ernst, E. K. M. (2015). History of the standards for birth centers. *AABC News, 29*(1), 6–8. Retrieved from http://www.birthcenters.org/global_engine/download.asp?fileid=ED11C5A8-1C62-41D8-AFE8-4F4CF1553FA9&ext=pdf

Herdmon, B. (1987). A hospital perspective on birthing center quality assurance. *AABC News* 4(All), 28–32. Retrieved from http://www.birthcenters.org/global_engine/download.asp?fileid=A59499B6-63CB-4439-8186-C5A0DB21F010&ext=pdf

Institute of Medicine and National Research Council Committee on Assessing Alternative Birth Settings. (1982). *Research issues in the assessment of birth settings.* Washington, DC: National Academies Press. Retrieved from http://www.nap.edu/catalog/18297/research-issues-in-the-assessment-of-birth-settings-report-of

Lubic, R. W. (1979). *Barriers and conflict in maternity care innovation* (Doctoral dissertation). ProQuest Dissertations Publishing. (Accession No. 8022178.)

Lubic, R. W. (1985). Keynote address of first convention of birth centers: Where do we go from here? *AABC News, 3*(3). Retrieved from http://www.birthcenters.org/global_engine/download.asp?fileid=20A181AA-F3A1-4DCF-A8CE-779A4A458407&ext=pdf

Peck, S. (1987). The health insurers perspective on birth center accreditation. *AABC News,* 4(All), 26–28. Retrieved from http://www.birthcenters.org/global_engine/download.asp?fileid=A59499B6-63CB-4439-8186-C5A0DB21F010&ext=pdf

The Joint Commission. (2016). The Joint Commission: Over a century of quality and safety. Retrieved from https://www.jointcommission.org/assets/1/6/TJC-history-timeline_through_20161.PDF

CHAPTER 9

Birth Center Regulation in the United States

JILL ALLIMAN

LEARNING OBJECTIVES

Upon completion of this chapter, the reader will be able to:

1. Describe the history of birth center regulation in the United States
2. List components of state birth center regulation that impede access to birth center care
3. Describe reimbursement challenges with Medicaid and TRICARE
4. Describe the federally funded Strong Start project and its influence on access to birth center care

Freestanding birth centers have a history of more than 40 years in the United States, and progress toward becoming part of the mainstream maternity care system can be seen in regulations and policy changes over the years. Early leaders in the birth center movement went to great efforts to ensure the model would have standards for operation; high-quality, evidence-based care; and be integrated into the health care system for optimum safety and collaboration. Regulations and licensure were part of that effort early in the development of birth centers.

AMERICAN PUBLIC HEALTH ASSOCIATION DEFINITION AND MODEL REGULATIONS

The American Public Health Association (APHA) developed model birth center regulations in 1982 (APHA, 1982). The APHA defined the birth center as "any health facility, place, or institution which is not a hospital or in a hospital and where births are planned to occur away from the mother's usual residence following normal, uncomplicated pregnancy" (1982). This definition continues be a useful description of the modern birth center facility that meets American Association of Birth Centers (AABC) standards (AABC, 2014).

STATES ADOPT REGULATIONS

As birth centers developed in various states, licensure statutes and regulations were written and approved. Some birth center laws and regulations have not been modified since they were originally written in the 1980s. At that time, states modeled regulations after ambulatory surgery centers or other medical facilities with stringent requirements for construction, hallway width, and size of a birth room being the same as an operating room. As licensed health care facilities, birth centers in all states must comply with all environmental, health, safety, laboratory, sanitation, and professional licensure standards as required by authorities at the federal, state, and local levels.

DEFINITION IN FEDERAL LAW IN 2010

Birth centers have experienced inconsistent payment from state Medicaid agencies. In some states, the midwife provider was paid for professional services, but the facility was not recognized as a state health care facility, and therefore not reimbursed. In an effort to improve access for Medicaid beneficiaries, a bill to mandate facility fee coverage of freestanding birth centers by Medicaid was introduced in 2009 and included in the Affordable Care Act (ACA) when it was passed in 2010 (Patient Protection and Affordable Care Act [PPACA], 2010). The definition of freestanding birth center in this federal statute is "a health facility that is not a hospital or physician's office, where childbirth is planned to occur away from the pregnant woman's residence that is licensed or otherwise approved by the state to provide prenatal labor and delivery or postpartum care and other ambulatory services that are included in the plan" (Patient Protection and Affordable Care Act, 2010). This definition uses the APHA definition as its basis (APHA, 1982).

Additional language in the Medicaid law identifies birth centers as a mandated covered service, with separate payment for the professional services of any licensed birth-attendant and facility services as a part of the statute (Patient Protection and Affordable Care Act, 2010). Language mandating payment by Medicaid of any licensed birth attendant providing services was the first recognition by Medicaid of direct-entry midwives or midwives other than certified nurse-midwives (CNMs) in federal statute.

This federal birth center definition provides an additional level of credibility for birth centers when working with federal and state agencies to improve payment and to reduce other barriers to access for women and families. The definition can also be used for standardization when including birth centers in other proposed legislation or regulation.

UNDERSTANDING STATE REGULATION

Current Licensure and Regulation Status

Forty-one of the 50 states and the District of Columbia license or otherwise recognize birth centers under other regulation or statute. Two states, North Carolina and Louisiana, operate under Medicaid regulations that deem birth centers eligible for Medicaid reimbursement. Birth center licensure or recognition by the states is necessary for eligibility for Medicaid reimbursement. Since almost half of U.S. births are paid for by Medicaid, it is beneficial to be eligible for Medicaid payment. In a few states, Medicaid reimbursement is too low to cover birth center costs, so birth centers in those states are not able to accept clients covered by Medicaid or must limit their numbers.

Licensure on a State-by-State Basis

States with the largest numbers of birth centers have fewer restrictive regulations in place. Conversely, in states where regulations or licensure requirements are difficult to achieve, there are fewer birth centers (Figure 9.1). This is similar to regulations for advanced practice registered nurses (APRNs) and midwives (Yang, Attanasio, & Kozhimannil, 2016) where restrictive regulations decrease access. In 2014, AABC filed comments with the Federal Trade Commission (FTC) to draw attention to ways in which restrictive birth center regulations limit access to birth center care (AABC, 2014).

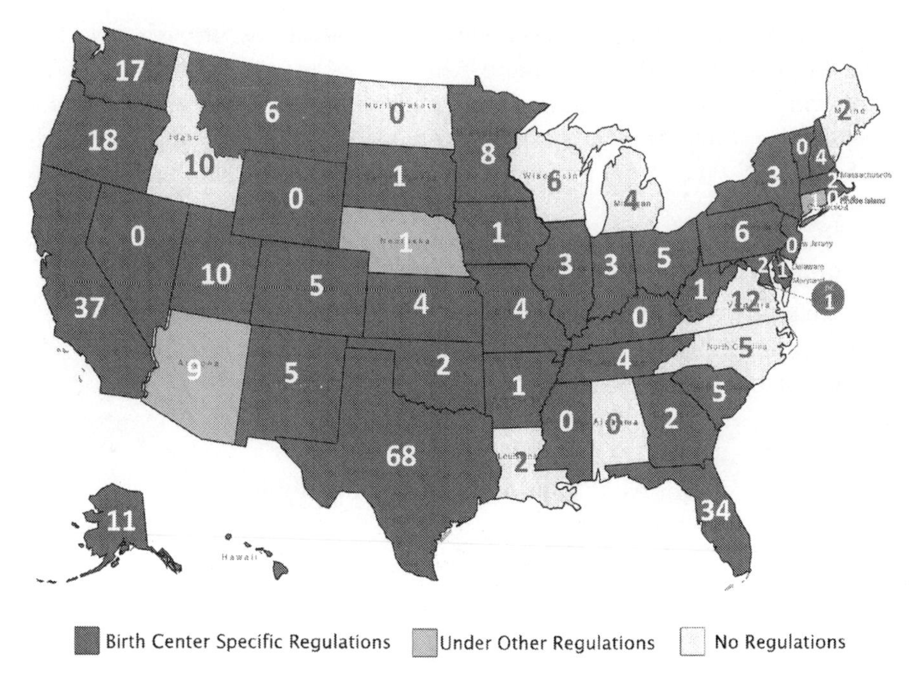

FIGURE 9.1 Numbers of birth centers and associated regulations
Source: AABC (2016a).

Best Model Regulation Components

Birth center regulations function best and support development of birth centers when certain components are present and others are not required (Table 9.1). AABC issued a Position Statement in 2016 outlining components of regulation that promote the effective regulation of birth centers and those that are restrictive (AABC, 2016b).

The Position Statement suggests that regulations are most effective when they are based on current evidence, such as the AABC standards and those that support accreditation by the Commission for the Accreditation of Birth Centers (CABC). Regulations should be limited to requirements for the birth center facility itself and not the providers who practice there. Regulations for providers should be separate from those for facilities. It is helpful if regulations require that guidelines be put in place with plans for transfers to hospitals with both maternal and newborn care capabilities when needed. Collaborative planning best occurs between birth centers and the hospitals in their communities so when transfers are necessary,

TABLE 9.1
Model Regulation Requirements

State Birth Center Regulations should:
Be based on standards and evidence
Include CABC accreditation
Be facility specific and have provider regulations be separate
Require birth centers to have policies or guidelines for transfer
Require business occupancy level of construction without costly building standards that do not increase safety
State Regulations should *not* require:
Written contract or agreement with transfer hospital
Certificate of Need (CON)
Physician as medical director
Written agreement with physician

CABC, Commission for the Accreditation of Birth Centers.
Source: AABC (2016b).

they can be safe and seamless for the women and/or their infants. Physical layout requirements for the birth center should be based on business occupancy codes, and requirements should not be added that increase cost without improving the safety of women and newborns utilizing the facility.

Those components of state regulations that impede the safe and effective operation of birth centers put restrictions in place without improving safety. Restrictive elements include requirements for written agreements with hospitals or physicians, Certificate of Need (CON), or requiring a physician be hired as medical director of the birth center. These components put control of the birth center in the hands of groups that can be seen as competitors and threaten the existence of birth centers and access to birth center care for women and families. Hospitals and birth centers should be required to participate in joint planning for transfers from birth centers, in the same way policies and procedures are put in place for transfers between hospitals when women or newborns require more complex levels of care than the facility where they are admitted offer (American College of Obstetricians and Gynecologists [ACOG], 2015).

Written Agreement With Hospital

All birth center staff desire good relationships with collaborating hospitals so when transfers are needed, they can be accomplished in a seamless manner that prioritizes the safety of the mother and infant. However, when a written agreement is a regulatory requirement and some hospitals refuse to enter into such agreements, the requirement becomes a barrier for access to birth center care. For example, 15 states have requirements for written transfer agreements with a local hospital; however, only 37 of the total 319 birth centers and 15% of birth center births occur in those states. More than 88% of all birth centers are located in the states that do not require a formal written transfer agreement with the receiving hospital. Similar findings exist for other restrictive regulations, such as CON and requiring a physician medical director for birth centers.

Certificate of Need

Sixteen states and the District of Columbia require that a CON be approved before a birth center can be opened in that state. CON laws were designed to contain costs of health care facilities by requiring coordinated planning of new services and construction, and avoiding duplication of services. In 1974, the federal Health Planning Resources Development Act was passed, leading many states to enact CON laws (National Conference of State Legislatures [NCSL], 2016). The federal law was repealed in 1987, followed by 14 states discontinuing their CON laws (NCSL, 2016). However, 36 states maintain some form of CON law. Current CON laws tend to focus on outpatient facilities that are in direct competition with hospital facilities (NCSL, 2016). According to AABC, 15 states and the District of Columbia have CON laws that impact the development of new birth centers (AABC, 2016e).

Access to freestanding birth center care can be improved by reducing barriers for women seeking maternity care services in freestanding birth centers. State regulations requiring CON can be a barrier to freestanding birth center care when other providers in direct competition with freestanding birth centers oppose CON applications. Freestanding birth centers have only two or three beds, which differ from hospital beds in that care is limited to low-risk childbirth and does not include surgery or regional or general anesthesia. AABC believes that due to their small size and services that are not comparable to hospital services, freestanding birth centers should be exempt from the CON process. Removal of the CON process for freestanding birth centers is one way to improve access to this high-quality care option. Access to freestanding birth center care increases when states do not require a CON.

Medical Director or Written Agreement With Physician

Birth centers in states requiring a physician as medical director are not associated with better outcomes (AABC, 2016b). The CABC recommends that birth centers have a clinical director, who can be a midwife or physician. All birth centers desire relationships with physicians and other service providers for consultation or referral when needed. However, requiring that birth centers hire a medical director adds a cost that cannot be recouped through billing, which threatens sustainability of the birth center.

An additional vulnerability to birth center sustainability is the difficulty in finding and keeping a medical director on staff in states with this requirement. If the medical director has to leave abruptly due to illness, moving, or other outside causes, the birth center is subject to immediate cessation of operations. In those situations, birth centers cannot continue to operate legally and must therefore send patients to the hospital for care. In rural communities or areas with limited medical support of the birth center, loss of a medical director can force closure.

Risk Criteria or Required Distance From Hospital

Some states may add specific risk criteria to their definitions within birth center regulations that identify women as being too high risk to be eligible for birth center care. Examples of risk criteria contained in state regulations include diabetes or heart disease. History of conditions such as postpartum hemorrhage requiring a transfusion, or low transverse cesarean incision, may require a consultation with a physician or prohibit birth center care. It is important to maintain broad categories of risk to avoid language that may unnecessarily restrict patient enrollment. Several states specify the distance a birth center is allowed to be located from the hospital, usually expressed in minutes of travel time (AABC, 2016c). Requiring minimum distance from hospitals can limit access in rural communities with no local hospital for maternity care.

Regulations That Include CABC Accreditation

Several states refer to CABC accreditation in licensing statute or regulation. The state of Minnesota passed birth center licensure later than most other states, and ruled that birth centers that are accredited by the CABC are deemed licensed by the state (Minnesota, n.d.). This decision was popular among lawmakers who understood that no significant cost would be incurred by the state in establishing licensure in this way. Accreditation is required for licensure in Minnesota and Illinois. Montana, California, and Florida regulations include a provision that if a birth center is CABC accredited, CABC site visits can take the place of state inspections, at least during the years that accreditation site visits occur. Two other states, North Carolina and Louisiana, deem birth centers eligible for Medicaid reimbursement if they are accredited by the CABC (AABC, 2016c). A few states require accreditation but do not specify the accrediting body.

UNDERSTANDING REIMBURSEMENT

Medicaid funding comes from federal and state dollars, is administered by each state, and pays for 44% of all births in the United States (Kaiser Family Foundation, 2010). The freestanding birth center is a licensed and often accredited health care facility. As such, birth centers are eligible for both Medicaid reimbursement for professional service fees and facility service fees (PPACA, 2010). Professional reimbursement pays for all care provided by the licensed health professional in the birth center including pregnancy, labor and birth, newborn care, or postpartum care. Depending on the scope of practice, gynecological and primary care services may also be covered. The health care professional is usually a midwife but sometimes a physician practicing in the midwifery model of care. According to the federal Medicaid statute, any midwife licensed within that state is eligible for professional reimbursement by Medicaid, inclusive of CNMs, certified midwives (CMs), certified professional midwives (CPMs), licensed midwives (LMs), or direct-entry midwives.

Federal statute also requires that separate payments be made to birth centers for professional and facility services (PPACA, 2010). Facility reimbursement covers the cost of the licensed health care facility and is similar to the costs incurred by a hospital. Facility costs may include rent, furnishings, medical equipment, utilities, nursing or birth assistant staff, insurance, administrative staff, maintenance, and all other costs of sustainability of the facility that are not part of the professional reimbursement coverage. Facility reimbursement is available in most states for labor, birth, and recovery time until discharge, and for at least partial reimbursement if the baby is not born in the birth center due to the need for a transfer during labor.

Several states currently reimburse a newborn facility fee as well as a payment for the mother's care, and others are seeking to add a newborn payment. Equipment and trained staff that are required to be available to provide neonatal resuscitation at birth if needed and normal newborn care during the birth center stay provide the justification. In a birth center, mother and baby are cared for together in the same birth room until discharge. The midwife and birth assistant or nurse must be dually trained to handle normal birth and postpartum care, as well as maternal or newborn emergencies should they arise.

State Medicaid and Medicaid Managed Care Organizations

Since passage of birth center Medicaid payment, implementation of mandated Medicaid payment of birth centers has been slow and inconsistent in some states. A review of State Plan Amendments (SPAs) filed with Centers for Medicare and Medicaid Services (CMS) finds that five states that recognize or license birth centers have no SPA on file (AABC, 2016d). Nine states have SPAs on file that are not in compliance with the mandate to pay licensed birth centers with separate payments to the licensed birth attendant and facility (AABC, 2016d).

Medicaid managed care organizations (MMCOs) administer all or part of Medicaid plans in 39 states (CMS, n.d.; Kaiser Family Foundation, 2013). MMCOs in some states have refused to contract with freestanding birth centers (AABC, 2015). In California, State Medi-Cal officials issued an "All Plan Letter" instructing the MMCOs to include birth centers in their plans (California Department of Health Care Services [DHCS], 2015). The letter states that all Medicaid health plans must provide access to birth centers in the state to be in compliance with federal law. Furthermore, health plans are encouraged to contract directly with birth centers, or at least to pay for their services as out-of-network providers (DHCS, 2015). According to communications with California birth centers, Medicaid health plans have not changed contracting or payment patterns in response to the letter (AABC, 2016d).

TRICARE Payment

Birth centers have been recognized and reimbursed by CHAMPUS/TRICARE since 1988 (TRICARE, 2008). To be an authorized TRICARE birth center, the center must be accredited by CABC, Accreditation Association for Ambulatory Health Care, or The Joint Commission (TJC), and care must be provided by CNMs at this time (TRICARE, 2008). Current challenges with TRICARE are that plans are now administered by private contractors who are affiliated with private health plans. These plans may refuse to contract with birth centers that have met requirements, stating that they have adequate networks of obstetric providers within hospitals. AABC is working with TRICARE administrators to encourage them to include birth centers in all their networks (AABC, 2016d).

CURRENT POLICY AND BIRTH CENTERS

ACA and Birth Centers

Other components of the ACA have the potential to affect access to birth center and midwifery care (PPACA, 2010). The Harkin Amendment to the ACA, Section 2706(a) of the Public Health Service Act, is codified in the U.S. Code as 42 U.S.C. §300gg-5 (Patient Protection and Affordable Care Act, 2010). The Harkin Amendment requires that group health insurers and individual health plans may not exclude a health provider from participation in a health plan if that individual is acting within the scope of his or her license or certification. The provision was put in place to prevent health plans from discriminating against nonphysician providers. The amendment also states that although health plans are not required to contract with or include in network all willing providers, they may not exclude an entire class or type of provider. The Harkin Amendment does not apply to Medicaid, but to commercial health plans that qualify under the ACA, and to Employee Retirement Income Security Act (ERISA) plans, also known as self-insured plans. Thus far, birth center efforts to point to the Harkin Amendment when negotiating with commercial health plans have not been helpful because no mechanism for enforcement is included in the measure (AABC, 2015).

CMS Issues New Guidance

In 2016, the CMS issued new guidance to all states in a state official letter (CMS, 2016). The guidance addresses problems with payment to Federally Qualified Health Centers (FQHCs) and Rural Health Centers (RHCs). The guidance also addresses MMCO network insufficiency with FQHCs, RHCs, and freestanding birth centers, which CMS abbreviates as FBCs. It reiterates that coverage of all these facility types is mandated in federal law. The guidance further requires that as of July 2017, every MMCO must contract with at least one birth center to be considered as having an adequate network of providers. In addition, the letter states that birth center services must be provided in birth centers, so MMCOs can no longer claim that those services are being provided by physician providers in a hospital (CMS, 2016). The impact of this guidance on access to birth center care for Medicaid beneficiaries remains to be seen and must be evaluated periodically.

FEDERAL RESEARCH AND INITIATIVES

Strong Start for Mothers and Newborns

In 2012, the Center for Medicare and Medicaid Innovation (CMMI, 2016) initiated the Strong Start for Mothers and Newborns Initiative with an announcement by Secretary Kathleen Sebelius at the DC Developing Families Center and Birth Center. Strong Start I was an initiative to work nationally via public and private partnerships to reduce elective induction of labor before 39 completed weeks (CMMI, 2017). Strong Start II is a project to study enhanced models of prenatal care to determine their effectiveness in reducing preterm birth and other complications of pregnancy that are associated with significant racial disparities in the United States.

AABC was awarded a grant to convene a group of 45 birth centers in 20 states to provide enhanced prenatal care and collect data on outcomes over the course of a 3-year period. Currently, AABC is in Year 3 of enrollment and data collection using the AABC Perinatal Data Registry (PDR). As of fall 2016, 8,300 women have been enrolled and more than 4,900 babies have been born to AABC Strong Start mothers (AABC, n.d.). Birth center prenatal care topics related to cost, quality, and satisfaction have been discussed in many other chapters in this book, including Chapter 10. The enhanced model of prenatal care is essentially midwifery-led care of low-risk women that is time intensive and relationship based. Prenatal visits are longer than in standard prenatal care, with time spent getting to know women and their individual needs and providing education and supportive care that is individualized for their unique situations.

The AABC sample of 8,376 participants enrolled in AABC Strong Start is much more diverse than the populations in previous large cohort studies of birth center care (AABC, n.d.; Rooks et al., 1989; Stapleton, Osborne, & Illuzzi, 2013). According to preliminary data, participants include 12.9% Black women and 22.8% Hispanic women in the study group (AABC, n.d.; Cross-Barnet & Clark, 2016). All participants must be Medicaid or

Children's Health Insurance Program (CHIP) beneficiaries. Demographic and risk characteristics of the AABC sample are comparable to the U.S. childbearing population overall (Jolles, Stapleton, & Langford, 2016).

Preliminary data for AABC Strong Start show an overall 8.77% primary cesarean rate, a preterm birth rate of 4.87%, and low birth weight rate of 3.1%, compared with national rates of 21.5% cesareans for low-risk women, a preterm birth rate of 9.6%, and low birth weight rate of 8% (AABC, n.d.; Leapfrog Group, 2016; Martin, Hamilton, Osterman, Curtin, & Mathews, 2015; Osterman & Martin, 2014). Breastfeeding rates are significantly higher for AABC participants than the other models being tested. Participants also express a higher rate of satisfaction with their care (AABC, n.d.).

Quality Indicators for Maternal and Infant Health

Quality outcome measures comparing data from Medicaid beneficiaries in birth center care with national baseline levels and benchmark levels demonstrate that birth center outcomes are significantly better (AABC, 2016, n.d.; Osterman & Martin, 2014). Quality indicators such as elective inductions prior to 39 weeks and low-risk cesarean rates are used to monitor how providers and facilities compare with national benchmarks set by groups, such as Leapfrog Initiative and the National Quality Forum (Leapfrog Group, 2016; National Quality Forum, 2012; see Figure 9.2).

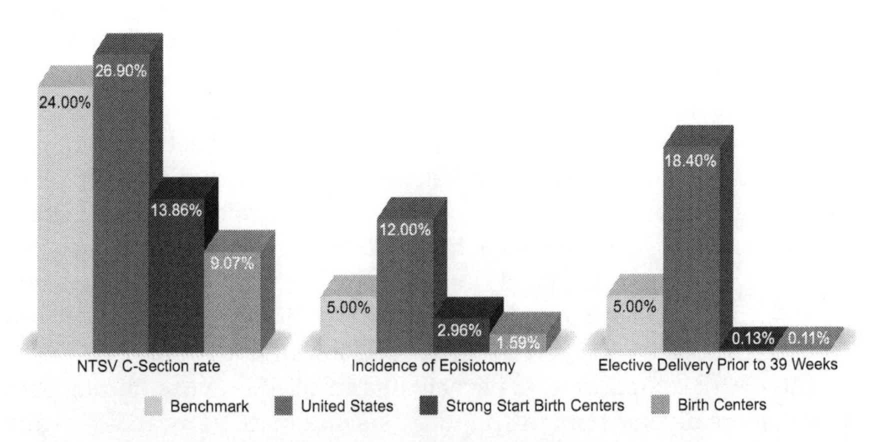

FIGURE 9.2 Birth center outcomes exceed quality benchmarks.

NTSVC, nulliparous, term, singleton, vertex

Sources: AABC (n.d.); Leapfrog Group (2016); Osterman & Martin (2014); and Stapleton et. al (2013).

CURRENT POLICY DEVELOPMENTS

American College of Obstetricians and Gynecologists Consensus Statement Levels of Maternal Care

In 2015, the Consensus Statement 2 was published by the American of College Obstetricians and Gynecologists (2015). It states that freestanding birth centers are a recognized level of maternity care within the U.S. health care system. The purpose of the document is to describe each level of maternal care, document types of providers required to provide care, and identify levels of risk appropriate to each level of care. Levels of care were first recognized in the 1970s with the development of regionalization of maternity care (American College of Obstetricians and Gynecologists, 2015).

The Levels of Maternal Care document states that for birth center care, every birth should be attended by at least two professionals. Primary maternal care providers shall include CNMs, CMs, CPMs, and LMs who are legally recognized to practice within the jurisdiction of the birth center; family physicians; and OB/GYNs. An appropriate number of qualified professionals with competence in Level 1 care criteria and ability to stabilize and transfer high-risk women and newborns should also be available (American College of Obstetricians and Gynecologists, 2015). Levels of risk appropriate to the birth center are described as singleton, vertex, and term pregnancies and women who are expected to experience low-risk labor and birth without complications (American College of Obstetricians and Gynecologists, 2015). Capabilities of a birth center under the Levels of Care document include having equipment to provide low-risk maternal care and a readiness at all times to initiate emergency procedures to meet unexpected needs of the woman and newborn within the center, and to facilitate transport to an acute care setting when necessary. In addition, the document recommends that birth centers have an established agreement with a transfer hospital and procedures in place that will facilitate timely transport, quality improvement programs, and data collection capabilities (American College of Obstetricians and Gynecologists, 2015).

Finally, the American College of Obstetricians and Gynecologists document recommends that medical consultation be available at all times. As birth centers have repeatedly indicated, the availability of medical consultation is required for the safe practice of primary maternity care (AABC comments to FTC; AABC, 2014). Relationships for consultation should be mutually respectful with open and trusting communication, which will contribute to the safety of the mother and newborn and provision of seamless transfers of care when needed.

Alternative Payment Models

Alternative payment models (APMs) are new ways to reimburse health care providers and facilities for health care services provided. The prevalent payment model currently used is fee for service (FFS), in which payment is made based on the number of medical procedures and tests that are done and leads to higher overall costs for health care without an improvement in quality of care (CMMI, 2016). In alternative models, payments to providers are based on quality measures and clinical outcomes, sometimes called pay for performance (CMMI, 2016). To change the usual payment model to be more in alignment with efforts to transform health care, the U.S. Department of Health and Human Services (USDHHS) began work to emphasize value over volume (CMMI, 2016). USDHHS set the goal of tying 30% of Medicare fee-for-service provider reimbursements to quality or value by 2016 and 50% of all reimbursements by 2018 (CMMI, 2016). CMS met the goal of 30% of Medicare payments being tied to value in early 2016 (Baird, 2016).

To support this work, USDHHS launched the Health Care Payment Learning and Action Network (HCP-LAN) as a centralized work group to advance the adoption of value-based payments and APMs. This network is made up of USDHHS staff, private health plans, not-for-profit groups, and individual stakeholders working toward reforming the payment system (CMMI, 2016).

Maternity care is one focus of APM work by the HCP-LAN with specific goals of increasing the percentage of full-term births and the percentage of vaginal births in the United States (HCP-LAN, 2016). A white paper demonstrating examples of this work was released in August 2016. The white paper proposed combining innovative models of care such as birth centers with APMs (HCP-LAN, 2016). Examples included a payment bundling model where birth centers would be one of a network of options low-risk women can choose for their maternity care setting. A set rate would be paid for each woman who completes full maternity care with birth at the birth center. One example offered by AABC would make incentive payments to birth centers for providing enhanced prenatal care. Providing care in the birth center is time intensive, which limits the number of prenatal appointments a midwife can complete in 1 day. However, this model of education- and relationship-based care is worthwhile to women and payers due to cost savings over the whole maternity episode of care. Enhanced care in the birth center leads to improved outcomes of fewer cesareans, fewer elective inductions of labor, and fewer unnecessary medical interventions, providing higher value for lower cost (HCP-LAN, 2016).

CONCLUSION

As the benefits of birth center care are more widely recognized, additional effort will be needed to reduce barriers to birth center care. Activity will be needed at the federal legislative and agency level, and in individual states. Many of the current barriers to birth centers include outdated regulations requiring CON, written agreements with physicians, or limiting the scope of practice of the midwives practicing in birth centers to less than what they are educated and trained to provide.

All midwives working in birth centers desire positive collaborative relationships with physicians and local hospitals. Birth centers should be able to establish transfer policies and procedures with receiving hospitals. To decrease risk to mothers and infants that may occur during a transfer, policies should emphasize clear communication, respect, and support of the mother and family, as well as seamless handoffs of care. There should be no associated increase in risk to physicians or hospitals for consulting with birth centers (Booth, 2007). Birth centers are recognized as a part of the levels of maternal care; therefore, organized planning for safe and seamless transfers should be part of staff preparation and training (American Congress of Obstetricians and Gynecologists, 2015). Policies and procedures for nonemergent and emergent transfer should be in place in both the birth center and receiving hospital, and communication should be professional and focused on mother and newborn safety. Hospitals and birth centers must partner together to improve the safety of transfers between levels of maternity care.

All states need regulation allowing birth centers to operate within a positive business and health care climate. Of the eight states that do not yet recognize or license birth centers, three are in the process of adding licensure or Medicaid recognition in regulation. At least four states are currently working on revising regulations to improve access to birth center care.

Advocates for access to birth center care will continue efforts to educate Medicaid payers at the state level and TRICARE administrators about the value of birth center care and steps needed to reduce barriers to that care. Data from large cohort studies and AABC Strong Start will be used to demonstrate the value of birth center care. In addition, birth center advocates will encourage payers to include birth centers in their networks to help improve maternal and infant health indicators, such as cesarean rates, episiotomy, elective induction of labor, and breastfeeding rates for their entire networks.

EXEMPLAR
BIRTH CENTER: Dar a Luz, Albuquerque, New Mexico

Year established: 2011

Type of building/square feet/architectural features: The oldest part of the building was a house. It was renovated with an outside building and was rezoned as commercial. It is about 3,500 square feet.

Location: Located outside of downtown Albuquerque in agricultural area

Business structure: Non-profit

Ownership: Non-profit

Licensed as: Licensing in process. Will be a freestanding birth center

Accredited by: Commission for the Accreditation of Birth Centers

Number of births to date/births per year: 477 total births/average 115 births per year

Services/enhanced services: Community support groups free to all community members, including breastfeeding, loss, birth trauma, new parents, Pappy Hour; GYN care

Providers: CNMs

Client mix: 35% Medicaid as primary or secondary, 55% private, 10% TRICARE; 75% White, 18% Hispanic, 7% mix of Native, Asian, Pacific, other

Dar a Luz opened in March 2011 with no facility license as there was not an option for licensure at that time and it was not illegal to operate without a facility license. It was initially told that if it wanted a license, it would be as a special hospital.

(continued)

EXEMPLAR *(continued)*

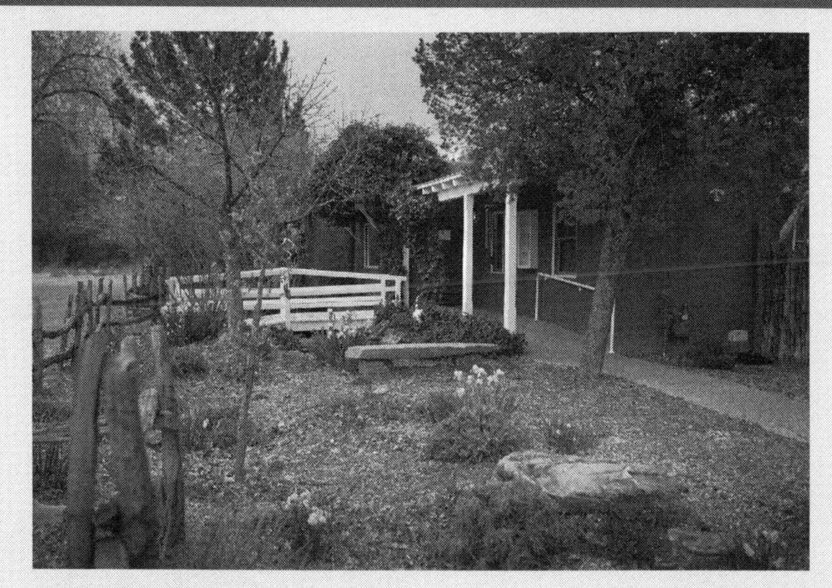

Photo courtesy of Abigail Eaves, Dar a Luz

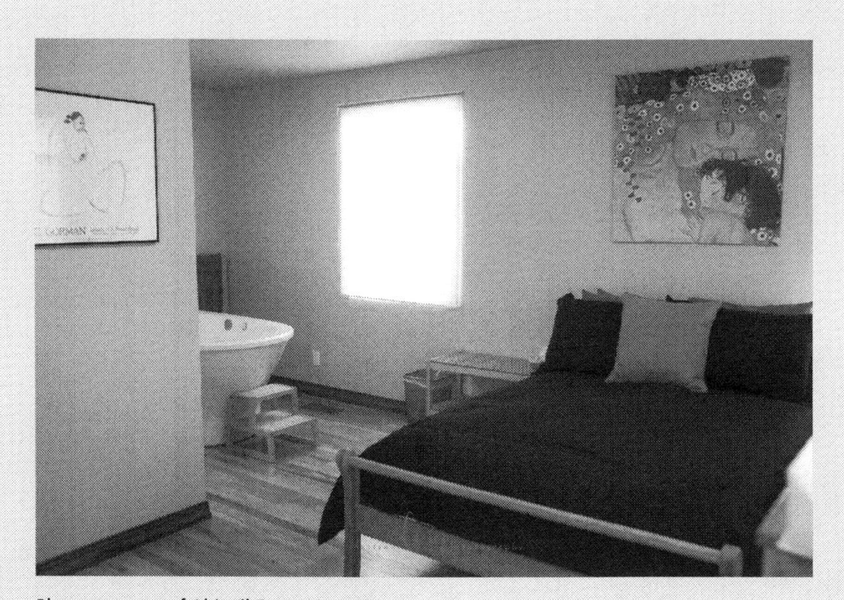

Photo courtesy of Abigail Eaves, Dar a Luz

(continued)

EXEMPLAR *(continued)*

At the end of 2011 and as the rules of the ACA were released regarding birth centers, a group of community birth workers and activists met with the New Mexico Department of Health (DOH). They decided that the DOH would regulate birth centers under outpatient facilities, which encompassed ambulatory surgical centers and diagnostic treatment facilities. There were immediate issues with birth centers being added to these regulations, namely the size of the birth suites. This was a stalemate.

In July 2013, midwives met with the New Mexico secretary of health, who listened to their issues. By late 2014, stakeholders decided to introduce a bill at the next legislative session to add birth centers to facilities that must be licensed. They met again with the DOH as well as the secretary of health. She mandated again that not only would DOH license birth centers, but they would write birth center-specific regulations with the help of the involved community stakeholders. She also agreed with the plan to introduce a bill.

The bill passed unanimously in both the House and the Senate and was signed by the governor on April 10, 2015. The regulations were finally complete on March 1, 2016. Dar a Luz achieved licensure as the first freestanding birth center to be licensed in New Mexico under the new regulations on January 20, 2017.

REFERENCES

American Association of Birth Centers (n.d.) AABC Perinatal Data Registry. Perkiomenville, PA: Author. (Unpublished data.)

American Association of Birth Centers. (2014). Comments to Federal Trade Commission. Retrieved from https://c.ymcdn.com/sites/aabc.site-ym.com/resource/collection/DCBDA72A-41EA-4AFE-A8D1-112542F4A0BC/FTC_Letter_-_4.30.14_with_appendices.pdf

American Association of Birth Centers. (2015). Comments to CMS on Medicaid MCO proposed regulations (File Code: CMS–2390–P. Medicaid and Children's Health Insurance Program (CHIP) Programs). Retrieved https://c.ymcdn.com/sites/aabc.site-ym.com/resource/collection/DCBDA72A-41EA-4AFE-A8D1-112542F4A0BC/AABC_Comment_-_CMS-2390-P_-_7.27.15_MedicaidMCO_Rule.pdf

American Association of Birth Centers. (2016a). Birth center regulations. Retrieved from http://www.birthcenters.org/?page=bc_regulations

American Association of Birth Centers. (2016b). Position paper on regulation and licensure of birth centers. Retrieved from https://c.ymcdn.com/sites/aabc.site-ym.com/resource/collection/DCBDA72A-41EA-4AFE-A8D1-112542F4A0BC/AABC_Comment_-_CMS-2390-P_-_7.27.15_MedicaidMCO_Rule.pdf

American Association of Birth Centers. (2016c). State birth center regulations worksheet (Unpublished data).

American Association of Birth Centers. (2016d). State Plan Amendment, MMCO compliance with ACA Section 2301 and TRICARE coverage (Unpublished data).

American Association of Birth Centers. (2016e). White paper: Improving access to freestanding birth centers. Retrieved from: http://www.birthcenters.org/?page=leg_library

American College of Obstetricians and Gynecologists. (2015). Levels of maternal care (Obstetric Care Consensus No. 2). *Obstetrical Gynecology, 125*, 502–515. Retrieved from http://www.acog.org/Resources-And-Publications/Obstetric-Care-Consensus-Series/Levels-of-Maternal-Care

American Public Health Association. (1982). APHA guidelines for licensing and regulating birth centers (Policy Statement Adopted by The Governing Council of The American Public Health Association, November 17, 1982). Retrieved from https://c.ymcdn.com/sites/www.birthcenters.org/resource/collection/028792A7-808D-4BC7-9A0F-FB038B434B91/9.APHA_Guidelines.pdf

Baird, C. (2016). Top healthcare stories for 2016: Pay-for performance. Committee for Economic Development, Arlington, VA. Retrieved from https://www.ced.org/blog/entry/top-healthcare-stories-for-2016-pay-for-performance

Booth, J. W. (2007). An update on vicarious liability for certified nurse-midwives/certified midwives. *Journal of Midwifery and Women's Health, 52*(2), 153–157.

California Department of Health Care Services. (2015). All Plan Letter 15–017. Provision of Certified Nurse Midwife and alternative birth center services. State of California Health and Human Services Agency. Retrieved from: http://www.dhcs.ca.gov/formsandpubs/Documents/MMCDAPLsandPolicyLetters/APL2015/APL15-017.pdf

Center for Medicare and Medicaid Innovation. (2016). Health care payment learning and action network. Retrieved from https://innovation.cms.gov/initiatives/Health-Care-Payment-Learning-and-Action-Network

Center for Medicare and Medicaid Innovation. (2017). Strong Start for Mothers and Newborns Initiative: General information. Retrieved from https://innovation.cms.gov/initiatives/strong-start/

Centers for Medicare and Medicaid Services. (n.d.). Managed care state profiles and enrollment data. Baltimore, MD. Retrieved from https://www.medicaid.gov/medicaid-chip-program-information/by-topics/delivery-systems/managed-care/managed-care-site.html

Centers for Medicare and Medicaid Services. (2016). *Guidance on FQHC and RHC supplemental payment requirements and FQHC, RHC, and FBC network sufficiency under Medicaid and CHIP Managed Care* (SHO #16-006). Baltimore, MD: Author.

Cross-Barnet, C., & Clark, W. (2016). Strong Start for Mothers and Newborns: Second annual evaluation report. Volume 2. Retrieved from https://downloads.cms.gov/files/cmmi/strongstart-enhancedprenatalcare_evalrptyr2v2.pdf

Health Care Payment Learning and Action Network. (2016). Accelerating and aligning clinical episode payment models: Maternity care white paper. Retrieved from https://hcp-lan.org/groups/cep/maternity-care

Jolles, D., Stapleton, S., & Langford, R. (2016). The birth center model of care and childbearing Medicaid beneficiaries: A comparison of national benchmarks and variations in care and quality (Manuscript in preparation).

Kaiser Family Foundation. (2010). Births financed by Medicaid: State health facts. Retrieved from http://kff.org/medicaid/state-indicator/births-financed-by-medicaid

Kaiser Family Foundation. (2013). Medicaid enrollment in managed care by plan type: State health facts. Retrieved from http://kff.org/medicaid/state-indicator/enrollment-by-medicaid-mc-plan-type

Leapfrog Group. (2016) Maternity care report. Leapfrog Hospital Survey. Retrieved from http://www.leapfroggroup.org/sites/default/files/Files/Castlight-Leapfrog%20Maternity%20Report_Final.pdf

Martin, J. A., Hamilton, B. E., Osterman, M. J. K., Curtin, S. C., & Mathews, T. J. (2015). Births: Final data for 2013. *National Vital Statistics Reports, 64*(1). Retrieved from http://www.cdc.gov/nchs/data/nvsr/nvsr64/nvsr64_01.pdf

Minnesota Statutes. (2011). Birth centers, Section 144.615. Office of the Revisor of Statutes, State of Minnesota.

National Conference of State Legislatures. (2016). Certificate of Need: State health laws and programs. Retrieved from http://www.ncsl.org/research/health/con-certificate-of-need-state-laws.aspx

National Quality Forum. (2012). Endorsement summary: Perinatal and reproductive health measures. Washington, DC: Author. Retrieved from http://www.qualityforum.org/Projects/n-r/Perinatal_Care_Endorsement_Maintenance_2011/Perinatal_and_Reproductive_Healthcare_Endorsement_Maintenance_2011.aspx

Osterman, M. J. K., & Martin, J. A. (2014). Trends in low-risk cesarean delivery in the United States, 1990–2013. *National Vital Statistics Reports, 63*(6). Retrieved from https://www.cdc.gov/nchs/data/nvsr/nvsr63/nvsr63_06.pdf

Patient Protection and Affordable Care Act. (2010). Nondiscrimination amendment to the PPACA. 42 U.S.C. § 300gg-5.

Rooks, J. P., Weatherby, N. L., Ernst, E. K. M., Stapleton, S., Rosen, D., & Rosenfield, A. (1989). Outcomes of care in birth centers: The national birth center study. *New England Journal of Medicine, 321*(26), 1804–1811.

Stapleton, S., Osborne, C., & Illuzzi, J. (2013). Outcomes of care in birth centers: Demonstration of a durable model. *Journal of Midwifery and Women's Health, 58*(1), 3–14. Retrieved from http://onlinelibrary.wiley.com/doi/10.1111/jmwh.12003/full

TRICARE Department of Defense. (2008). Birthing Centers. In TRICARE Policy Manual 6010-.57M (Chapter 11, Section 2.3). Aurora, CO: Defense Health Agency. Retrieved from manuals.tricare.osd.mil/DisplayManualPdfFile/TO08/194/AsOf/tp08/c11s2_3.pdf

Yang, Y. T., Attanasio, L., & Kozhimannil, K. (2016). State scope of practice laws, nurse-midwifery workforce, and childbirth procedures and outcomes. *Women's Health Issues, 26*(1), 6–13.

SECTION IV

Envisioning the Future of the Freestanding Birth Center

CHAPTER 10

Enhanced Care Services and Health Homes

ALISHA H. WILKES AND JILL ALLIMAN

LEARNING OBJECTIVES

Upon completion of this chapter, the reader will be able to:

1. Define enhanced care services (ECSs) in relation to midwifery-led care at freestanding birth centers in the United States
2. Describe elements of ECSs currently offered by freestanding birth centers in the United States
3. Describe elements of the patient-centered medical home (PCMH) model that are common to the freestanding birth center model
4. Explain ways in which freestanding birth centers can meet the diverse needs of health care consumers in the United States

Despite advancing technologies and increased spending in the United States, the needs of women and families, particularly in maternity care, are not being met (WHO, UNICEF, UNFPA, the World Bank, and United Nations Population Division Maternal Mortality Estimation Inter-Agency Group, 2013). For example, from 2000 to 2012 the maternal mortality rate in the United States increased from 13 per 100,000 to 15.9 per 100,000 (Centers for Disease Control and Prevention [CDC], 2016). Improved models of health care delivery are needed to better meet the needs of health care consumers. The federal Affordable Care Act (ACA) has called for the implementation of collaborative, integrated models of health care delivery (U.S. Department of Health and Human Services [USDHHS], 2014). The PCMH model, birth center model, and midwifery model of care have been shown to decrease health care costs, improve outcomes, and improve patient satisfaction (Neilson, Langner, Zema, Hacker, & Grundy, 2012; Sandall et al., 2013). Adapting and blending elements of the freestanding birth center models and PCMH models provides an opportunity to create a synchronistic, sustainable model, better equipped to provide evidence-based care and improve outcomes. Although there is little data available, we explore the integration of ECSs and collaborative, integrated care with the freestanding birth center model and propose such a model.

ENHANCED CARE SERVICES

ECSs are defined as those services beyond the scope of standard midwifery-led maternity care most often provided in freestanding birth centers (Wilkes, 2015). Services such as mental health, men's health, pediatric care, nonpregnant women's health, and some maternity services, including ultrasound and genetic testing/counseling, may be considered ECSs. Standard midwifery-led maternity care generally includes prenatal, labor and birth, newborn, and postpartum care, although the scope and details of these services vary. The scope of midwifery-led maternity care differs from state to state and depends on the type of midwife providing services and the individual state laws. Professional organizations outline scope of practice for their membership, including the American College of Nurse-Midwives (ACNM, 2011), the National Association of Certified Professional Midwives (NACPM, 2014), and the American Association of Birth Centers (AABC, 2016).

ENHANCED CARE SERVICES IN FREESTANDING BIRTH CENTERS

As of 2015, no data were available regarding services provided by freestanding birth centers beyond the scope of standard midwifery-led maternity care (Wilkes, 2015). In order to determine if birth centers could function as health homes and/or collaborative, integrated health centers, several questions needed to be answered:

- *Are freestanding birth centers providing services beyond maternity care?*
- *What services are they providing?*
- *What types of providers are providing the services?*
- *Who is using the services?*

In order to begin addressing these questions, this author (Dr. Alisha H. Wilkes) conducted an online survey of freestanding birth centers in the United States (Wilkes, 2015). Elements of this survey and discussion of its implications are presented.

About the Survey

An in-depth literature review revealed no relevant articles or research regarding ECSs offered by freestanding birth centers or linking freestanding birth centers and the PCMH model. A web engine search for "primary care at freestanding birth centers" resulted in five relevant links to birth centers providing some type of care beyond maternity services. Information from these websites indicated that freestanding birth centers were likely providing some types of ECSs and that there was a need to gather data regarding the services provided.

An online survey consisting of 63 questions covering freestanding birth center demographics and funding, patient demographics, and various types of services was created. A list of 301 known freestanding birth centers in the United States was obtained from the AABC. An introductory letter containing a link to the online survey was sent to the 267 with e-mail addresses included in the AABC list. Twenty-five e-mails were returned undeliverable, leaving a total of 242 e-mails assumed to have been delivered. Forty-eight freestanding birth center representatives began the survey and 45 finished the survey, resulting in a 19.8% response rate and a 93.7% completion rate of those who responded. Respondents were able to skip questions as desired and many questions allowed for multiple responses. Institutional review board (IRB) approval was obtained and participating freestanding birth centers provided informed consent (Wilkes, 2015).

Survey Results

Freestanding Birth Center Demographics

Respondents were located in 20 states. Nine were in Texas; three were in each of Florida, Oregon, Utah, and Virginia; two in Alaska, California, Colorado, Idaho, Maryland, New Mexico, New York, and Washington State; and one was from each of Georgia, Minnesota, Montana, North Carolina, South Carolina, Wyoming, and West Virginia. The highest percentage of birth centers were located in suburban areas (44%) and the lowest percentage were rural centers (21%). Accreditation had been achieved by 56% of the centers, and 71% were state licensed (Wilkes, 2015). Eight percent of respondents identified their birth center as part of a larger organization, whereas 44% selected independent and 94% identified as collaborative organizations. One freestanding birth center identified as a federally qualified health center and one as a PCMH, whereas 13% were not-for-profit organizations, and 54% were for-profit. The majority indicated clients paid for services with private insurance or self-pay, whereas 7% indicated use of federal funding. Of the respondents, 55.8% accepted Medicaid, 25.6% accepted Medicare, and 32.6% accepted TRICARE. For all of the questions, respondents could select more than one answer (Wilkes, 2015).

Patient Demographics

Respondents were asked to indicate the income categories and ethnicities/races of the populations they served. The majority served moderate (84%) and low-income (59%) populations, followed by those below the poverty level (25%) and high income (23%). The majority of respondents served Caucasians (96%) followed by Hispanics (67%) and African Americans (64%; Wilkes, 2015).

Maternity Services Provider Types

Respondents were asked to indicate which types of providers offered maternity services at their freestanding birth centers and were able to select multiple provider types. Figure 10.1 shows the percentage of freestanding birth centers with certain provider types offering maternity services (Wilkes, 2015).

Enhanced Maternity Services

Respondents were asked if their freestanding birth center provided maternity services beyond the scope of standard midwifery-led maternity care. The following statement was provided to participants to describe ECSs:

> Enhanced care includes anything outside of standard midwifery-led maternity care which includes: Antepartum care: surveillance of maternal and fetal well-being within the midwifery scope of care. *Intrapartum care: in a free-standing birth center, within the midwifery scope of care. Postpartum care: within the midwifery scope of care. (Wilkes, 2015, p. 71)

It is possible respondents had differing interpretations of the scope of maternity care. More precise definitions of standard maternity care and ECSs in birth centers will assist researchers and policy makers in the future. Of the respondents, 70% indicated they provided some type of

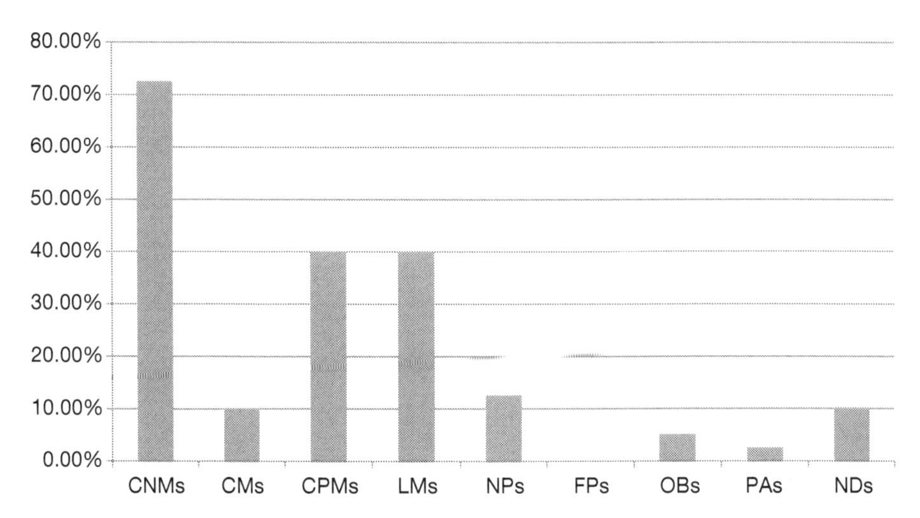

FIGURE 10.1 Percentage of freestanding birth centers with certain types of maternity services providers.

CNMs (certified nurse-midwives) = 72.5%; CMs (certified midwives) = 10%; CPMs (certified professional midwives) = 40%; LMs (licensed midwives) = 40%; NPs (nurse practitioners) = 12.5%; FPs (family practice physicians) = 0%; OBs (obstetricians) = 5%; PAs (physician assistants) = 2.5%; NDs (naturopathic doctors) = 10%.

enhanced maternity services. Table 10.1 shows the percentage of freestanding birth centers offering certain enhanced maternity services; respondents were able to select multiple services.

Enhanced Care Services

Of the respondents, 56% offered community resources, 52% offered women's health services, 42% offered mental health services, 35% offered pediatric services, 30% offered adjunct/alternative health services, and 28% offered men's health services. These services were not defined within the survey, leaving them open to interpretation by respondents. Tables 10.2 and 10.3 show the percentage of freestanding birth centers offering certain types of services and Table 10.4 shows the percentage of freestanding birth centers using certain types of alternative/adjunct service providers.

Sustainability and Profitability

Interestingly, most respondents indicated the majority of the ECSs they provided were sustainable and/or profitable. Enhanced maternity services, women's health services, and adjunct/alternative health services were all indicated as sustainable and/or profitable by greater than 70% of

TABLE 10.1
Enhanced Maternity Services Offered by Freestanding Birth Centers

Service	Percentage of Freestanding Birth Centers Providing Service (n = 30)
Lactation services	93.3
Laboratory services	73.3
Fetal monitoring	66.7
Nutrition services	63.3
Individual postpartum support	60
Home birth	53.3
Ultrasound	50
Infant care classes	43.3
Postpartum classes	36.7
Parenting classes	36.7
Other group prenatal classes	33.3
Hospital birth	26.7
Centering pregnancy	3.3

respondents. More than 50% of respondents indicated pediatric and mental health services were sustainable and/or profitable. Neither sustainable nor profitable were specifically defined within the survey, so both were open to interpretation by respondents.

The fact that ECSs are regarded as sustainable and/or profitable is encouraging. For birth centers to reasonably and responsibly offer ECSs, the services need to be integrated into a functional business plan. Knowing that other birth centers have been financially successful in doing so is vital to this process.

Understanding the Survey and Its Implications

Results of this survey indicate birth centers are offering a wide array of services beyond standard midwifery-led maternity care. It is likely they

TABLE 10.2
Percentage of Freestanding Birth Centers Offering Certain Types of Women's and Men's Health Services

Women's Health Service	Percentage of Freestanding Birth Centers	Men's Health Service	Percentage of Freestanding Birth Centers
Family planning	96	Nutrition/diet	71.4
Contraception	92	Annual exams	57.1
Miscarriage management	84	Preventative care	57.1
Primary care	80	Screenings	42.9
Preventative care	80	Weight management	42.9
Breast health	80	Education/classes	28.6
Screenings	76	Prostate exams	28.6
Adolescent care	72	Adolescent care	28.6
Nutrition/diet	60	Diabetes care	14.3
Fertility services	60	Elder care	14.3
Urgent care	56	Fertility care	14.3
Weight management	36	Vasectomy	0
Education/classes	36		
Diabetes care	24		
Elder care	16		
Colposcopy	12		
Abortion	12		
Breast imaging	8		

are working to better meet the health care needs of the communities they serve via the addition of these services and perhaps improve the financial viability of the birth center model. As with so many undertakings, the results of this survey lead to further questions and possibilities. In-depth case studies of freestanding birth centers known to provide ECSs may

TABLE 10.3
Percentage of Freestanding Birth Centers Providing Certain Types of Pediatric and Mental Health Services

Pediatric Service	Percentage of Freestanding Birth Centers	Mental Health Service	Percentage of Freestanding Birth Centers
Primary care	100	Pediatric counseling	50
Urgent care	33.3	Independent counseling	35
Preventative care	44.4	Family counseling	15
Immunizations	11.1	Education/classes	15
Screenings	55.6	Treatment plans	10
Education/classes	22.2		
Nutrition/diet support	55.6		
Weight management	33.3		
Diabetes care	11.1		
Infant male circumcision	22.2		

provide important information regarding the development, sustainability, and feasibility of an expanded model of birth center care. Consumer forums and focus groups addressing the desires and expectations of freestanding birth center consumers, such as the types of services they desire, conditions that would cause them to choose ECSs at a freestanding birth center rather than at another location, and their feelings, thoughts, and opinions on ECSs offered by freestanding birth centers would provide valuable insights and information (Wilkes, 2015).

The survey had several strengths and limitations. Limitations included a relatively low response rate of 19.8% and allowing respondents to skip questions, making the survey user-friendly but creating challenges for data management. Another limiting factor was the lack of clear definitions of services (e.g., women's health, alternative/adjunct, leaving the terms open to interpretation by respondents). Strengths included a 93.7%

TABLE 10.4
Percentage of Freestanding Birth Centers With Certain Types of Alternative/Adjunct Service Providers

Alternative/Adjunct Provider	Percentage of Freestanding Birth Centers
Midwives	42.9
Naturopathic doctors	28.6
Massage therapists	28.6
Herbalist	28.6
Yoga instructor	28.6
Nurse practitioners	14.3
Chiropractor	14.3
Diabetes educator	14.3
Social worker	14.3
Nutritionist/dietician	14.3
Acupuncturist	14.3
Aromatherapist	14.3
Craniosacral therapist	14.3

completion rate by respondents and the generation of data and information not previously available. Clearly there *are* freestanding birth centers providing services in addition to standard midwifery-led care in the United States. The survey represented the first step in understanding ECSs and their role in the freestanding birth center model of care.

Birth center leaders may use the data generated from this survey to plan care services to better meet the needs of their communities via the addition of ECS, including creating sustainable and profitable models of care. If the staff of a freestanding birth center provides primary care services, as well as maternity, birth, and postpartum services, outcomes may improve, health care costs may decrease, and access to care for women, children, and families may increase. The data indicating that most survey participants accepted Medicaid may help those pursuing increased payment for birth centers to also increase payment for primary care and ECSs.

Further research is needed to more clearly understand the ECSs being provided by FSCBs. This survey provides some key building blocks for the foundational evidence informing us about the enhanced services being offered by birth centers to provide sustainable, affordable, and safe care to families in the United States. In addition, the survey provides information helpful in exploring the possibility of birth centers as midwifery-led maternity health homes.

BIRTH CENTERS AS MIDWIFERY-LED MATERNITY HEALTH HOMES

Despite evidence that birth center care is associated with improved health outcomes, cost savings, and increased patient satisfaction with care, the care model is underutilized in the United States. Reasons that freestanding birth centers are underutilized include regulatory barriers and inadequate payment for services, both low reimbursement and unwillingness of many payers to contract with birth centers (Alliman, Jolles, & Summers, 2015).

A potential solution to these problems is for qualified birth centers to be designated as patient-centered health homes (PCHHs) or midwifery-led health homes (Alliman et al., 2015). The PCHH was originally known as the patient-centered medical home (PCMH). The PCHH is a model of care recognized by policy makers and payers as deserving increased reimbursement for enhanced patient care (Burton, Devers, & Berenson, 2012). PCHHs are associated with improved health outcomes, decreased utilization of the emergency department (ED), increased utilization of preventive care services, and fewer visits for sick care (Hoff, Weller, & DePuccio, 2012; Homer et al., 2008; Long, Bauchner, Sege, Cabral, & Garg, 2011; Savage, Lauby, & Burkard, 2013). Improved outcomes are related to quality of preventive and chronic care, access to care for adults, and increased adherence to health-promoting behaviors and improved health care utilization patterns for children (Long et al., 2011). These outcomes have been reported in primary care settings and in the management of chronic disease (Hoff et al., 2012; Savage et al., 2013). However, the PCHH model has had only minimal application in the maternity care setting. Significant policy change will be required to achieve the PCHH designation for birth centers.

Background

In 2007, a group of medical associations including the American Academy of Family Physicians (AAFP), American Academy of Pediatrics, American College of Physicians, and American Osteopathic Association issued a joint statement describing the principles to be included in the PCMH model (American Academy of Family Physicians, American Academy of Pediatrics, American College of Physicians, and American Osteopathic Association, 2007; Patient-Centered Primary Care Collaborative, 2007). Since that time, many payers, including states, Medicaid programs, and commercial payers, have established demonstration projects to test the application of PCHH principles to improve outcomes of primary care (Burton et al., 2012). The PCHH is team-based care with patient-centered clinical practice patterns, continuity of care, and the adoption of health information technology and decision support systems (Carrier, Gourevitch, & Shah, 2009). Several principles of the health home model are central to the birth center model of care and predate the development of the PCHH. Those include building a relationship with the primary care provider or midwife, care with a focus on the whole person, use of evidence-based guidelines for care, shared decision making, and enhanced access to midwives outside of regular office hours (Hoff et al., 2012; Miller, Crabtree, Nutting, Stange, & Jaen, 2010).

Outcomes of Birth Center Care Similar to Health Home Goals

Birth centers have been shown to achieve outcome improvements similar to those sought in implementing the health home model. Similarities in some elements of the two models justify establishing a midwifery-led health home model in birth centers. Women who give birth in birth centers have significantly improved outcomes compared with women in standard hospital-based care (Alliman & Phillippi, 2016; Benetar, Garrett, Howell, & Palmer, 2013; Jackson et al., 2003; National Perinatal Epidemiology Unit [NPEU], 2011; Overgaard, Fenger-Gron, & Sandall, 2012; Rooks, Weatherby, & Ernst, 1992; Stapleton, Osborne, & Illuzzi, 2013). Research comparing the outcomes of birth center care with standard maternity care has demonstrated that women giving birth in birth centers were significantly more likely to have a spontaneous vaginal birth, less likely to experience a cesarean birth, and likely to have equivalent neonatal outcomes compared with women in standard care (Alliman & Phillippi, 2016; Jackson et al., 2003; NPEU, 2011; Overgaard et al., 2012; Stapleton et al., 2013). Improved outcomes including lower cesarean rates, fewer preterm births, and less use of costly medical interventions were also found in studies that evaluated the outcomes of vulnerable populations, such as women with low income and less education (Alliman & Phillippi, 2016; Benetar et al., 2013; Jackson et al., 2003; Overgaard et al., 2012).

In addition to the improved health outcomes associated with birth center care, significant cost savings have been observed resulting from lower intervention rates and fewer cesarean births (Jackson et al., 2003; Truven Health Analytics Marketscan Study, 2013). Immediate cost savings are related to the use of fewer interventions at the time of birth. Longer term cost savings are due to the impact of the lower cesarean birth rates on future pregnancies and maternal health (Stapleton et al., 2013).

Women receiving birth center care also report increased satisfaction with care compared with women in hospital-based maternity care (Birthrights, 2013). In a randomized controlled study with random assignment to birth setting, women in birth center care expressed greater satisfaction with all aspects of care, especially the psychological aspects such as respect and parental involvement, compared with women in the standard care (Waldenström & Nilsson, 1993). In a review of multiple qualitative studies of women's experiences of birth center care, it was found that women reported feelings of empowerment, being a partner in their care, and increased confidence in their ability to parent following birth center care (Alliman & Phillippi, 2016).

Developing the Patient-Centered Health Home Designation for Birth Centers

Developing a strategic plan to expand the PCHH designation to birth centers by applying the Triple Aim of improved patient experience, improved population health, and decreased cost, all associated with birth center care, may be effective in health-related policy and/or legislative changes (Berwick, McFadden, & Whittington, 2008). The goals of adding the PCHH designation to birth centers would be to (a) improve health outcomes related to childbirth by increasing options for evidence-based, lower cost, and satisfying maternity care for women and families by making birth center care more widely available; and (b) improve reimbursement for birth center care by achieving the designation of PCHH for birth centers.

Alignment of the birth center model with other innovative health care delivery systems such as the PCHH may promote increased access to birth center care. The PCHH model of care is recognized by policy makers and payers as deserving increased reimbursement for enhanced patient care in primary care and chronic disease management settings (Burton et al., 2012). Enhanced care in a PCHH includes such services as patient care coordination, in-house mental health services, nutrition, and health education (Hoff et al., 2012). Patients also learn how to provide better self-care for chronic conditions to decrease emergency department visits (Hoff et al., 2012). Primary health care practices achieve the PCHH designation through application to organizations such as the National Committee for Quality Assurance (NCQA) or The Joint Commission (TJC; Burton et al., 2012).

Many birth centers have already expanded services in these areas. In addition, the Center for Medicare and Medicaid Innovation (CMMI) is currently examining a model of maternity care called the *Maternity Health Home* as a part of the Strong Start for Mothers and Newborn Initiative. Only preliminary data are available at this time (Cross-Barnet & Clarke, 2016).

Implementation of the PCHH designation for birth centers would require significant policy change. Currently, the PCHH is used for primary and chronic disease care, and funding was included in the ACA to facilitate implementation of the model in more states (Burton et al., 2012). To be eligible for this particular funding, patients enrolled in the PCHH must have at least one chronic health condition (USDHHS, 2013). Birth center clients are reasonably healthy and low risk, so most would not have a chronic disease diagnosis that would qualify for this particular funding mechanism (USDHHS, 2013).

Birth centers have incorporated principles similar to the PCHH for many years, including woman-centered comprehensive coordinated primary maternity care within a larger network of specialty consultant providers, developing relationships with clients and families, and shared decision making (Martin, 2014; Palmer et al., 2010). Policy change leading to the designation of birth centers as PCHH could significantly increase public and commercial payer funding support to promote access to birth center care for women. Designation of the birth center as a health home could be identified as midwifery-led maternity health homes (Alliman, et al., 2015). This designation can be achieved by a change in federal law, regulation, or administrative rule making. If a specialty PCHH designation for childbearing women made birth centers eligible for increased reimbursement and more visible in the health care system, more women could have the option of birth center maternity care.

Community Assessment

For birth centers to function as health homes, staff would need to understand the needs of their consumers. Conducting a community assessment, including identifying and engaging with consumers and other stakeholders, gathering and utilizing local data, and determining key findings, is an important initial step. Those desiring to develop birth centers as health homes will need to investigate the needs of their communities and to define their service populations. Questions to be addressed may include:

- Who will our birth center serve as a health home? Who is our population?
- What particular health needs are apparent in our population?
- What types of services/providers are accessed by our population?
- What types of services/providers does our population need and/or desire?
- What issues affect our population's ability to access care (e.g., transportation, insurance, culture, socioeconomic status, and so forth)?
- How can we best meet the needs of our population (e.g., services, providers, pay structures, and so forth)?

CONCLUSION

Birth centers have repeatedly demonstrated quality maternity and infant care outcomes, but remain consistently underutilized in the United States. Many birth centers are providing ECSs, such as women's reproductive health, pediatric care, and mental health services, improving access to health care services within their communities and meeting the broader needs of consumers. Providing ECSs is often profitable for birth centers, contributing to sustainability, and has the possibility to lower overall health care expenditure in the United States.

Birth center leaders have access to more and better evidence supporting the integration of various elements of the health home model than ever before. The potential to further improve health care outcomes and satisfaction with care, access to care, and decrease overall health care expenditure is great. The expansion of the birth center model to include elements of primary care via the addition of services that meet the unique needs of local communities is within reach.

The PCHH is a model that shares many common elements with the birth center model of care. Shared elements include woman-centered comprehensive coordinated primary maternity care within a larger network of specialty consultant providers, developing relationships with clients and families, and shared decision making. We have an opportunity to create the policy change necessary to develop the midwifery-led maternity health home and improve access to comprehensive woman-centered care.

EXEMPLAR BIRTH CENTER
Lisa Ross Birth and Women's Center, Knoxville, Tennessee

Year established: 1991

Year Closed: 2017

Type of building/square feet/architectural features: Medical office stand-alone 4,000-foot structure, built in 1989

Location: Urban

Business structure: Not-for-profit

Ownership: Community-owned not-for-profit

Licensed as: Birth center

Accredited by: Commission for the Accreditation of Birth Centers

Number of births to date/births per year: 121 births in 2016; 2,950 total births at birth center over the span of the 25-year operation of the center

Services/enhanced services: Breastfeeding center, pediatrics birth to age 12, CenteringPregnancy, Strong Start Program, case management, mental health counseling, Mom's café, Walk and Wear support groups

Providers: Certified nurse midwives, family nurse practitioners, lactation consultants

Client mix: 78% Caucasian, 7% African American, 14% Hispanic, 1% other or unspecified **Payer mix:** 44% Medicaid (TennCare in Tennessee), 56% commercially insured

Lisa Ross Birth and Women's Center (LRBWC) was started in 1991 as the second accredited freestanding birth center in Tennessee by two physicians, a nurse, and the son of a public health nurse. The name of the center was changed from the Maternity Center of East Tennessee to the LRBWC in 1999 to honor one of the first midwives practicing at the center who also led the efforts to finally obtain birth center regulation in the state of Tennessee. Lisa died at age 44.

With a public health mission, the center has always sought to respond to the needs of the community. It was found that the zip code the birth center was located in had the highest rates of preterm birth and prematurity in the larger Knoxville area. An outreach program was started to get women into care and soon after that a CenteringPregnancy® program was started to address these

(continued)

EXEMPLAR BIRTH CENTER *(continued)*

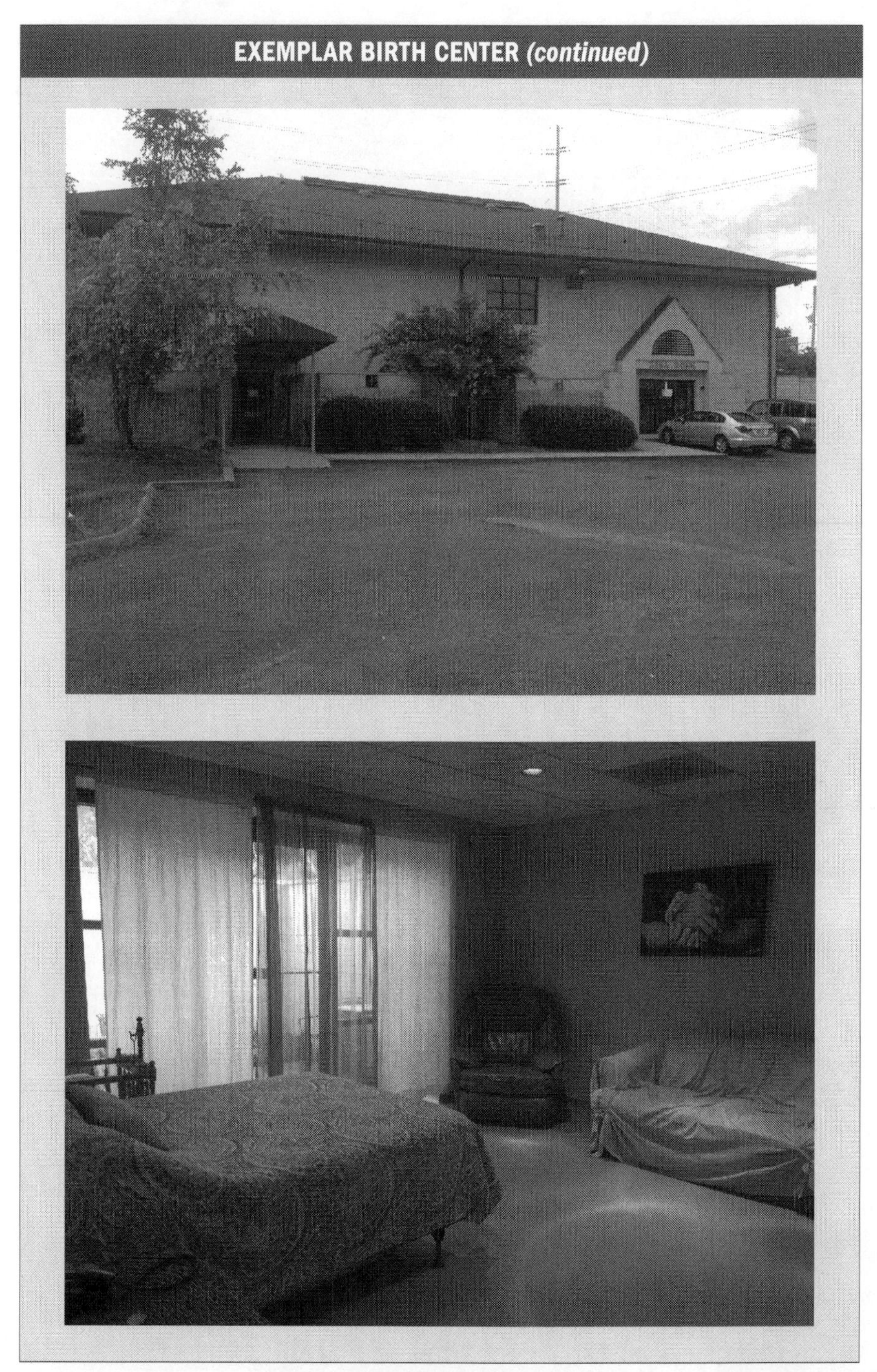

(continued)

EXEMPLAR BIRTH CENTER *(continued)*

poor perinatal outcomes in the community. A breastfeeding center was started after realizing that so many women needed lactation support. Translation services were added when the local health department stopped providing prenatal care and a large number of Spanish-speaking women began seeking care at the center. The addition of case management and counseling services was made to address the psychosocial needs of the population and a pediatric program for ages birth to 12 years was added so that seamless care in the centering model could be continued long after birth.

Maintaining birth center accreditation was always of utmost importance to the management and staff of the center, understanding that with the addition of many ECSs, quality of that care must be assured. Meeting the needs of the community, while managing growth and staying true to the mission of the organization, requires strong leadership and a common vision among stakeholders.

REFERENCES

Alliman, J., Jolles, D., & Summers, L. (2015). The innovation imperative: Scaling freestanding birth centers, CenteringPegnancy, and midwifery-led maternity health homes. *Journal of Midwifery and Women's Health, 60*(3), 244–249. doi:10.1111/jmwh.12320

Alliman, J., & Phillippi, J. C. (2016). Maternal outcomes in birth centers: An integrative review of the literature. *Journal of Midwifery and Women's Health, 61*(1), 21–51. doi:10.1111/jmwh.12356

American Academy of Family Physicians, American Academy of Pediatrics, American College of Physicians, and American Osteopathic Association. (2007). Joint principles of the patient-centered medical home. Retrieved from http://www.aafp.org/dam/AAFP/documents/practice_management/pcmh/initiatives/PCMHJoint.pdf

American Association of Birth Centers. (2016). Standards for birth centers. Retrieved from http://www.birthcenters.org/resource/resmgr/AABC_STANDARDS-RV2016.pdf

American College of Nurse-Midwives. (2011). Definition of midwifery and scope of practice of certified nurse-midwives and certified midwives. Retrieved from http://www.midwife.org/ACNM/files/ACNMLibraryData/UPLOADFILENAME/000000000266/Definition%20of%20Midwifery%20and%20Scope%20of%20Practice%20of%20CNMs%20and%20CMs%20Dec%202011.pdf

Benetar, S., Garrett, A. B., Howell, E., & Palmer, A. (2013). Midwifery care at a freestanding birth center: A safe and effective alternative to conventional maternity care. *Health Services Research, 48*(5), 1750–68. doi:10.1111/1475-6773.12061

Berwick, D. M., McFadden, A., & Whittington, J. (2008). The Triple Aim: Care, health and cost. *Health Affairs, 27*(3), 759–769. doi:10.1377/hlthaff.27.3.759

Birthplace in England Collaborative Group. (2011). Perinatal and maternal outcomes by planned place of birth for healthy women with low risk pregnancies: The birthplace in England national prospective cohort study. *British Medical Journal, 343*. doi:10.1136/bmj.d7400

Birthrights. (2013). The Dignity Survey 2013: Women's and midwives' experiences of dignity in UK maternity care. Retrieved from http://www.birthrights.org.uk/wordpress/wp-content/uploads/2013/10/Birthrights-Dignity-Survey.pdf

Burton, R. A., Devers, K. J., & Berenson, R. A. (2012). *Patient-centered medical home recognition tools: A comparison of ten surveys' content and operational details.* Washington, DC: Health Policy Center, Urban Institute.

Carrier, E., Gourevitch, M. N., & Shah, N. R. (2009). Medical homes: Challenges in translating theory into practice. *Medical Care, 47*(7), 714–722. doi:10.1097/MLR.0b013e3181a469b0

Centers for Disease Control and Prevention. (2016). Pregnancy mortality surveillance system. Retrieved from http://www.cdc.gov/reproductivehealth/maternalinfanthealth/pmss.html

Cross-Barnet, C., & Clark, W. (2016). Strong Start for Mothers and Newborns: Second annual evaluation report. Volume 2. Retrieved from https://downloads.cms.gov/files/cmmi/strongstart-enhancedprenatalcare_evalrptyr2v2.pdf

Hoff, T., Weller, W., & DePuccio, M. (2012). The patient-centered medical home: A review of recent research. *Medical Care Research and Review, 69*(6), 619–644.

Homer, C., Klatka, K., Romm, D., Kuhlthau, K., Bloom, S., Newacheck, P., . . . Perrin, J. (2008). A review of the evidence for the medical home for children with special health care needs. *Pediatrics, 122*(4), e922–e937.

Jackson, D., Lang, J., Swartz, W., Ganiats, T., Fullerton, J., Ecker, J., & Nguyen, U. (2003). Outcomes, safety, and resource utilization in a collaborative care birth center program compared with traditional physician-based perinatal care. *American Journal of Public Health, 93*(6), 999–1006.

Long, W., Bauchner, H., Sege, R., Cabral, H., & Garg, A. (2011). The value of the medical home for children without special health care needs. *Pediatrics, 129*(1), 87–98.

Martin, D. M. (2014). Interprofessional teams in the patient-centered medical home. *Nursing Administration Quarterly, 38*(3), 214–220.

Miller, W., Crabtree, B., Nutting, P., Stange, K., & Jaen, C. (2010). Primary care practice development: A relationship-centered approach. *Annals of Family Medicine, 8*(Suppl. 1), s68–s79. doi:10.1370/afm.1089

National Association of Certified Professional Midwives. (2014). Professional standards and competencies. Retrieved from http://nacpm.org/about-cpms/professional-standards

Neilson, M., Langner, B., Zema, C., Hacker, T., & Grundy, P. (2012). Benefits of implementing the primary care patient-centered medical home: A review of cost & quality results [Entire issue]. *Patient-Centered Primary Care Collaborative.* Retrieved from http://www.pcpcc.org/guide/benefits-implementing-primary-care-medical-home#sthash.QoMcLJb1.dpuf

Overgaard, C., Fenger-Gron, M., & Sandall, J. (2012). Freestanding midwifery units versus obstetric units: Does the effect of place of birth differ with level of social disadvantage? *BMC Public Health, 12,* 478. doi:10.1186/1471-2458-12-478

Palmer, L., Cook, A., & Courtot, B. (2010). Comparing models of maternity care serving women at risk of poor birth outcomes in Washington, DC. *Alternative therapies in health and medicine, 16*(5), 48.

Patient-Centered Primary Care Collaborative. (2007). Joint principles of the patient-centered medical home. Retrieved from http://www.aafp.org/dam/AAFP/documents/practice_management/pcmh/initiatives/PCMHJoint.pdf

Rooks, J. P., Weatherby, N. L., & Ernst, E. K. M. (1992). The National Birth Center Study. Part II—Intrapartum and immediate postpartum and neonatal care. *Journal of Nurse-Midwifery, 37*(5), 301–330.

Sandall, J., Soltani, H., Gates, S., Shennan, A., & Devane, D. (2013). Midwife-led continuity models versus other models of care for childbearing women. *Cochrane Database of Systemic Reviews, 8.* doi:10.1002/14651858.CD004667

Savage, A. I, Lauby, T., & Burkard, J. F. (2013). Examining selected patient outcomes and staff satisfaction in a primary care clinic at a military treatment facility after implementation of the patient-centered medical home. *Military Medicine, 178*(2), 128–134.

Stapleton, S. R., Osborne, C., & Illuzzi, J. (2013). Outcomes of care in birth centers: Demonstration of a durable model. *Journal of Midwifery and Women's Health, 58*(1), 3–14. doi:10.1111/jmwh.12003

Truven Health Analytics Marketscan Study. (2013). *The cost of having a baby in the United States.* Ann Arbor, MI: Truven Health Analytics. Retrieved from http://transform.childbirthconnection.org/wp-content/uploads/2013/01/Cost-of-Having-a-Baby1.pdf

U.S. Department of Health and Human Services. (2013). Interim report to Congress on the Medicaid health home state plan option. Retrieved from https://www.medicaid.gov/Medicaid-CHIP-Program-Information/By-Topics/Long-Term-Services-and-Supports/Integrating-Care/Health-Homes/Health-Homes.html

U.S. Department of Health and Human Services. (2014). Key features of the affordable care act by year. Retrieved from http://www.hhs.gov/healthcare/facts/timeline/timeline-text.html

Waldenström, U., & Nilsson, C. A. (1993). Women's satisfaction with birth center care: A randomized, controlled study. *Birth, 20*(1), 3–13.

World Health Organization, United Nations Children's Fund, United Nations Population Fund, the World Bank, and United Nations Population Division Maternal Mortality Estimation Inter-Agency Group. (2013). Maternal mortality 1999–2013. Retrieved from http://www.who.int/gho/maternal_health/countries/usa.pdf?ua=1

Wilkes, A. H. (2015). *Freestanding birth centers and enhanced care services in the United States* (Doctor of Nursing Capstone Project). Retrieved from http://cdm16161.contentdm.oclc.org/cdm/ref/collection/dc/id/540

CHAPTER 11

The Role of Birth Centers in Promoting Physiologic Birth

MELISSA D. AVERY

LEARNING OBJECTIVES

Upon completion of this chapter, the reader will be able to:

1. Define birth center care as a physiologic approach to pregnancy, labor and birth, and postpartum/newborn care
2. Describe common care practices and additional therapies/approaches to support physiologic labor and birth in the freestanding birth center care context
3. Analyze the birth center as the ideal learning environment for physiologic pregnancy and birth

DEFINITIONS

Physiologic birth and birth center care are synonymous—two sides of the same coin. Physiologic birth refers to care in which the normalcy and state of health represented by pregnancy and birth is respected and supported; the freestanding birth center is the formal care location in which that approach is most appropriately implemented. In fact, the birth center standards defined by the American Association of Birth Centers (AABC) include that assertion in the definition of a birth center (AABC, 2016a). Birth center care has been shown to be a model that results in less use of medical interventions and fewer cesareans when compared with a risk-adjusted group of women, thus demonstrating it is the care approach, and not a low-risk designation contributing to outcomes (Jackson et al., 2003; Stapleton, Osborne, & Illuzzi, 2013). Common practices consistent with a physiologic approach to pregnancy, labor, and birth employed in birth centers are discussed in this chapter, and the birth center as the ideal location for learning about physiologic birth is explored.

BACKGROUND ON PHYSIOLOGIC BIRTH AND BIRTH CENTER CARE

Physiologic birth has received a good deal of attention in the past two decades as an ideal approach to maternity care for healthy women (American College of Nurse-Midwives [ACNM], Midwives Alliance of North America (NAMA), and National Association of Certified Professional Midwives (NACPM), 2012; International Confederation of Midwives [ICM], 2014; WHO, 1996). Current birth outcome statistics in the United States suggest that a modified maternity care model is needed to reverse current harmful and embarrassing trends. Maternal mortality has increased in the United States since 2000 (MacDorman, Declercq, Cabral, & Morton, 2016) and is greater than in most other industrialized countries (Save the Children, 2015). The United States spends 17.5% of gross domestic product (GDP) on health care, more than any other country (Healthcare Cost and Utilization Project [HCUP], 2016). "Live newborn" is the third most expensive reason for hospitalization when considering all payers (Medicare, Medicaid, private insurance); it ranks as the top condition billed to Medicaid (23% of stays) and was second for private insurance (16.2% of stays) in 2013 in the United States. The cesarean rate has declined slightly and was 32% in 2015 (Martin, Hamilton, Osterman, Driscoll, & Mathews, 2017) and 23% of women (with singletons) experienced induction of their labor, a number finally starting to slowly decline (Osterman & Martin, 2014). Defined initially by Rosenblatt (1989), we continue the perinatal paradox of spending more and getting less value for our health care dollars. Continued efforts to reduce the use of unnecessary interventions are needed to improve care outcomes and reduce expenditures.

Normal or physiologic birth has been defined by a number of groups, recognizing that pregnancy and birth are normal physiologic events for women, not an illness to be treated. In 1996, the World Health Organization defined a normal birth as "spontaneous in onset, low-risk at the start of labour and remaining so throughout labour and delivery. The infant is born spontaneously in the vertex position between 37 and 42 completed weeks of pregnancy. After birth mother and infant are in good condition" (WHO, 1996, p. 4). The ACNM, Midwives Alliance of North America (MANA), and National Association of Certified Professional Midwives (NACPM) issued a joint statement defining physiologic birth simply as "one that is powered by the innate human capacity of the woman and fetus" (ACNM, MANA, and NACPM, 2012, p. 2). The ICM defines normal birth as "where the woman commences, continues and completes labour with the infant being born spontaneously at term, in the vertex position at term, without any surgical, medical, or pharmaceutical intervention" (ICM, 2014, p. 1).

Research supports a physiologic approach to labor and birth for low-risk women (Romano & Lothian, 2008); physiologic approaches can also be incorporated into care for women who require a higher level of care and monitoring as appropriate to their situation. A recently published summary of the research on the physiology of the childbearing period supports the benefits of nonintervention unless needed. Buckley (2015) reviewed more than a thousand studies and suggested that interruptions to the normal hormonal physiology that occur in later pregnancy and labor may make labor more difficult, increase the likelihood of fetal distress requiring additional interventions, interrupt maternal–newborn bonding, and make breastfeeding more difficult. Newborns may experience disrupted thermoregulation and glycemic regulation. Disruptions to breastfeeding could have longer term effects on infant/child health. Additional research in many of these areas to further explain physiologic phenomena and the effects of intervening in normal processes is needed.

BIRTH CENTER APPROACH TO CARE

Birth center philosophy is consistent with promoting normal physiology during pregnancy, labor, and birth, which are considered normal family events unless the specific situation suggests otherwise (AABC, 2016b). Birth center care offers a model of a physiologic approach throughout pregnancy and birth, which is evident in preconception planning, antenatal care, intrapartum care, and the postpartum/newborn periods. The setting has been referred to as a maximized home setting, thus demonstrating the approach of woman-centered care, a focus on health and wellness, and links to an existing broader system of care (AABC, 2016c).

Preconception and Antenatal Care

Preconception and antenatal care set the stage for the focus on health promotion throughout pregnancy and planning for a physiologic birth. Although preconception care is not routinely sought by women, it provides an opportunity to plan in advance for a healthy pregnancy (Delissaint & McKyer, 2011). Women seeking a freestanding birth center experience for their pregnancy may be more likely to visit care settings and examine their options prior to pregnancy. In addition, some women will already be familiar with a birth center after receiving well-woman care there, and thus it is a natural extension to continue to receive prenatal and birth care during pregnancy. Prenatal care in a birth center is consistent with traditional care including baseline laboratory screening, ongoing risk assessment and measurement to assure safety for mother and fetus, and prenatal education related to healthy lifestyle and pregnancy-related topics. In addition, birth center care is specifically focused on helping women prepare for physiologic birth because labor and birth care in the freestanding birth center rely on human presence and nonpharmacological support techniques to achieve spontaneous labor and birth. Although the research on preparing women prenatally for physiologic birth is limited, the factors gleaned from a systematic review reflect the birth center approach to care including providing information to women and supporting their participation in care decisions in a relationship with a trusted care provider (Avery, Saftner, Larson, & Weinfurter, 2014).

Labor and Birth Care

Following an emphasis on healthy lifestyle and detailed planning for physiologic labor and birth during the pregnancy, supporting spontaneous onset and progression of labor becomes the focus with women's preferences respected and modified as needed. Evidence-based resources highlighting physiologic care practices during labor are numerous (ACNM, n.d.; ACNM, 2014; Lamaze International, 2016). In addition, the Mother-Friendly Childbirth Initiative, built on the principles of normalcy of the birthing process, empowerment, autonomy, do no harm, and responsibility, includes 10 steps that birthing sites can follow to provide appropriate care (CIMS, 2015; Box 11.1). Admission to the birth center is planned to occur during active labor and thus communication and support in early labor while a woman remains at home is essential. Common approaches include encouraging adequate hydration and good intake with sufficient calories, ambulation to support labor progression balanced with rest as needed, presence of support persons, and being alert to ongoing fetal movement and signs of healthy labor progress. When planning to give birth in a hospital, women may need to include regular food and fluids, avoidance of an intravenous line, ambulation, intermittent auscultation of the fetal heart rate, and water immersion in their birth preferences. However,

BOX 11.1
Mother-Friendly Steps That Are Most Applicable to Birth Centers

- Offer women unrestricted access to birth companions of their choice, skilled continuous labor support, and professional midwifery care
- Provide unbiased information about birth practices and outcomes
- Provide culturally sensitive care
- Provide women freedom of movement in labor; avoid the lithotomy position
- Have clear policies for consultation, transfer, and communication; provide access to community resources
- Do not use labor practices unsupported by evidence such as routine intravenous lines, restricting oral intake, or artificial rupture of membranes; limit use of induction and episiotomy
- Educate staff in nonpharmacological pain relief methods
- Aim to achieve the baby-friendly steps

Source: Adapted from Coalition for Improving Maternity Services (2015).

in the birth center these are the standard of care and methods employed to support physiologic labor.

These care principles and approaches continue when a woman is admitted to the birth center with her family and important support persons. Singata, Tranmer, and Gyte (2013) reviewed existing studies examining the restriction or use of food and fluids in labor. Neither harms nor benefits were found for restricting fluids and food in labor for women at low risk of needing general anesthesia; the authors recommended that women be allowed the flexibility to determine their intake in labor. Ambulation in labor, particularly upright positioning, has been well studied. Systematic reviews of both first- and second-stage labor have demonstrated that upright positions during first-stage labor result in shorter labor, less use of epidural analgesia, and fewer cesareans (Lawrence, Lewis, Hofmeyr, & Styles, 2013). During second-stage labor for women without epidurals (22 trials, more than 7,000 women), upright positions were associated with reduced assisted births, reduced episiotomies, an increase in second-degree lacerations, and a nonsignificant reduction in second-stage duration. An increase in the incidence of blood loss greater than 500 mL was also observed, and thus must be considered in caring for women using upright positions in second-stage labor (Gupta, Hofmeyr, & Shehmar, 2012). More and better research is needed in all of these areas to improve the evidence for practice.

Intermittent auscultation of the fetal heart rate is standard in birth center care. Admission monitoring of the fetus by continuous cardiotocography (Devane, Lalor, Daly, McGuire, & Smith, 2012) and during labor (Alferivic, Devane, Gyte, & Cuthbert, 2017) has not been shown to improve outcomes and may increase cesarean and instrumental birth rates. Continuous cardiotocography in labor was associated with reduced neonatal seizures and no reduction in cerebral palsy or infant mortality, as well as an increase in cesarean and instrumental births (Alfirevic et al., 2017). The physiologic approach in birth centers of appropriate use of intermittent auscultation has been suggested as a way to reduce cesarean births (Cahill & Spain, 2015; Cox & King, 2015). Commission for the Accreditation of Birth Centers (CABC) accredited birth centers are required to demonstrate that they do not use continuous fetal monitoring once women are admitted in active labor (AABC, 2016a; CABC, 2016). ACNM (2015) provides a defined approach to intermittent auscultation that may be used in labor and birth settings.

Physiologic labor progress is supported while staying alert to any change in status that might indicate transfer to a hospital where higher levels of care are available. The most common reasons for transfer include lack of labor progress or need for pharmacological pain relief not available in the birth center (see Chapter 4).

Additional Care Practices to Promote Relaxation and Pain Relief in Labor

A number of integrative therapies have been used to support relaxation and thus improve coping and responses to labor pain for women who prefer to avoid pharmacological interventions. These care practices fit well with the woman-centered and physiologic approach to care in the birth center. Relaxation techniques were first formally taught to parents during childbirth education classes decades ago; Leggitt (2013) shares some simple techniques to promote relaxation during labor, such as appropriate use of language and focusing attention on the laboring woman as well as using music, progressive relaxation techniques, imagery, breathing, heat/cold, positioning, and more. These techniques along with ongoing presence of supportive persons are recommended. The research in these areas is not well developed and additional research is needed.

Intentional touch therapies including therapeutic touch, healing touch, reiki, and massage therapy are techniques that can be learned and may be useful during pregnancy or labor to aid relaxation and stress reduction, as well as reduce pain (Ringdahl, 2013). Smith, Levett, Collins, and Crowther (2011) conducted a systematic review of studies of relaxation methods (11 trials, 1,374 women) used to help women cope with labor pain. Relaxation techniques and yoga were shown to reduce pain in latent and active labor as well as increase satisfaction with the birth experience. These techniques may be helpful in labor; there was no evidence of effect for music or audio-analgesia.

Aromatherapy is another technique that may be utilized in labor to promote relaxation and stress reduction. Defined as "the intentional evidence-based application of plant essential oils for preventive or therapeutic purposes" (Halcon, 2013, p. 174), aromatherapy (excluding ingestion) is believed to be safe in appropriate doses in the second and third trimesters of pregnancy. Lavender, mandarin, frankincense, clary sage, and Roman chamomile are some essential oils that have been used. Research is limited and the few studies of aromatherapy for pain relief are not adequate to make clinical recommendations (Smith, Collins, & Crowther, 2011).

Water immersion is a common relaxation and pain relief technique used in birth centers and other birthing units. Water immersion during labor has been reviewed and shown to reduce the use of epidural analgesia and the duration of first-stage labor (Cluett & Burns, 2011). Water birth may also be requested by women for their childbirth experience. The majority of water immersion and water birth studies are descriptive or observational studies with small samples; few randomized controlled trials have been conducted. Authors of a recent integrative review of water birth studies concluded that although the research evidence has many limitations, outcomes are at least equivalent to conventional birth. Offering women a complete explanation of potential risks as well as benefits and considering the best information available along with their preferences is essential (Nutter, Meyer, Shaw-Batista, & Marowitz, 2014). Jones and colleagues (2012) conducted a review of systematic reviews of pain management techniques for women in labor, including 15 Cochrane reviews (255 trials) and three non-Cochrane systematic reviews (55 trials). Of therapies that could be used in a birth center, the authors concluded that water immersion, relaxation, massage, and acupuncture may relieve pain and increase satisfaction. Evidence was insufficient about the efficacy of hypnosis, biofeedback, transcutaneous electrical nerve stimulation (TENS), aromatherapy, and sterile water injections. Additional research is needed for most of these techniques to more fully assess efficacy.

Postpartum Care

Immediately following the birth, physiologic transition of the newborn and new mother continues. Mother and baby are encouraged to be skin to

BOX 11.2
Baby-Friendly Steps Most Applicable to Birth Centers

Provide information to pregnant women about breastfeeding benefits.

- Support initiation of breastfeeding within the first hour of life.
- Support mothers in breastfeeding and maintaining lactation.
- Assist mothers in providing breast-milk only, unless a medical indication to do otherwise.
- Do not separate mothers and infants.
- Encourage mothers to breastfeed on demand.

Adapted from Babyfriendlyusa (https://www.babyfriendlyusa.org/about-us/baby-friendly-hospital-initiative/the-ten-steps).

skin as the newborn is dried and breastfeeding is encouraged. Consistent with research demonstrating benefits of delayed cord clamping, this practice is standard in birth center care (McDonald, Middleton, Dowswell, & Morris, 2013). Commonly accepted baby-friendly principles are applied; some birth centers have achieved the baby-friendly designation (see Box 11.2). Maternal vital signs, bleeding, and newborn transition and vital signs are monitored carefully. Discharge from the birth center, to facilitate family transition to the home environment, occurs typically between 4 and 12 hours postpartum after assuring stability of mother and baby and initiation of breastfeeding. Birth center staff members stay in touch with the family to assure ongoing stable transition; home visits are made in the early days following the birth by most birth centers. Accredited birth centers are required to describe their plan for monitoring women and their newborns during the initial 48 to 72 hours post birth (AABC, 2016a; CABC, 2016).

BIRTH CENTER AS IDEAL LOCATION TO TEACH PHYSIOLOGIC BIRTH

Just as physiologic pregnancy and birth are synonymous with birth centers, the birth center is the ideal setting to teach an approach to undisturbed birth. High induction, epidural, and cesarean rates seen in hospitals can reduce the chances of nursing and medical students as well as family medicine and OB/GYN residents truly experiencing physiologic labor and birth. Midwifery students experience the majority of their student births with a qualified midwife and thus experience physiologic pregnancy and birth care, although in settings with high induction, epidural, and cesarean rates, that care might be more difficult to provide (see Chapter 4).

The birth center is a perfect location for midwifery education. Although 98% of births occur in hospitals, they are typically places for sick care; staff are prepared to act when problems occur versus supporting the normal process and being prepared for more complex care as needed. Where birth centers are able to support midwifery education, increasing the number of students who can have this experience is important. Birth centers can provide midwifery students with opportunities to learn physiologic labor support and birth techniques in a location where there is not an epidural right down the hall. Being "with woman" and learning the "art of doing 'nothing' well" (Kennedy, 2000) are the options available for labor support. In addition, increasing student opportunities in birth centers will increase the number of midwives prepared to practice in the growing number of birth centers.

Interprofessional practice opportunities can be ideally located in a birth center. Family medicine and obstetric/gynecological residents can learn about physiologic birth from midwives and partner in providing this model of care. If they have experience in a birth center during residency, physicians will be better prepared to provide consultation to birth center clinicians in a respectful and collaborative manner; some may even decide to practice in a birth center. Clinical experiences in a birth center can also be invaluable to nursing and medical students interested in maternity care as they are considering areas of specialization for practice. One option for including nursing and medical students is to provide instruction in labor support techniques so they can assist in providing labor support to women. Avery, Jennings, and O'Brien (2013) suggested a possible curriculum for learners about physiologic birth that may be used in these settings.

Transfer of care from the birth center to the hospital is another situation that provides learning opportunities for interprofessional care, collaborative practice, and promoting good communication strategies. A series of summits on home birth held between 2011 and 2014 resulted in a set of best practice guidelines for transfer from home to hospital during labor (Home Birth Summit, n.d). Responsibilities of the midwife, the hospital clinicians, and policies to have in place are all identified. Although the focus is on home birth, the document provides a model to consider for transfers from a birth center and is described as such. Accredited birth centers are required to have a robust plan for care transfer at any time during pregnancy and particularly during labor when more complex care is required (AABC, 2016a). Opportunities to learn about birth center care and the timely, respectful transfer of women, whether working on the transferring or receiving side, will educate all providers on the integration of the birth center into the broader care system and thus enhance the transfer of a physiologic approach from birth center to hospital when possible.

CONCLUSION

Care providers including midwives, nurses, and physicians recognize that the predominant U.S. model of maternity care must change and there are signs that this is happening (Richards et al., 2016). The cesarean rate has declined somewhat in recent years (Martin et al., 2017), emphasis on avoiding nonmedical induction before 39 weeks has increased (American College of Obstetricians and Gynecologists [ACOG], 2013), although the number of early term births (37–38 weeks) increased 2% from 24.76% to 24.99% from 2014 to 2015 and full term births (39–40 weeks) declined from 58.72 to 58.47. These changes in 2015 followed a decline in early term and increase in term birth rates between 2007 and 2014 (Martin et al., 2017). However, amid these mostly promising trends, recent news reports have highlighted a $16 million settlement to a woman who chose a hospital for its promise of natural birth practices and then found her preferences were not supported (Cosmopolitan, 2016) and another woman who sued her obstetrician for performing an episiotomy after she specifically refused the procedure (National Public Radio, 2016).

Birth centers are defined as the initial level of maternal care by major medical groups (ACOG, 2015), and women's choice of birth location should be supported (Stark, Remynse, & Zwelling, 2016). For some time, we have seen certain types of health care move out of hospitals into more community-based settings, including surgical centers, testing centers, urgent care clinics, hospice, and more. A 2011 report by the American Hospital Association (AHA, 2011), *Hospitals and Care Systems of the Future,* described unprecedented changes in health care and recommended that hospitals must use evidence-based practices improving quality and safety, improve population health by pursuing the triple aim, and implement patient-centered and integrated care among other strategies and competencies. Trends in reductions in in-patient care along with corresponding increases in out-patient and ambulatory services are expected to continue. A focus on population health will aim to keep individuals out of the hospital except those most needing in-patient services

(Adamopoulos, 2013). The same trends are occurring in maternity care as out-of-hospital births increase (Martin et al., 2017). The birth center is an opportunity for continued growth as we shift the focus of maternity care in this country from what might go wrong to what is healthy, physiologic, and will most often go right. Supporting that approach in a healthy, supportive, and collaborative environment such as the freestanding community-based birth center is the growth opportunity in maternity care.

REFERENCES

Adamopoulos, H. (2013). The future of hospitals: Visions of the healthcare landscape in 2035. Retrieved from http://www.beckershospitalreview.com/hospital-management-administration/the-future-of-hospitals-visions-of-the-healthcare-landscape-in-2035.html

Alfirevic, Z., Devane, D., Gyte, G. M. L., & Cuthbert, A. (2017). Continuous cardiotocography (CTG) as a form of electronic fetal monitoring (EFM) for fetal assessment during labour. *Cochrane Database of Systematic Reviews, 2017*(2). doi:10.1002/14651858.CD006066.pub3

American Association of Birth Centers. (2016a). Birth center standards. Retrieved from https://aabc.site-ym.com/?page=Standards

American Association of Birth Centers. (2016b). The birth center experience. Retrieved from http://www.birthcenters.org/?page=bc_experience

American Association of Birth Centers. (2016c). What is a birth center? Retrieved from http://www.birthcenters.org/?page=bce_what_is_a_bc

American College of Nurse-Midwives. (n.d.). BirthTools. Retrieved from http://www.birthtools.org

American College of Nurse-Midwives. (2014). Pearls of midwifery. Retrieved from http://www.midwife.org/Evidence-Based-Practice-Pearls-of-Midwifery

American College of Nurse-Midwives. (2015). Intermittent auscultation for intrapartum fetal heart rate surveillance. *Journal of Midwifery and Women's Health, 60*(5), 626–632.

American College of Nurse-Midwives, Midwives Alliance of North America, and National Association of Certified Professional Midwives. (2012). Supporting healthy and normal physiologic childbirth: A consensus statement by the American College of Nurse-Midwives, Midwives Alliance of North America, and the National Association of Certified Professional Midwives. *Journal of Midwifery and Women's Health, 57*(5), 529–532.

American College of Obstetricians and Gynecologists. (2016). Practice bulletin: Induction of labor. No. 107. Washington, DC: Author.

American College of Obstetricians and Gynecologists. (2015). Levels of maternity care. Retrieved from http://www.acog.org/Resources-And-Publications/Obstetric-Care-Consensus-Series/Levels-of-Maternal-Care

American Hospital Association. (2011). *Committee on Performance Improvement, Jeanette Clough, Chairperson. Hospitals and care systems of the future.* Chicago, IL: Author.

Avery, M. D., Jennings, J., & O'Brien, M. (2013). Educating health professionals for collaborative practice in support of normal birth. In M. Avery (Ed.), *Supporting a physiologic approach to pregnancy and birth: A practical guide* (pp. 275–299). Ames, IA: Wiley-Blackwell.

Avery, M. D., Saftner, M. A., Larson, B., & Weinfurter, L. V. (2014). A systematic review of maternal confidence for physiologic birth: Characteristics of prenatal care and confidence measurement. *Journal of Midwifery and Women's Health, 59*(6), 586–595. doi:0.1111/jmwh.12269

Buckley, S. J. (2015). *Hormonal physiology of childbearing: Evidence and implications for women, babies, and maternity care*. Washington, DC: Childbirth Connection Programs, National Partnership for Women & Families.

Cahill, A. G., & Spain, J. (2015). Intrapartum fetal monitoring. *Clinical Obstetrics and Gynecology, 58*(2), 263–268. doi:10.1097/GRF.0000000000000109

Cluett, E. R., & Burns, E. (2011). Immersion in water in labour and birth. *Cochrane Database of Systematic Reviews*, (2), Art. No.: CD000111. doi:10.1002/14651858.CD000111.pub3

Coalition for Improving Maternity Services. (2015). Mother-friendly childbirth initiative. Retrieved from http://www.motherfriendly.org/MFCI

Commission for the Accreditation of Birth Centers. (2016). *CABC indicators* (R.Ed. v.1.1. CABC). Hamburg, PA: Author.

Cosmopolitan. (August 10, 2016). Another nurse held my baby's head into my vagina to prevent him from being delivered. Retrieved from http://www.cosmopolitan.com/lifestyle/news/a62592/caroline-malatesta-brookwood-childbirth-lawsuit

Cox, K. J., & King, T. L. (2015). Preventing primary cesarean births: Midwifery care. *Clinical Obstetrics and Gynecology, 58*(2), 282–293. doi:10.1097/GRF.0000000000000108

Delissaint, D., & McKyer, E. L. (2011). A systematic review of factors utilized in preconception health behavior research. *Health Education and Behavior, 38*(6), 603–616. doi:10.1177/1090198110389709

Devane, D., Lalor, J. G., Daly, S., McGuire, W., & Smith, V. (2012). Cardiotocography versus intermittent auscultation of fetal heart on admission to labour ward for assessment of fetal wellbeing. *Cochrane Database of Systematic Reviews*, (2), CD005122. doi:10.1002/14651858.CD005122.pub4

Gupta, J. K., Hofmeyr, G. J., & Shehmar, M. (2012). Position in the second stage of labour for women without epidural anaesthesia. *Cochrane Database of Systematic Reviews, 2012*(5). doi:10.1002/14651858.CD002006.pub3

Halcon, L. (2013). Aromatherapy in pregnancy and childbirth. In M. Avery (Ed.), *Supporting a physiologic approach to pregnancy and birth: A practical guide* (pp. 173–195). Ames, IA: Wiley-Blackwell.

Home Birth Summit. (n.d.). Best practice guidelines: Transfer from planned home birth to hospital. Retrieved from http://www.homebirthsummit.org/best-practice-transfer-guidelines

International Confederation of Midwives. (2014). Keeping birth normal. Retrieved from http://www.internationalmidwives.org/who-we-are/policy-and-practice/icm-position-statements-general

Jackson, D. J., Lang, J. M., Swartz, W. H., Ganiats, T. G., Fullerton, J., Ecker, J., & Nguyen, U. (2003). Outcomes, safety, and resource utilization in a collaborative care birth center program compared with traditional physician-based perinatal care. *American Journal of Public Health, 93*(6), 999–1006.

Jones, L., Othman, M., Dowswell, T., Alfirevic, Z., Gates, S., Newburn, M., . . . Neilson, J. P. (2012). Pain management for women in labour: An overview of systematic reviews. *Cochrane Database of Systematic Reviews*, (3), Art. No.: CD009234. doi:10.1002/14651858.CD009234.pub2

Kennedy, H. P. (2000). A model of exemplary midwifery practice: Results of a Delphi study. *Journal of Midwifery and Women's Health, 45*, 4–19.

Lamaze International. (2016). Healthy birth practices. Retrieved from http://www.lamaze international.org/healthybirthpractices

Lawrence, A., Lewis, L., Hofmeyr, G. J., & Styles, C. (2013). Maternal positions and mobility during first stage labour. *Cochrane Database of Systematic Reviews*, (10), Art. No.: CD003934. doi:10.1002/14651858.CD003934.pub4

Leggitt, K. (2013). Techniques to promote relaxation in labor. In M. Avery (Ed.), *Supporting a physiologic approach to pregnancy and birth: A practical guide* (pp. 105–117). Ames, IA: Wiley-Blackwell.

MacDorman, M. F., Declercq, E., Cabral, H., & Morton, C. (2016). Recent increases in the U.S. maternal mortality rate: Disentangling trends from measurement issues. *Obstetrics and Gynecology, 128*, 1–10.

Martin, J. A., Hamilton, B. E., Osterman, M. J., Driscoll, A. K., & Mathews, T. J. (2017). Births: Final data for 2015. *National Vital Statistics Report, 66*(1). Hyattsville, MD: National Center for Health Statistics.

McDonald, S. J., Middleton, P., Dowswell, T., & Morris, P. S. (2013). Effect of timing of umbilical cord clamping of term infants on maternal and neonatal outcomes. *Cochrane Database of Systematic Reviews*, (7), Art. No.: CD004074. doi:10.1002/14651858.CD004074 .pub3

National Public Radio. (2016). Episiotomies still common during childbirth despite advice to do fewer. Retrieved from http://www.npr.org/sections/health-shots/2016/07/04/ 483945168/episiotomies-still-common-during-childbirth-despite-advice-to-do-fewer

Nutter, E., Meyer, S., Shaw-Batista, J., & Marowitz, A. (2014). Waterbirth: An integrative analysis of peer-reviewed literature. *Journal of Midwifery and Women's Health, 59*(3), 286–319.

Osterman, M. J. K., & Martin, J. A. (2014). *Recent declines in induction of labor by gestational age* (NCHS Data Brief No. 155). Hyattsville, MD: National Center for Health Statistics.

Richards, J. L., Kramer, M. S., Deb-Rinker, P., Rouleau, J., Mortenson, L., Gissler, M., . . . Kramer, M. R. (2016). Temporal trends in late preterm and early term birth rates in 6 high-income countries in North America and Europe and association with clinician-initiated obstetric interventions. *Journal of the American Medical Association, 316*(4), 410–419. doi:10.1001/jama.2016.9635

Ringdahl, D. (2013). Touch therapies in pregnancy and childbirth. In M. Avery (Ed.), *Supporting a physiologic approach to pregnancy and birth: A practical guide*. Wiley Blackwell.

Romano, A. M., & Lothian, J. A. (2008). Promoting, protecting, and supporting normal birth: A look at the evidence. *Journal of Obstetric, Gynecologic, and Neonatal Nursing, 37*, 94–105. doi:10.1111/j.1552-6909.2007.00210

Rosenblatt, R. A. (1989). The perinatal paradox: Doing more and accomplishing less. *Health Affairs, 8*(3), 158–168.

Save the Children. (2015). State of the World's Mothers 2015. Retrieved from https://www .savethechildren.net/state-worlds-mothers-2015

Singata, M., Tranmer, J., & Gyte, G. M. L. (2013). Restricting oral fluid and food intake during labour. *Cochrane Database of Systematic Review*, (8), Art. No.: CD003930. doi:10.1002/ 14651858.CD003930.pub3

Smith, C. A., Collins, C. T., & Crowther, C. A. (2011). Aromatherapy for pain management in labour. *Cochrane Database of Systematic Reviews*, (7), Art. No.: CD009215. doi:10.1002/ 14651858.CD009215

Smith, C. A., Levett, K. M., Collins, C. T., & Crowther, C. A. (2011). Relaxation techniques for pain management in labour. *Cochrane Database of Systematic Reviews*, (12), Art. No.: CD009514. doi:10.1002/14651858.CD009514

Stapleton, S. R., Osborne, C., & Illuzzi, J. (2013). Outcomes of care in birth centers: Demonstration of a durable model. *Journal of Midwifery and Women's Health, 58*(1), 3–14. doi:10.1111/jmwh.12003

Stark, M. A., Remynse, M., & Zwelling, E. (2016). Importance of the birth environment to support physiologic birth. *Journal of Obstetric, Gynecologic & Neonatal Nursing, 45*(2), 285–294.

World Health Organization. (1996). Care in normal birth: A practical guide. Retrieved from http://www.who.int/maternal_child_adolescent/documents/who_frh_msm_9624/en

CHAPTER 12

Preparing the Workforce

BARBARA A. ANDERSON, LINDA J. COLE, AND
JESSE S. BUSHMAN

LEARNING OBJECTIVES

Upon completion of this chapter, the reader will be able to:

1. Discuss the global and national workforce shortage of qualified midwives
2. Explain the concept of task shifting as it applies to freestanding birth centers
3. Identify three key strategies for preparing the midwifery workforce for practice in birth centers

CURRENT STATE OF THE MATERNAL CHILD WORKFORCE

A functional health care system is comprised of fluid interactions among all the components (Riley, 2016). Building capacity for these interactions is dependent upon a sufficient and appropriately distributed workforce (Fullerton & Anderson, 2017). Currently, one of the most critical issues facing health care systems globally, including the United States, is the inadequate number and maldistribution of the health care workforce (World Health Organization [WHO], 2015a).

Maternal and child health is particularly vulnerable to the large gap in health care providers, driving the need for adequate number and appropriate distribution of the midwifery workforce across the globe, collaboration among providers of varying skill levels, and accessible, safe venues for birth. Although the highest maternal mortality still remains in

Sub-Saharan Africa (Zureick-Brown et al., 2013), the United States has a shocking number of maternal deaths given its level of economic development. In the United States, maternal mortality has risen rapidly between 1990 and 2013 (Kassebaum et al., 2014). Other countries, including both high- and low-resource nations, have seen appreciable declines. The United States now ranks 60th (out of 180 nations) in maternal mortality, the highest among developed countries (Kassebaum et al., 2014).

The 2014 *Lancet* series on midwifery focused on the potential impact of midwifery services on reducing maternal and newborn mortality worldwide. Funded by the Gates Foundation, this report brought attention to the critical contribution that midwives make in improving the health of women and children globally. Examining care needs across all settings, the authors identified more than 50 short-, medium-, and long-term goals to improve the health of this population. This framework of quality care by midwives who are properly educated, trained, licensed, and regulated has been shown to decrease maternal mortality, improve outcomes, and decrease cost. These findings were applicable to high- and lower income countries and settings (Renfrew et al., 2014). Future maternal child workforce development planners should take these findings into consideration and choose to focus on the expansion of midwifery in those plans.

Authors of another article in the *Lancet* series reported finding that 83% of maternal deaths, stillbirths, and neonatal deaths worldwide would be prevented with the scaling up of the midwifery workforce. It was only when specialists were removed from the primary care of women and babies, and instead positioned within a system to accept referrals and transfers from midwives of women who need their services, that these improvements in outcomes could be observed (Homer et al., 2014). Similarly, freestanding birth centers in the United States, positioned in communities within integrated health systems, may improve health outcomes and serve as clinical sites for midwives and student midwives to learn to practice in this needed practice model.

The American College of Nurse-Midwives (ACNM) and the Accreditation Commission for Midwifery Education (ACME) published a joint statement in 2015 pointing to the global pattern of midwifery as the default profession caring for women anticipating normal birth, the extreme variance seen in this pattern in the United States, and the projected forecast by the U.S. Bureau of Labor Statistics for 31% growth in the market for midwifery care from 2012 to 2022. In a 7-year span between 2007 and 2014, the number of graduated certified nurse-midwives (CNMs) and certified midwives (CMs) approximately doubled, not due to an expansion in the number of educational programs for midwives but an increasing number of students in certain programs (ACNM & ACME, 2015).

The Strong Start for Mothers and Newborns Initiative grants, under the auspices of the Centers for Medicare and Medicaid Services (CMS), have provided impetus for midwifery practice, specifically within the context of birth center care (Alliman, Jolles, & Summers, 2015; American Association of Birth Centers [AABC], 2013). (See Chapter 9 for further discussion of the Strong Start program.) Opportunity for the advancement of midwifery within the venue of the birth center has never been greater. Preparing the midwifery workforce for the anticipated growth in freestanding birth centers is the challenge. A sufficient number of midwives must be educated and prepared for employment in this expanding care model.

U.S. Maternity Care Provider Balance

In the U.S. context, there are many more obstetrician/gynecologists than midwives; therefore, it is important to understand trends in the OB/GYN workforce when considering women's access to a skilled maternity care provider and the anticipated role midwives will play going forward. The number of medical school graduates in the United States entering an OB/GYN residency has remained basically flat, at about 1,200 per year, for the past 30 years. In addition, the proportion of first-year OB/GYN residents who are female has changed substantially in that time period. At the beginning of that period, OB/GYN residents were almost all male, whereas at the time of this writing more than 80% of first-year OB/GYN residents are female (Association of American Medical Colleges [AAMC], 2014; Rayburn, 2011). Thus, the OB/GYN profession has transitioned from a primarily male to a largely female profession.

Natural increases in the number of pregnancies in the United States and flat entries into the obstetric profession, coupled with this demographic shift, have important ramifications for workforce capacity. Female physicians balance their lives differently than their male colleagues, working fewer hours per week across nearly their entire careers, retiring from obstetric practice several years earlier, and working part time much more frequently (Rayburn, 2011). In addition, the profession is experiencing an increasing number of residents subspecializing in fields that do not involve maternity care (e.g., gynecological oncology, pelvic reconstructive surgery; Rayburn, Gilstrap, & Williams, 2012). As a result of these factors, the American College of Obstetricians and Gynecologists (ACOG) has estimated that by 2050, the United States will face a shortage of between 15,723 and 21,723 OB/GYNs (Rayburn, 2011).

Educating more midwives is an excellent solution to this situation because their education is less expensive and more rapid than that of obstetricians. Midwives could attend a much larger percentage of uncomplicated births in the United States, taking significant pressure off the obstetric workforce. There is not a universally acknowledged estimate of the proportion of pregnant women who fall into low- or moderate-risk categories, the type of births that midwives most commonly attend. However, Centers for Disease Control and Prevention (CDC) assumptions and data can be used to estimate that 83% of first-time mothers are at low risk for a cesarean birth (Osterman & Martin, 2014) and the National Institutes of Health (NIH) has published statements about the prevalence of certain risk factors among pregnant women (National Institute of Child Health and Human Development, 2013). Furthermore, the United Nations Population Fund has estimated that properly trained midwives could provide 87% of maternity care needs (United Nations Population Fund, 2014).

It is a reasonable assumption that most women in the United States are likely to experience an uncomplicated birth and thus are good candidates for midwifery care. Because of this reality, many countries have structured their maternity care workforce so that the number of midwives exceeds that of obstetricians. A review of data on 20 high-resource countries shows that the median midwife-to-obstetrician ratio was 2.5 to 1. In the United States, for various reasons, this ratio is inverted; there are 0.28 midwives per obstetrician (American Midwifery Certification Board [AMCB], 2014; AAMC, 2014; Eguchi, 2009; Emons & Luiten, 2001; Rowland, McLeod, & Froese-Burns, 2012).

The assertion that midwives could attend a larger proportion of U.S. births is supported by actual data as well. For example, in several developed countries midwives attend between 70% and 80% of all births (Emons, 2001). In the United States, CNMs/CMs attended 8.33% of all births in 2014; however, in several states CNMs/CMs attended between 20% and 25% of births (CDC, 2014). Data on hospitals in New York and Massachusetts show that midwives attend between 30% and 70% of births in many facilities in those states (Bebinger, 2016; New York State Department of Health, 2014).

Parallel Growth of Midwives and Birth Centers

The case for a parallel scaling up of midwives and birth centers can be made. Improving the care experience and health outcomes for a population while at the same time reducing the costs fulfills the Triple Aim promoted by the Institute for Healthcare Improvement (IHI, n.d.; Berwick,

Nolan, & Whittington, 2008). In order to meet these needs, a plan for educating more midwives must be put into place. Increasing the number of midwives educated along with the number of freestanding birth centers in the United States would help solve both workforce issues and lower the cost of care with a demonstrated quality care clinician and care model.

If policy makers take steps to promote midwifery education, mainly by supporting efforts to support clinical preceptors, the midwifery workforce in the United States could be rapidly grown to address the slowly evolving, but critical shortage of maternity care providers in our country. In addition, policy changes removing barriers to birth center growth would allow this underused care model to increase and provide access for women who would choose this physiologic approach to labor and birth in the United States.

TASK SHIFTING TO PROMOTE PHYSIOLOGIC BIRTH

In 2012, ACNM, Midwives Alliance of North America (MANA), and the National Association of Certified Professional Midwives (NACPM) released a consensus statement supporting physiologic birth (ACNM, MANA, & NACPM, 2012). In 2015, the promotion of physiologic birth was identified as a national priority by the National Partnership for Women and Families (2015). Birth centers are a care setting where physiologic birth is actively promoted, in contrast to hospital settings, which typically have high rates of medical intervention. This signature strength of birth centers has been described for more than 25 years (Rooks et al., 1989). Yet, less than 1% of births in the United States occur in freestanding birth centers (U.S. Department of Health and Human Services, Centers for Disease Control and Prevention [CDC], and National Center for Health Statistics, 2014). Preparing the workforce to manage more births in birth centers, thus offering greater opportunity for physiologic birth, requires a thoughtful analysis of the concept of task shifting.

The Origins of the Task-Shifting Concept

Task shifting is a global strategy addressing the workforce shortage. It involves critical analysis of necessary tasks and delineating these tasks, within a community framework, to the most available health care workers. It often entails a shifting of skills and skill upgrading to less skilled workers in order to maximize health care coverage for populations at risk (Fullerton & Anderson, 2017). This concept was first proposed by the

Joint United Nations Programme on HIV/AIDS (UNAIDS), a division within the WHO, in response to the critical shortage of health care workers available to manage community-based HIV/AIDS programming (Piot, 2012; WHO, 2008a). The concept was rapidly adopted in international development planning and has been adapted to community-based care in both high- and low-resource nations (WHO, 2008b). By 2012, task shifting was endorsed by WHO as a strategy to disseminate essential care for mothers and newborns (WHO, 2015b). In a recent publication, O'Malley Floyd and Brunk (2016) examined this concept in the provision of rural, community-based midwifery care in Haiti, using exemplars from the organization *Midwives for Haiti.*

Task Shifting as a Strategy for Birth Center Care

Task shifting as a strategy to address limited human resources in maternity care can be extrapolated to improving access to safe birthing venues. Shifting the task of safe, affordable, and available care during childbearing to community-based birth centers is supported by the Affordable Care Act (ACA), evidenced by mandating Medicaid payment for services in state-licensed birth centers (Patient Protection and Affordable Care Act, 2009). Cost analysis and microcosting of task-shifting birth to community-based birth centers is currently being explored (Cole, Osborne, & Xu, 2015).

PREPARING THE MIDWIFERY WORKFORCE

For the birth center model to grow and function as anticipated, an adequate and well-trained workforce is required. In the United States, birth centers are primarily staffed by midwives with a range of educational backgrounds and preparation. This educational landscape for midwifery preparation is in variance to most other nations. In some nations, all nurses are trained in midwifery skills as part of basic nursing education. In other nations, midwifery is a specialty following nursing education or midwifery is a separate profession, unrelated to prior preparation as a nurse.

Pathways to Midwifery Education

In the United States, there are multiple pathways to becoming a midwife, some of which are not regulated or licensed.

Certified Nurse-Midwife

The predominant pattern is entry into midwifery education following completion of the bachelor's degree in nursing (BSN). Preparation for becoming a CNM is at the master's level in nursing or may lead directly to the doctor of nursing practice (DNP) degree. It culminates with eligibility to sit for the midwifery certification exam conducted by the AMCB. Nurses holding a master's or higher degree may complete a midwifery certification program without repeating the graduate-level courses in nursing (AMCB, 2015).

Another pathway is the accelerated master's or doctoral program for persons coming from a non-nursing background. Graduate programs such as these, in schools of nursing, prepare persons with other educational backgrounds (minimally baccalaureate level and often higher level degrees) for the nursing profession and for the advanced practice profession of nurse-midwifery. This preparation results in eligibility to sit for the national registered nurse licensure examination and then the AMCB midwifery certification exam. Additionally, those nurses who hold an associate degree can enter what is termed a "bridge" program, directly entering a master's program without earning a bachelor's degree, with the same eligibility to sit for state licensure and national certification exams. Some CNMs are choosing to pursue doctoral education in either a research or practice capacity. A growing workforce requires a growing pool of educators, and education at the doctoral level may be required by educational institutions to teach rising professionals in the midwifery field. CNMs have the legal authority to practice in all 50 states and U.S. territories (AMCB, 2015).

Certified Midwife

Preparation for the CM credential does not require preparation as a registered nurse. The candidate for this certification must already hold a graduate degree or earn one in the process of midwifery preparation, meet the same standards applicable to nurse-midwifery education, graduate from an ACME-accredited program, and take the same AMCB-administered midwifery certification exam.

Two programs in the United States currently offer preparation as a CM. CMs can legally practice in five states with a sixth anticipated soon. In contrast, 40 programs offer nurse-midwifery education. All graduates of CNM and CM preparation programs meet the standards of the WHO-sponsored International Confederation of Midwives (ICM), which requires a 3-year midwifery education program, or an 18-month program if nursing is prerequisite, with both didactic and clinical education (ICM,

2013). According to AMCB, the number of CNMs and CMs continues to rise (AMCB, 2014).

Direct-Entry Midwife

There are no degree requirements for the direct-entry midwife (DEM) with self-study and apprenticeship as the predominant learning modes. DEMs may be eligible to take the North American Registry of Midwives (NARM) examination, resulting in certification as a certified professional midwife (CPM). Eligibility is established by documenting self-study and apprenticeship or by completion of a direct-entry midwifery educational program accredited by the Midwifery Education Accreditation Council (MEAC; Cheyney et al., 2015; NARM, 2016). Some states require DEMs to be licensed and 28 states authorize practice (MANA, 2015). Oregon has provided leadership in the licensure of DEMs (Oregon Health Licensing Agency, 2015). It is possible to practice as a licensed midwife (LM) if a state has that provision without also requiring certification as a CNM, CM, or CPM.

U.S. Midwifery Education, Regulation, and Association

The U.S. Midwifery Education, Regulation, and Association (USMERA) developed as a coalition of the various midwifery organizations in the United States seeking to build collaboration, promote physiologic birth, and create a common understanding of meeting ICM standards (USMERA, 2015). The landscape for entry into the midwifery profession in the United States is quite complex; most other nations have government-regulated midwifery education; however, consistency with ICM standards is quite variable (Bharj et al., 2016). Those practicing outside of this formal midwifery framework are identified as *traditional birth attendants* (TBAs) and usually do not have legal status.

The Birth Center Workforce

When considering the educational preparation of the birth center workforce, an examination of who comprises that workforce naturally follows. (For a more complete discussion of providers of birth center care, see Chapter 7.) In the United States, clinicians attending births in birth centers may include CNMs, CMs, CPMs, LMs, obstetricians, family practice physicians, or naturopathic physicians. In addition, other cadres of personnel function in support capacities in birth centers including nurse practitioners, registered nurses, and administrative and office managers. The most common birth attendant is the midwife. In 2013, government statistics indicated that the majority of births in birth centers were attended by CNMs and CMs. Of 16,913 births that occurred in birth centers in that year, 53% were attended by CNMs or CMs (Martin, Hamilton, Osterman, Curtin, & Mathews, 2015).

Most CNMs and CMs do not receive clinical experience in birth centers during their education. Their clinical experience occurs primarily in the hospital setting. Although their education meets ICM standards, they rarely have the opportunity to participate in community-based births, in a birth center or at home. Conversely, the education of CPMs and LMs, while not always consistent with ICM standards, provides experience in home and/or birth center settings. There is a need to increase the clinical experience of all categories of midwives in the United States in the birth center setting in order to reach the imperative of safe, affordable, and available community-based care. The experience is especially lacking in CNM and CM educational programs, creating barriers to adequate preparation of the workforce in birth center care and scaling up the availability of birth center care.

SCALING UP MIDWIFERY EDUCATION FOR BIRTH CENTER COMPETENCE

Barriers to Birth Center Education for Midwives

The United States lacks a national system of planning for health care professional education. The projections of retirement, attrition, and entrance into the health professions have been haphazard compared with more centrally planned economies. The popular press regularly publishes dire predictions, especially related to the impending nursing shortage. The fact that midwifery education in the United States is closely tied to the nursing pipeline can exacerbate the low availability of midwives. An idea to recruit more nurses to midwifery is to introduce midwifery in a more prominent way in undergraduate nursing programs with more content related to midwifery. This might ignite an earlier passion for the nursing route to midwifery. Furthermore, unlike most developed nations, the United States does not have a seamless system of referral from community-based systems of birth to high-acuity settings in an emergency transfer. The highly litigious environment surrounding health care and the lack of a well-coordinated referral system from community to hospital-based care in many communities can create an environment of fear around educating student midwives in birth centers.

In some midwifery education programs, the birth center model is promoted as a community-based model. Although there are more birth centers than ever before and the number increases every year, there are simply not enough birth centers to meet the demand for clinical placements. With 375 birth centers known to exist in the United States (S. Stapleton, personal communication, March 31, 2016) and with only approximately one fourth of those having attained accreditation, often a requirement for student program placement, it is easy to see the deficit this presents. Many more accredited birth centers are needed in order to create these clinical experiences for midwifery students.

Establishing the Conversation About Birth Center Education

A critical need in midwifery education is a broad-based conversation about ways to scale up the birth center experience. This conversation needs to include stakeholders from multiple backgrounds, not just educators. Creating a community-based learning environment includes public health workers, community citizens, hospital administrators, health professional cadres operating in hospitals, emergency room personnel, and first responders, among others. "Effective collaborations between midwifery education providers and clinical partners to adequately prepare students for their future midwifery practice should be promoted" (Bharj et al., 2016, p. 3).

Creating Communities of Practice

Setting up "communities of practice" as described by Bharj et al. (2016) is an essential first step. Educational institutions should offer faculty status to community-based birth center practitioners in order to empower their role as educators. Practitioners need to open clinical placements for students as future birth center practitioners and owners. One way to bridge this practice–education chasm is for educational programs to invest in university-linked birth centers. Such a facility not only provides a service for the community and a learning environment for midwifery students, but is also an excellent site for faculty practice. Modeling through faculty practice with a student at one's elbow is a powerful learning strategy for deep learning during midwifery education.

A key element in fostering collaborative communities of practice is providing interprofessional education (IPE). WHO and the Institute of

Medicine (IOM) have both promoted this approach to health professional learning (IOM, 2003; WHO, 2010). The IOM document, *Health Professions Education: A Bridge to Quality* (2003), is regarded as a mandate for improving quality of care. A central premise in both WHO and IOM documents is creating a culture of respectful teamwork (IOM, 2003; WHO, 2010). The Interprofessional Education Collaborative (IPEC), a coalition of health professionals from multiple disciplines, convened an expert panel to frame the competencies for IPE, first published in 2011 and updated in 2016 (IPEC, 2016). The basic assumption is that health professional students learning together in a community of collaboration will develop essential competencies and skills for bridging levels of care that they can use or build on following their education programs.

Designing Curricular Approaches to Promote Birth Centers

The AABC regularly conducts a workshop, "How to Start a Birth Center," which addresses the business of midwifery and how to create a community-based practice (AABC, 2015). The workshop is currently offered five times per year in locations around the United States. It is attended by nurses, midwives, physicians, hospital administrators, and others considering starting a birth center, as well as midwifery students required by their educational program to take the course. The workshops fill up quickly, and require a substantial expense, which is often challenging for students who must typically travel to the workshop location. Ideally, this workshop would be included in midwifery education programs as an integral part of the curriculum. A possible opportunity to increase the number of programs offering this preparation would be to offer the workshop as an online course with self-paced modules, making it available to more students.

Another curricular approach is to use high-fidelity simulation techniques in portraying and critically reviewing birth center scenarios. This approach is powerful in exemplifying physiologic birth, teamwork, and the judgment and management required for referral to higher acuity care and hospital settings. These simulations can occur on a continuum of least to most complex and from early labor to postpartum and newborn care. Examples of simulations based on care delivered at a birth center are included in Table 12.1. The clinical scenarios displayed can occur in any setting, but the processes of assessment and clinical decision making are unique in the birth center setting, given the limited resources and possible need for transfer to a hospital. Of note is that even though the predominant practitioner in birth centers is the midwife, nursing students

TABLE 12.1
Clinical Simulations for Birth Center Professionals

Simulation Scenario	Relevance to Birth Center Care	Skills Learned
Early labor phone call notification	Birth centers usually not staffed 24/7; good stewardship of staff resources requires timing of triage visits to the birth center for labor admission Since admission is typically in active labor, it is important to be in touch and provide phone support in early labor	Listening to key words, and through a contraction Asking the right questions Developing plan to call back or come in Deciding whether to call in other staff prior to woman's arrival
Intermittent auscultation monitoring in different positions	Not the standard in all hospital settings, even for women without risk factors IA is primary method of monitoring in BC so skill essential	Keeping woman's comfort in mind vs. provider convenience Key phrases to use to help woman move if she needs to
Birth in different positions and in tub	Limited toolbox in birth center setting for comfort measures. Ambulation, upright positioning, and water immersion are frequently used Women in birth centers expect to choose their position for delivery	Fetal presentation in relation to maternal position Respecting woman's choice and not compromising safety Knowing when position needs to change based on fetal response and descent
FHR decelerations in second stage with multiparous woman	Critical judgment needed to understand and interpret safety of continued care in BC vs. the need to transfer to higher level care, which may be a distance away	What is likely normal Interventions to employ When to activate EMS How to arrange for emergency transfer and notify receiving facility staff and provider
Prolonged pushing with primigravid woman	Fatigue must be guarded against in order for woman to maintain stamina—use of rest, oral hydration, and nutrition are very important IVs not used routinely in birth centers	Normal vs. abnormal limits Referring to clinical guidelines When/how to consult

(continued)

TABLE 12.1
Clinical Simulations for Birth Center Professionals *(continued)*

Simulation Scenario	Relevance to Birth Center Care	Skills Learned
Labor dystocia and transfer to the hospital	Pitocin not used for labor augmentation in the birth center Toolkit for labor augmentation is limited Major change in birth plan for woman—emotional support is necessary during this transition	Referring to clinical guidelines When/how to consult and arrange for transfer How to transfer? Ambulance? Family car? Receiving team SBAR reporting Maintaining woman's birth plan as much as possible Examination of best practices and tools for transfer
Retained placenta without bleeding	No access to anesthesia Employment of natural remedies such as breastfeeding, squatting	Appropriate out-of-hospital interventions When/how to consult
Retained placenta with bleeding	No access to anesthesia or operating room Distance from hospital and time involved to transfer	Manual removal skills Activating EMS Arranging for transfer/referral
Postpartum hemorrhage	Pharmacological and nonmedical therapy options Evaluation of patient status and likelihood for resolution, critical assessment of safety in BC vs. need to transfer Emotional support for change in PP recovery plan	Medical interventions Activating EMS Arranging for transfer/referral

BC, birth center; EMS, emergency medical services; FHR, fetal heart rate; IA, intermittent auscultation; IV, intravenous; PP, postpartum; SBAR, situation, background, assessment, recommendation.

can learn by being involved with many of these simulations, as well as medical students and residents. Although most physicians will not practice in a birth center, they would benefit by learning more about physiologic birth as well as how complications and transfers are handled in the birth center setting. Ultimately, with IPE will come an increased understanding of the birth center environment and respect for each other's profession and scope of practice.

The Case for Establishing Fellowships in Birth Centers

Fellowships that bridge the gap between students and practitioners are another way to address the lack of clinical opportunities in birth centers for students. An early example is the fellowship program at Holy Family Services Birth Center, the oldest known birth center in Texas, founded by Sister Angela Murdaugh (see Chapter 1). The Midwife Center for Birth and Women's Health in Pittsburgh, Pennsylvania, the exemplar birth center at the conclusion of this chapter, provides another example of a birth center fellowship program. A fellowship is a contractual agreement for a specified period of time, designed to immerse the new graduate in birth center practice with structured orientation and mentoring in place. In addition to providing support for new graduates assuming their professional role, a fellowship also benefits the birth center by adding professional staff when needed and allows other midwives in the practice to assume expanded roles including leadership or administrative activities (McCarthy, 2015). Even if the midwifery fellow or the birth center choose not to continue employment at the conclusion of the fellowship, the new midwife has learned the art of midwifery care in a supportive birth center environment, and can carry that anywhere into future practice; in addition, the birth center has at least temporarily filled a staffing need.

CONCLUSION

Increased attention to the role midwifery plays in positively impacting health outcomes for women and children internationally has brought an awareness of the need to increase the number of midwives to meet the gap in access to care. Scaling up of midwifery educational programs and community-based clinical sites is needed to adequately increase the maternity workforce. Task shifting of the existing workforce is called for immediately to meet critical national and international need.

The integration of systems of education and practice are essential for quality of care and the promotion of population-based health. This is especially true when considering the needs of women and families in the United States for patient-centered, cost effective maternity care. The birth center setting offers a substantial opportunity to extend the task-shifting concept in the United States for the promotion of physiologic birth and population-based health and meeting the triple aim. It is an essential step toward the creation of a system that places individual resiliency and empowerment at the core of health care (Anderson, 2012).

Major barriers to this public health initiative are the absence of a seamless approach to care between community-based and acute care systems and an insufficiently prepared workforce to lead this initiative. Task shifting the care of normal, low-risk birth to birth centers, increasing the number of midwives educated in the United States, and exposing other clinicians to the birth center model is in line with these public health principles. Preparing the midwifery workforce for competence in community-based birth center care through creatively integrating content and skills particular to birth center practice into basic midwifery education is the first step to removing these barriers.

EXEMPLAR BIRTH CENTER
The Midwife Center for Birth and Women's Health, Pittsburgh, Pennsylvania

Year established: 1982

Type of building/square feet/architectural features: 5,000 square foot brownstone

Location: Urban

Business structure: Not-for-profit

Ownership: Board of directors

Licensed as: Birth center

Accredited by: Commission for the Accreditation of Birth Centers

Number of births to date/births per year: Almost 6,000 total to date and about 450 per year

Services/Enhanced services: Primary GYN; lactation consultant and classes

(continued)

EXEMPLAR BIRTH CENTER *(continued)*

Providers: CNMs and CRNP

Client mix: 85% private insurance and 15% Medicaid; 50% from City of Pittsburgh and 50% from surrounding suburban and rural areas

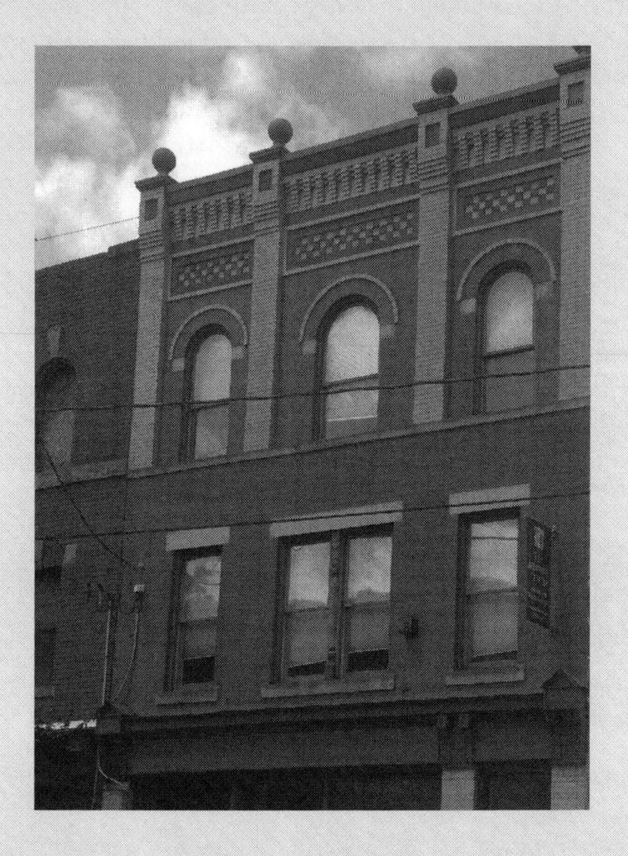

Opened in 1982, the Midwife Center (TMC) remains the only licensed, freestanding birth center in Western Pennsylvania. In 2000, TMC incorporated as an independent not-for-profit practice and has worked to increase public awareness of the many benefits of its services and raise additional funds to create innovative programs for women who experience barriers to care, make facility and technology upgrades, and expand programs to mentor new health care professionals. TMC provided more than 1,500 primary care appointments and had 454 babies born in the practice in 2015.

(continued)

EXEMPLAR BIRTH CENTER *(continued)*

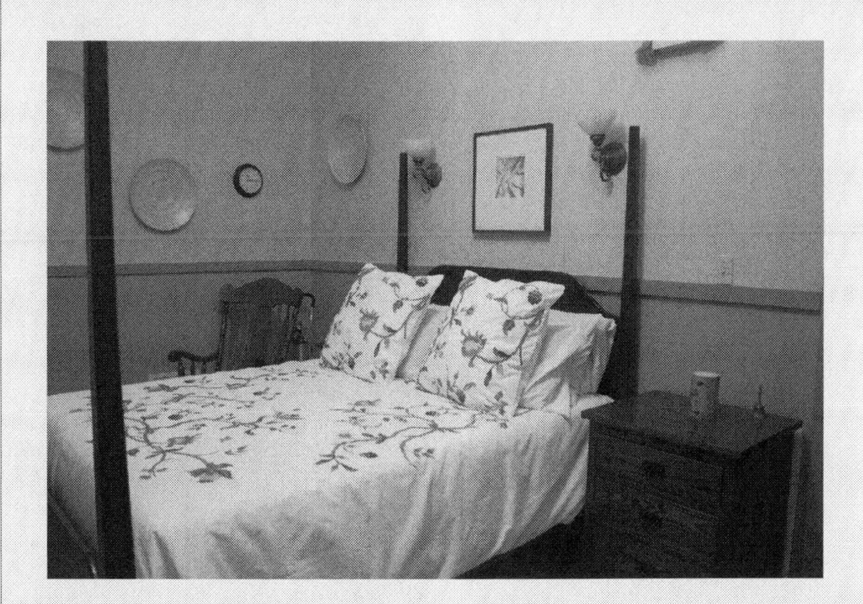

TMC combines evidence-based and compassionate care to provide high-quality primary gynecological, pregnancy, and birthing services to women in Southwestern Pennsylvania, and a safe, cost-effective, personal alternative to having a baby in a hospital. The midwives care for women in labor and attend births at the birth center as well as University of Pittsburgh Medical Center Mercy, TMC's primary referral hospital since late 2009. This relationship allows TMC midwives to call upon medical specialists for consultation, collaboration, and referral when necessary.

In 2010, TMC developed the Ruth B. Stifel fellowship for new graduate nurse-midwives. The program was designed to attract midwives to out-of-hospital birth, while serving the staffing needs of the center. The program has graduated 10 fellows and hired four of them. Other birth centers have also adopted similar fellowship programs. The fellowship lasts for up to 1 year and includes an orientation time of up to 4 months to allow for close mentorship and training by TMC senior midwives and medical director (MD). The fellowship includes outside educational experiences and attending one conference, such as the AABC's Birth Institute.

REFERENCES

Alliman, J., Jolles, D., & Summers L. (2015). The innovation imperative: Scaling freestanding birth centers, CenteringPregnancy, and midwifery-led maternity health homes. *Journal of Midwifery and Women's Health, 60*(3), 244–249. doi:10.1111/jmwh.12320

American Association of Birth Centers. (2013). AABC leads successful national grant award with 48 local birth center sites [Press Release March 1, 2013]. Retrieved from http://www.birthcenters.org/news/news.asp?id=229197&terms=%22strong+and+start+and+mothers%22

American Association of Birth Centers. (2015). How to start a birth center workshop. Retrieved from http://www.birthcenters.org/?page=hsbc_workshops

American College of Nurse-Midwives and Accreditation Commission for Midwifery Education. (2015). Midwifery education trends report 2015. Retrieved from http://www.midwife.org/ACNM/files/ACNMLibraryData/UPLOADFILENAME/000000000295/ACNM-Midwifery-Ed-Trends-Report

American College of Nurse-Midwives, Midwives Alliance of North America, and National Association of Certified Professional Midwives. (2012). Supporting healthy and normal physiologic childbirth: A consensus statement by ACNM, MANA, and NACPM. Retrieved from http://mana.org/pdfs/Physiological-Birth-Consensus-Statement.pdf

American Midwifery Certification Board. (2014). American Midwifery Certification Board annual report. Retrieved from https://www.midwife.org/2014AnnualReport

American Midwifery Certification Board. (2015). Why AMCB certification? Retrieved from http://www.amcbmidwife.org/amcb-certification/why-amcb-certification-

Anderson, B. (2012). Healthy communities and vulnerability: Enhancing curricula for teaching population-based nursing. In M. deChesnay & B. Anderson (Eds.), *Caring for the vulnerable: Perspectives in nursing theory, research, and practice* (3rd ed., pp. 455–463). Boston, MA: Jones & Bartlett.

Association of American Medical Colleges. (2014). *2014 Physician specialty data book*. AAMC Center for Workforce Studies: Washington, DC. Retrieved from https://members.aamc.org/eweb/upload/14-086%20Specialty%20Databook%202014_711.pdf

Bebinger, M. (2016). Midwives handle 16 percent of Mass. births, and there's a wide range among hospitals. Retrieved from http://www.wbur.org/commonhealth/2016/03/03/midwives-massachusetts

Berwick, D. M., Nolan, D. W., & Whittington, J. (2008). The Triple Aim: Care, health and cost. *Health Affairs, 27*(3), 759–769. doi:10.1377/hlthaff.27.3.759

Bharj, K. K., Luyden, A., Avery, M., Johnson, P., O'Connell, R., Barger, M., & Bick, D. (2016). An agenda for midwifery education: Advancing the state of the world's midwifery. *Midwifery, 33*, 3–6. Retrieved from doi:10.1016/j.midw.2016.01.004

Centers for Disease Control and Prevention. (2014). VitalStats—births. Retrieved from https://www.cdc.gov/nchs/data/nvsr/nvsr64/nvsr64_12.pdf

Cheyney, M., Olsen, C., Bovbjerg, M., Everson, C., Darragh, I., & Potter, B. (2015). Practitioner and practice characteristics of certified professional midwives in the United States: Results of the 2011 North American Registry of Midwives survey. *Journal of Midwifery and Women's Health, 60*(5), 534–545. doi:10.1111/jmwh.12367

Cole, L., Osborne, K., & Xu, X. (2015). Micro-costing analysis of a freestanding birth center: Development of a data collection tool. In B. A. Anderson, J. M. Knestrick, & R. Barroso (Eds.), *DNP capstone projects: Exemplars of excellence in practice* (pp. 79–85). New York, NY: Springer Publishing.

Eguchi, N. (2009). Do we have enough obstetricians? A survey of the Japan Medical Association in 15 countries. *Japan Medical Association Journal, 52*(3), 150–157.
Emons, J. K., & Luiten, M. I. J. (2001). *Midwifery in Europe: An inventory in fifteen EU-member states.* Retrieved from http://www.deloitte.nl/downloads/documents/website_deloitte/GZpublVerloskundeinEuropaRapport.pdf
Fullerton, J. T., & Anderson, B. A. (2017). The midwifery workforce: Issues globally and in the United States. In B. A. Anderson, J. P. Rooks, & R. Barroso (Eds.), *Best practices in midwifery: Using the evidence to implement change* (2nd ed., pp. 3–22). New York, NY: Springer Publishing.
Homer, C., Friberg, I., Bastos Dias, M., Hoope-Bender, P., Sandall, J., Speciale, A., & Bartlett, L. (2014). The projected effect of scaling up midwifery. *Lancet, 384*(9948), 1146–1157. doi:10.1016/S0140-6736(14)60790-X
Institute for Healthcare Improvement. (n.d.). Triple Aim for populations. Retrieved from http://www.ihi.org/Topics/TripleAim/Pages/Overview.aspx
Institute of Medicine. (2003). *Health professions education: A bridge to quality.* Washington, DC: National Academies Press. Retrieved from http://iom.nationalacademies.org/Reports/2003/Health-Professions-Education-A-Bridge-to-Quality.aspx
International Confederation of Midwives. (2013). *Global standards for midwifery education, with companion guidelines* (ICM Core Document 2010, amended 2013). Retrieved from http://www.internationalmidwives.org/assets/uploads/documents/Global%20Standards%20Comptencies%20Tools/English/MIDWIFERY%20EDUCATION%20PREFACE%20&%20STANDARDS%20ENG.pdf
Interprofessional Education Collaborative. (2016). *Core competencies for interprofessional collaborative practice: 2016 update.* Washington, DC: Author. Retrieved from http://www.aacn.nche.edu/education-resources/IPEC-2016-Updated-Core-Competencies-Report.pdf
Kassebaum, N. J., Bertozzi-Villa, A., Coggeshall, M. S., Shackelford, K. A., Steiner, C., Heuton, K. R., . . . Lozano, R. (2014). Global, regional, and national levels and causes of maternal mortality during 1990–2013: A systematic analysis for the Global Burden of Disease Study. *Lancet, 384*(9947), 980–1004. doi:10.1016/S0140-6736(14)60696-6
Martin, J. A., Hamilton, B. E., Osterman, M. J., Curtin, S. C., & Mathews, T. J. (2015). Births: Final data for 2013. *National Vital Statistics Reports, 64*(1), 1–65.
McCarthy, A. M. (2015). Benefits and challenges of a nurse-midwife fellowship: A review of the Ruth B. Stifel Fellowship Program at the Midwife Center for Birth and Women's Health. *Journal of Midwifery and Women's Health, 60*(3), 263–266.
Midwives Alliance of North America. (2015). Legal status of U.S. midwives. Retrieved from http://mana.org/about-midwives/legal-status-of-us-midwives
National Institute of Child Health and Human Development. (2013). How many people are at risk of having a high-risk pregnancy? Retrieved from https://www.nichd.nih.gov/health/topics/high-risk/conditioninfo/Pages/risk.aspx
National Partnership for Women and Families. (2015). Transforming maternity care: Improvement tools. Retrieved from http://transform.childbirthconnection.org/resources
New York State Department of Health. (2014). NYS health profiles: Attended by midwife. Retrieved from https://profiles.health.ny.gov/measures/all_state/16523
North American Registry of Midwives. (2016). Written exam questions and scoring. Retrieved from http://narm.org/testing/written-exam-questions-and-scoring
O'Malley Floyd, B., & Brunk, N. (2016). Utilizing task shifting to increase access to maternal and infant health intervention: A case study of Midwives for Haiti. *Journal of Midwifery and Women's Health, 61*(1), 103–111. doi:1111/jmwh.12396

Oregon Health Licensing Agency. (2015). Direct entry midwifery legend drugs and devices. Continuing education (renewal). Retrieved from http://www.oregon.gov/OHLA/DEM/docs/DEM_continuing_education/Education_Curriculum_-_Continuing.pdf

Osterman, M. J. K., & Martin, J. A. (2014). Trends in low-risk cesarean delivery in the United States, 1990–2013. *National Vital Statistics Reports, 63*(6). Retrieved from http://www.cdc.gov/nchs/data/nvsr/nvsr63/nvsr63_06.pdf

Patient Protection and Affordable Care Act of 2009, H.R. 3590, 111th Cong. (2009). Retrieved from http://www.govtrack.us/congress/bill.xpd?bill=h111-3590

Piot, P. (2012). *No time to lose: A life in pursuit of deadly viruses.* New York, NY: W. W. Norton.

Rayburn, W. F. (2011). *The obstetrician gynecologist workforce in the United States: Facts, figures, and implications.* Washington, DC: American Congress of Obstetricians and Gynecologists.

Rayburn, W. F., Gilstrap, G. N., & Williams, E. E. (2012). Pursuit of accredited subspecialties by graduating residents in obstetrics and gynecology, 2000–2012. *Obstetrics and Gynecology, 120,* 619–625.

Renfrew, M. J., McFadden, A., Bastos, M. H., Campbell, J., Channon, A. A., Cheung, N. F., . . . Declercq, E. (2014). Midwifery and quality care: Findings from a new evidence-based informed framework for maternal and newborn care. *Lancet, 384*(9948), 1129–1145. doi:10.1016/S0140-6736(14)60789-3

Riley, P. (2016). Health systems and human resources for health: New dimensions in global health nursing. In M. deChesnay & B. A. Anderson (Eds.), *Caring for the vulnerable: Perspectives in nursing theory, research, and practice* (4th ed., pp. 573–598). Burlington, MA: Jones & Bartlett.

Rooks, J. P. (1997). *Midwifery and childbirth in America.* Philadelphia, PA: Temple University Press.

Rooks, J. P., Weatherby, N. L., Ernst, E. K. M., Stapleton, S., Rosen, D., & Rosenfield, A. (1989). Outcomes of care in birth centers: The national birth center study. *New England Journal of Medicine, 321*(26), 1804–1811.

Rowland, T., McLeod, D., & Froese-Burns, N. (2012). Comparative study of maternity systems. Retrieved from http://www.health.govt.nz/publication/comparative-study-maternity-systems

United Nations Population Fund. (2014). The state of the world's midwifery 2014. Retrieved from http://www.unfpa.org/sowmy

U.S. Department of Health and Human Services, Centers for Disease Control and Prevention, and National Center for Health Statistics. (2013). National Vital Statistics Information 2013. Retrieved from https://www.cdc.gov/nchs/births.htm

U.S. Midwifery Education, Regulation, & Association. (2015). Creating the future of midwifery in the U.S. Retrieved from https://www.usmera.org

World Health Organization. (2008a). First global conference on task shifting. Retrieved from http://www.who.int/healthsystems/task_shifting/en

World Health Organization. (2008b). Task shifting: Global recommendations and guidelines. Retrieved from http://www.who.int/workforcealliance/knowledge/resources/taskshifting_guidelines/en

World Health Organization. (2010). Framework for action on interprofessional education and collaborative practice. Retrieved from http://apps.who.int/iris/bitstream/10665/70185/1/WHO_HRH_HPN_10.3_eng.pdf

World Health Organization. (2015a). World health statistics. Retrieved from http://www.who.int/gho/publications/world_health_statistics/EN_WHS2015_Part2.pdf?ua=1

World Health Organization. (2015b). Global strategy for women's, children's and adolescent's health, 2016–2030. Retrieved from http://www.who.int/life-course/partners/global-strategy/global-strategy-2016-2030/en/?utm_source=MHTF+Subscribers&utm_campaign=97a8a8fb80-MH_Buzz_Sept_29_2015&utm_medium=email&utm_term=0_8ac9c53ad4-97a8a8fb80-183740093

Zureick-Brown, S., Newby, H., Chou, D., Mizoguchi, N. M., Say, L., Suzuki, E., & Wilmoth, J. (2013). Understanding global trends in maternal mortality. *International Perspectives on Sexual and Reproductive Health, 39*(1), 32–41. doi:10.1363/3903213

CHAPTER 13

Launching a Birth Center

CYNTHIA FLYNN AND
BRIANNA HONEA BENNETT

LEARNING OBJECTIVES

Upon completion of this chapter, the reader will be able to:

1. Assess community need and create a mission statement for a new birth center
2. Understand the different kinds of business structures
3. Explain the elements of a business plan
4. Project start-up utilization, revenue, and expenses for a new birth center
5. Anticipate the unique business challenges that birth centers may face

This chapter is a brief summary of the process of getting a birth center launched. The material is divided into three major sections. The Early Planning section describes a process for assessing the community's need for a birth center and identifying and addressing any regulatory, financial, or other barriers to starting the birth center. Next, the Start-Up section identifies all of the resources needed before the birth center opens for business. Finally, the Business Plan section describes how the revenue and expenditures of the birth center will be accumulated and dispersed during the first 5 years of operation. After 5 years, the birth center's volume of business has either reached its breakeven or, in some cases, the volume and profitability of the center are large enough to warrant creating a larger or second center.

EARLY PLANNING

Community Assessment

Starting a birth center requires an assessment of the community's readiness to accept and grow the center. The Commission for the Accreditation of Birth Centers (CABC) has compiled a list of indicators that can be helpful in assessing the community (CABC, 2015). These include:

- Definition of the expected area that will be served by the birth center. Consider both distance and travel time at different times of the year in estimating the service area.
- Demographics and vital statistics of the population served, including race, ethnicity, cultural and religious background, socioeconomic status, education, and immigration status. Data from the National Vital Statistics Reports for 2013 showed that the percentage of non-Hispanic White births that occurred in a birth center was 0.66%, whereas the percentage of Hispanic births that occurred in a birth center was only 0.17%, or about a quarter of the rate for Whites (Martin, Hamilton, Osterman, Curtin, & Mathews, 2015). Understanding how demographic subgroups in the service area view birth center care and assessing their access to care is critical to sound planning for sustainability and growth (see Chapter 5).
- Current availability of and access to maternal and newborn services, including practitioners, hospital obstetrical and newborn services, home birth services, family-centered maternity care programs, birth rooms/suites, and clinics for underserved families, that is, a complete picture of services available for pregnant women. As these data are compiled, it is also useful to assess the availability of potential collaborators and assess whether there are other new services in planning stages.
- Availability of ancillary services, such as ambulance, ultrasound, laboratory, and medical waste disposal services. These services should be easily available to support the operations of a birth center.
- Total birth volume in the service area, perinatal outcome data. Nationally, birth center births comprise about 0.5% of the 4 million births each year. In some smaller communities, birth centers may accommodate as many as 30% of the births. However, now it is more common that after 5 years, the birth center(s) midwives in a community will be attending at most 1% to 3% of the births (2–6 times the national average of birth

center births), depending upon community receptivity. For planning purposes, calculating 3% of the total volume of births in an area gives a rough estimate of the likely maximum demand for birth center services. In communities with a single hospital that has a very high cesarean rate, the demand for birth center care may be greater.

It is also useful to consider whether women are choosing to leave the area in order to receive midwifery and/or birth center services, whether women currently choosing home birth would prefer birth center birth, or whether women are receiving suboptimal care due to the high cost of accessing currently available services; these factors can indicate that there is a need for a birth center in the community. At the national level, a well-designed study showed that about a quarter of women who gave birth in the hospital definitely want a birth center for their next birth and an additional 39% would consider it (see Chapter 5). However, there are not easy ways to gather such helpful information for a specific community; focus groups or formal surveys may be needed to obtain these data.

Taking the time to do a thorough community assessment will ensure that the assumptions made in the business plan will have a sound basis in reality. The assessment will also be helpful in preparing for accreditation. Periodic updates of the community assessment make it more likely that the birth center staff will continue to be aware of any changes that may occur in the service area.

Mission Statement

A mission statement is a statement describing the purpose of the birth center and what it intends to accomplish. Typically, it will appear on the birth center's web page, Facebook page, press releases, and similar sources available to the public (see Box 13.1). The mission statement also forms the basis of the strategic plan, which includes specific, measurable, attainable, realistic, and time-specific (SMART) goals and a design for achieving them.

McMurry University (n.d.) suggests nine components to consider in constructing a mission statement:

1. *Customers:* Who are the birth center's customers?
2. *Products or services:* What are the birth center's major services and/or products?

3. *Markets:* Where does the firm compete?
4. *Technology:* What is the firm's basic technology (For birth centers: What is the basic approach to caring for women, especially at the time of birth?)
5. *Concern for survival, growth, and profitability:* What is the birth center's commitment toward economic objectives?
6. *Philosophy:* What are the basic beliefs, core values, aspirations, and philosophical priorities of the birth center?
7. *Self-concept:* What are the birth center's major strengths and competitive advantages?
8. *Concern for public image:* What is the birth center's public image?
9. *Concern for employees:* What is the birth center's attitude/orientation toward employees?

Structure of the Business

In most jurisdictions, a business license and/or occupancy permit is required before the business opens. In order to apply for a business license, decisions must be made about the legal structure of the business. In addition, programmatic decisions should be made about how the birth center will operate.

BOX 13.1
Sample Mission Statement

Anytown Birth Center provides maternity services in the greater AnyCounty area for women who are expecting a normal pregnancy. Services include prenatal care, including childbirth education, childbirth at the birth center in a homelike environment, breastfeeding support, and postpartum care, including a home visit. We are committed to spending the necessary time throughout the maternity period to ensure that women feel supported to have a healthy pregnancy, safe delivery, and successful parenting experience. We strive to have the best maternity outcomes in the area for healthy women by providing personalized care for each woman using the midwifery model of care. We provide excellent care not only to our clients, but to our staff as well, with a generous benefit package and adequate time for them to be with their own families.

Types of Legal Structure

The broad types of legal structure used by birth centers, some with several subcategories, are a sole proprietorship, an S-corporation, a partnership, a limited liability company, and a not-for-profit or for-profit corporation (C-corporation). Some states have an additional structure, a benefit corporation, which is a hybrid between a not-for-profit and a for-profit company whose success is measured both by sustainability and by the specific benefits it provides to society, rather than monetary returns to its investors (B-corporation).

The Small Business Administration (SBA) has extensive, user-friendly information about each type of structure, which legal structures will work best in a specific situation (requirements, advantages and disadvantages), and how to get started with each one (SBA, n.d.-a).

A question asked by many start-ups is whether to be for-profit or not-for-profit. The primary advantages of a not-for-profit are that they do not pay ordinary income taxes, and they can accept tax-deductible donations from individuals and grants from foundations. The primary challenges of not-for-profits are that there must be a board of directors that has final responsibility for all decisions, including employment of the senior management team—that is, the founder—and, in exchange for not paying income taxes, a 990 form must be filed each year. The 990 is a public document that includes detailed financial and other information about the firm, and verification that guidelines about the percentage of income that is used for various functions (including salaries) are being met. The primary advantages of a for-profit are that the founder retains control of the firm, its financials are not public documents, and the allocation of the company's resources is determined by the center's management team. The tax implications for the various forms of for-profit companies are discussed in the SBA monographs for each type of business structure (SBA, n.d.). Another resource is "Should Your Business Be Nonprofit or For-Profit?" (Chen, 2013).

Board of Directors

If the birth center is organized as a not-for-profit organization, a board of directors is required. Many for-profit corporations also have a board that serves similar functions. Selecting directors who possess the skill set necessary to do the job is important. Skills include being able to read and analyze financial statements, understanding contracts and the health care system, the willingness to be politically engaged on behalf of the birth center, and the ability to think about long-term goals and strategies. In the case of not-for-profits, board members are expected to make an annual contribution to the birth center. In the case of for-profits, boards frequently include the investors.

Professionals with the skills for the board of directors may include accountants, lawyers, people with master of business administration degrees (MBAs), business owners, and other seasoned business professionals. Although business people can be immensely helpful, one of the most important attributes of a good board member is mission buy-in and understanding of the birth center culture. Choosing board members who are supportive and offer compassion, insight, and sound guidance is most important. Board members who have been a client or family member of a birth center client have a quicker learning curve than those who have not, and are often more invested in the mission of the organization.

Birth centers are also encouraged to have a citizen's advisory group composed of clients of the center, especially if they lack a board of directors. This group can provide feedback to management regarding marketing, client care, ease of use of the facility, and trends in the community that affect the birth center.

Open and Closed Models

Most birth centers are "closed models," which means that the providers who practice at the birth center are its owners or employees. This model is advantageous because everyone provides care using the same protocols; the clients are all clients of the birth center, and therefore known to the providers and birth center management; and employees are required to participate in emergency drills and quality improvement initiatives as part of their job descriptions.

Some birth centers use an "open model." This means that providers who are not employees of the birth center can attend births at the facility. This model is particularly helpful in communities that already have several independent practitioners, especially early on before the birth center is filled to capacity. These independent providers would bill insurers separately. However, the birth center can bill a service fee for the use of the facility, just as a hospital would, which is a supplemental source of income.

Open model birth centers do require additional management skills. Each midwife must be credentialed as a birth center provider, and it is recommended that they sign a contract with the birth center stating their mutual obligations. In order to ensure that space is available for everyone planning to use the birth center, outside practitioners need to apprise birth center management of their clients planning a birth center birth by 30 weeks of pregnancy. Birth center management should review the prenatal record at about 36 weeks for consistency with birth center risk assessment policies, and start a birth center record for the client. Original records of the period from admission to discharge remain at the birth center. When the mother and newborn are discharged from the practitioner's care at about 6 to 8 weeks postpartum, notes from the postpartum period should be provided to the birth center so that the birth center has a record of the full episode of maternity care. All practitioners should participate in regular fire and emergency drills for mother and fetus/baby, and in quality improvement/ peer review activities. A process should be documented for suspension or termination of privileges.

Finally, decisions must be made about any enhanced services that are planned (see Chapter 10). Examples of such services offered by birth centers include childbirth education and related classes (e.g., parenting, car seat safety, and so forth), retail store, breastfeeding support for women who are not clients, milk bank, doulas, patient navigators, peer counselors, massage or chiropractic care, acupuncture, yoga or prenatal exercise, nutrition counseling, and social work. Choosing which services to offer, and deciding whether to contract for the services or hire employees, depends both on the space available and community demand, as well as the availability of management time to ensure the quality of such services.

Space Considerations

Licensure

If the birth center is located in a state that requires licensure, there may be regulations about spaces the facility must include and their size. A common criterion is that birth rooms must be larger than a minimum square footage and the smallest dimension (width) must be at least a certain size. Although a birth center is a "maxi-home" rather than a "mini-hospital," some states do require that hallways between the door that an ambulance would use and each birth room be a certain width. There may be Americans With Disabilities Act (ADA) requirements for the size of the bathroom, and other access factors. When choosing a space for the birth center, all such regulations need to be taken into consideration.

Accreditation

The CABC has indicators for space that show that the birth center is in compliance with the American Association of Birth Centers' (AABC) Standards for Birth Centers. For example, birth centers must have adequate space for families, including a kitchen and a family room, with a place for children to play while awaiting the birth. Exam rooms must be large enough to accommodate family members. Most birth centers have at least one large room that can be used for classes, a reception area, a lending library, the family room, and/or staff meetings. Space is also provided for clean and dirty utility areas, laboratory equipment and supplies, a staff lounge, work areas for all staff and contractors, secure records storage, plenty of storage for supplies, medicines and equipment, adequate hand-washing facilities, and bathrooms. Some centers have one exam room large enough to include a rocking chair and supplies for breastfeeding support.

Other Space Guidelines

The American Institute of Architects (AIA) has specific building guidelines for birth centers that are different from either a midwifery office or a hospital (American Institute of Architects Academy of Architecture for Health & Facility Guidelines Institute, 2011). Another resource is the National Fire Protection Association (NFPA) Life Safety Codes, available at no cost by registering at their website (www.nfpa.org). Beginning in section 3.3.33, the Code states that birth centers that do not provide sleeping facilities, and have fewer than four patients at a time (not including infants) be classified as business occupancies (NFPA, 2015). Therefore, they do not require the same fire protection controls as hospitals and ambulatory surgery centers. Some state or local jurisdictions require adherence to AIA and/or NFPA recommendations for licensure or occupancy permits, or they have developed their own guidelines. Learning what is required in advance facilitates the constructing or remodeling of the intended space and prevents rework and delays.

Planning for Growth

Expected Volume at Capacity

The community assessment gives a good indication of the potential demand for birth center services in the service area. Consider having one birth room for approximately 100 births. If the facility is built to fire standards for a birth center (business occupancy), there will be at most three birth rooms (~300 births/year at full capacity) and possibly a "swing" room that is ordinarily used another purpose, such as breastfeeding support, and that can be used before admission for women in early labor on busy days. Some birth centers that do not provide well-woman care use birth rooms for prenatal and postpartum visits. Exam rooms can be smaller than birth rooms and do not need showers and/or tubs, or emergency and other birth equipment. It is usually more cost-efficient to plan for at least one exam room per two birth rooms. If the birth center provides well-woman care for its clients, consider one exam room for each birth room.

Number of Employees and Contractors at Capacity

Many birth centers begin with a single entrepreneurial midwife who has no employees or contracted help. Although this model provides a needed service to the community while containing costs, it can limit the growth of the center because the management burden in the early years is especially large. Hiring independent contractors during the early growth phase can help to provide flexibility and increased capacity until there is sufficient volume to hire regular employees. Examples of tasks that can be contracted include billing, answering service, childbirth education, doula services, birth assistants, and accounting. As the birth center grows, it becomes cost-efficient to bring some services in-house.

Birth centers that only offer prenatal and birth care can anticipate each provider will attend about six to seven births per month, or up to 75/year per midwife. Beyond this volume, quality care may be diminished. If the birth center also offers home birth, the annual number of births will likely need to be reduced in order to account for travel time to homes and the necessity to provide coverage in multiple locations. If the birth center also offers hospital birth, the need to cover two locations and to attend women who have longer than usual labors (such as induction) may again necessitate a reduction in volume per midwife.

Location

Ideally, the birth center would be located near a hospital in case there is a need for an emergency transport. Access by public transportation is a plus, as is street visibility. Parking is important and some jurisdictions have requirements about the number of parking places needed based on the square footage of the facility.

Own Versus Lease

Once an approximate idea of the space required is calculated, a decision must be made about whether to lease office space, purchase an existing structure, or build a new facility. The primary advantage of leasing space is that the initial capital necessary for getting started is significantly less than purchasing or building. Also, many amenities may already be in place, such as ADA bathrooms, parking, and floor covering, and the landlord may also be willing to make certain tenant improvements as a part of the contract. Longer leases ensure that the birth center will not need to renegotiate its lease or move frequently, but there will be a penalty for terminating the lease early. In considering the cost of the lease, it is important to understand which costs, such as housekeeping, maintenance, security, and utilities, are the responsibility of the landlord versus the tenant, and the conditions under which these expenses can increase. If the space is leased, the primary asset of the business is the equipment and furniture.

Purchasing an existing building or house provides a "hard" asset for the business that may prove useful if a loan is needed for construction/remodeling in order to get started, or a line of credit later. However, purchasing ties up cash that could be used as a reserve for the inevitable variations in monthly income that occur with a new business, and the asset cannot necessarily be sold easily when necessary.

Building a new facility is similar to purchasing an existing building. One difference is that it is likely to be more expensive per square foot, since it is new. Also, the time from purchase of the land to opening is longer than the time from purchase of an existing building to opening in the best of circumstances. On the positive side, a new facility can be built so as to ensure that all licensing and accreditation requirements are met, and that the desired amenities are included.

Zoning

A critical consideration in choosing property is the zoning. In most jurisdictions, commercial zoning is required for a birth center, so most residences cannot be used as a birth center. Rezoning a residential property can be a lengthy, time-consuming, expensive process with uncertain results. When a properly zoned house in a good location that meets budget constraints is found, applying the previous considerations ensures that the space is adequate and that it can be licensed and accredited. The budget will need to include all of the normal expenses of home ownership, such as taxes, insurance, yard work, pest control, repairs and maintenance, and any other local fees, such as for irrigation.

Most office space is zoned commercial, so leasing space for a birth center is not straightforward. However, some local jurisdictions have several types of commercial zoning, which may restrict where the birth center can be located. The local zoning regulations should be examined prior to negotiating the lease. With new construction, it is best to have the local zoning office provide a letter in writing that the property that is being considered can be used for a birth center.

Early Planning Budget

Producing a complete financial plan requires time, energy, and resources, all of which require a budget. For the early planning budget, most of the time and expense budgets relate to gathering data. Formal surveys or focus groups, or the engagement of a consultant to gather information, may require cash expenditures. An example of an early planning budget worksheet is shown in Table 13.1.

TABLE 13.1
Early Planning Budget Worksheet

Activity	Time	Expense	Other
Community Market Research			
Demographics of birth population			
Readiness of current providers of care for a birth center			
Consumer preferences			
Services available (primary/secondary areas)			
Identify Certificate of Need (CON) requirements (if applicable)			
Readiness of payer market for a birth center			
Investigation of Relevant Regulations			
Birth center licensure regulations			
Midwifery regulations			
Facility regulations (construction, zoning, fire, building, and so forth)			
Estimation of Needs for Space			
Locating Suitable Site			
Checking zoning and other local regulations			
Investigation of Liability Insurance Coverage Options			
Assembling the Board of Directors (If Applicable)			
Identifying Financing Options			
TOTAL		$	

START-UP

Introduction to the Financial Plans

Building a realistic budget for a birth center presents challenges because the industry is still small and there are many variations from center to center in terms of local costs for the major expenses, the amount reimbursed by payers in different areas, the design of the space, and the programs offered. Budgeting also involves making assumptions regarding growth, inflation, staffing, payer mix, and service mix. Therefore, it is important to be clear about the assumptions that are being made. As soon as possible, these assumptions should be tested against actual experience and adjusted accordingly.

Following is an example of the process used to construct a financial plan for launching a birth center in Anytown, USA. Once the thought processes behind the elements of the plan are described, examples of spreadsheets can be constructed to incorporate these elements. Spreadsheets should be constructed using formulas that allow the assumptions to be modified as needed.

Start-Up Expenses

Expenses that will be incurred *before* the first day that clients are seen are grouped as start-up expenses. In the best of circumstances, once the early planning is completed, there are usually still at least 3 months of work to do prior to opening.

Certificate of Need

Many states have a Certificate of Need (CON) program . These programs were originally developed to ensure that hospitals did not overbuild, and then charge more for beds that were used in order to cover the costs of empty beds. More information about CONs and a map of the states that require a CON for health care facilities is available from the National Conference of State Legislatures (2016). Some of these states have a CON process for other health care facilities, but do not require that birth centers go through this process. Each state's regulations have to be checked to know whether a CON is needed and the specific requirements to obtain one.

Ordinary Business Expenses

Setting up a birth center is similar to setting up any other business. Space must be purchased or leased, and constructed or built out for birth center use, all according to federal, state, and local regulations and AABC's Standards for Birth Centers so that CABC accreditation is possible. Regulatory fees for incorporation, occupancy, licensure, and accreditation must be paid. Accounts need to be set up to pay local, state, and federal taxes, along with workers' compensation and unemployment taxes. Some types of revenue received by the birth center prior to opening must be treated as income for tax purposes. An accountant can help with setting up a chart of accounts and a cost accounting system. Bank accounts with appropriate signatories need to be opened. Business insurance such as property insurance (e.g., fire, hazards), general liability insurance (e.g., slip and fall), and directors and officers insurance must be purchased. An insurance broker can advise about other types of business insurance that are available, such as employee theft, data breaches, or income maintenance in case of natural disaster. AABC membership dues for a developing birth center may be paid by the time of opening, or may be paid sooner in order to be able to access the wealth of helpful information contributed by experienced birth center owners.

Preparing the Space to Do Business

A telephone system must be chosen, and accounts set up with a telephone carrier, water and sewer providers, an electricity provider, an Internet provider, garbage disposal, and a hazardous waste disposal provider. The space must be equipped with furniture, fixtures, furnishings, office equipment, medical equipment, office supplies, medical supplies, and information technology (IT) equipment. Examples of "shopping lists" for such items for a birth center with three birth rooms are provided in a sample worksheet in Table 13.2.

Hiring Staff

Once a certificate of occupancy is obtained from the local planning office, employees may be recruited and hired.

Salary Determination

For the business to be successful and sustainable, everyone—including the founder(s)—needs to be paid a fair market wage. Undercapitalized

TABLE 13.2
Supplies and Equipment Worksheet

Capital Equipment Detail	Budget
Furniture/Fixtures	
Tubs (3)	
Beds/mattresses (3)	
Exam table	
Linens/pillows	
Washer/dryer	
Kitchen equipment	
Rugs, lamps, décor items	
Total	
Office Equipment	
Desks	
Chairs	
Telephone system	
Work spaces	
Copier/Fax (or lease)	
Postage meter	
Filing cabinets/safe storage	
Computers	
Total	
Medical Equipment	
Rocking chairs (3)	
Birth instruments (5 sets)	
Autoclave (reconditioned)	
Microscope	
Birth stool	
Infant scales	
Adult scale	
Blood pressure cuffs (3)	
Stethoscopes (3)	

(continued)

TABLE 13.2
Supplies and Equipment Worksheet *(continued)*

Capital Equipment Detail	Budget
Dopplers (3)	
Oto/ophthalmoscope	
Oxygen tanks with regulators	
Laryngoscope	
IV pole	
Fire extinguishers (4)	
Glucometer	
Total	
Medical Supplies	
Disposable infant bag & mask (3)	
Laryngeal mask airways (3)	
Medications	
Suture	
IV solutions	
IV tubing/catheter/needles	
Amnihooks	
Syringes	
Bulb syringes	
DeLee mucous traps	
Gloves (sterile and nonsterile)	
U/A strips	
Lancets	
Doppler gel	
Exam lubricating gel	
Autoclave bags	
Cleaning solutions for instruments, counters, tubs	
Exam table paper	
Patient drapes	
Underpads	

(continued)

TABLE 13.2
Supplies and Equipment Worksheet *(continued)*

Capital Equipment Detail	Budget
Gauze pads	
Misc. supplies	
Total	

IV, intravenous; U/A, urinalysis

birth centers are often tempted to "defer" the salary of the founder indefinitely and/or expect staff to work for less than they are worth. A better strategy is to time-limit any deferral and create a believable strategy for repaying the "loan," and ensure that enough capital is in place to pay staff adequately. If job advertisements state that the birth center is offering competitive wages, some idea of what those wages should be can be inferred from the current wages of the applicants. Median salaries and the range for most jobs in most market areas can be found at this website (www.salary.com).

Consider how salary increases and bonuses will be determined from the start. Besides cost of living and merit increases, consider "step" increases for longevity and/or total years of experience as a mechanism for encouraging staff retention. Providing raises for well-trained, productive, loyal employees is preferable to the higher costs of replacing an employee, especially a midwife. Employees earning less than $50,000/year cost about 20% of their annual salary to replace, and a physician or executive director costs more than 200% of their annual salary to replace. Registered nurses and midwives fall somewhere in between (Boushey & Glynn, 2012).

Benefit Determination

Most birth centers offer the same benefits to all employees. Exceptions are the vacation and continuing education benefits for the clinical provider staff, which are often larger than for the administrative staff, in order to compensate for the fact that providers will be required to work weekends and holidays, and their licenses require continuing education. Birth centers that offer a health savings account (HSA) allow the employee to have some choice in how benefit dollars are spent. It is wise to state both the salary and the approximate current combined value of the benefits in a formal job offer. Few start-ups can afford to have the combined value of the benefits exceed 20% of the salary. Examples of benefits provided by birth centers include:

- Health, vision, and dental insurance coverage/health savings account
- Short/long-term disability insurance/life insurance
- Vacation, sick, and parenting leave
- Retirement contribution
- Malpractice insurance/tail insurance
- Continuing education
- Licensing fees/Drug Enforcement Administration (DEA)-controlled substance license
- Profit sharing
- Bonuses
- Cell phone subsidy

In addition, the birth center will be responsible for paying workers' compensation and payroll taxes, which may amount to as much as 14% of the salary, depending on the state.

Administrative Staff

Prior to opening a new birth center, the administrative staff will be responsible for tasks associated with ordinary business expenses mentioned earlier, purchasing to build out and equip the space, marketing, hiring, and devising the personnel policies in the employee handbook. Since these tasks are critical to the success of the birth center, they should be performed professionally, either by employed staff with experience in these areas or contracted staff.

At a minimum, the personnel files for all administrative staff should contain a new hire letter, signed by the employee; signed documentation that they have read, understood, and intend to comply with the employee handbook and that their questions have been answered; a job description signed and dated by the employee; evidence that they have successfully completed Health Insurance Portability and Accountability Act (HIPAA) and Occupational Safety and Health Administration (OSHA) training; and evidence that they are at least minimally competent on charting and billing. In addition, the birth center may wish to require some of the additional items that are required of clinicians, such as immunizations.

Midwives

Midwives generally take the most time to hire. If a midwife is currently employed elsewhere, she or he would normally be expected to give

3 months' notice. Hiring midwives who lack birth center experience is challenging. Midwives who only have hospital experience may be somewhat more likely to transport mothers who could be cared for at the birth center, which reduces the income of the birth center and may result in dissatisfied clients. Midwives with home birth experience are somewhat less likely to be used to working within the parameters of strict protocols, and may have less experience with quality control processes. It is wise to use the interview and reference check processes to ascertain the fit-for-birth center practice. AABC members have privileges to download "How to Hire a Midwife: More Than a Gut Feeling," which contains examples of questions useful for screening midwives by accessing the Birth Center Forum Archive section of the AABC website. Appropriate orientation with an experienced birth center midwife is also important.

Attracting midwives who are a good fit for the birth center is obviously critical for a start-up. Their energy and enthusiasm can help to grow the birth center and establish its good reputation in the community. A competitive salary, a good benefit package, good working conditions, and a reasonable call schedule can help create stability. The AABC website contains two documents that may prove helpful: (a) a PowerPoint presentation, "Negotiating Contracts With Birth Center Staff," provides details about elements to include in contracts with midwives and other staff; and (b) "Optimal Call Scheduling," which provides suggestions for creating a call schedule that promotes quality of life for the midwife. Changing the usual call schedule that begins in the morning to one that better matches the midwives' circadian rhythm, that is, beginning and ending the call shift in the evening, can significantly increase the effectiveness of the midwives and their job satisfaction. Both of these are available to members at no charge.

Malpractice Insurance

All of the midwives, other clinicians, and the birth center itself need professional liability insurance prior to the first day that clients are seen. There are two common types and a hybrid, not all of which are available in all areas. The most common type today is "claims made." A *claims-made policy* is one that provides coverage for any adverse outcome that occurred while the policy was in effect *and* the accompanying lawsuit was filed during the policy period. Any adverse outcome that occurred prior to when the policy began is not covered *unless* the policy has a "prior acts" clause back to a date before the adverse outcome occurred. The claims-made policy also does not cover adverse outcomes that occurred during the policy period without the lawsuit being filed during the policy period *unless* "tail coverage" is purchased. Although policies vary, typically the "tail" lasts until the baby is of age (usually age 18) plus the statute of limitations for that state (usually 3 years). Tail coverage is expensive, usually 1.5 to 2.0 times the annual charge for the policy, and typically must be paid within 30 to 60 days after the termination of the policy. This can become a significant burden to birth centers with high turnover of their provider staff, as a "tail" needs to be paid each time a midwife leaves the practice.

An *occurrence policy* in effect includes both coverage for adverse acts (and possibly prior acts) that occur during the time when the policies is in effect *plus* the "tail" for as long as the insured lives. Most midwives coming from employment in the hospital setting are used to having occurrence coverage. Because of the additional expense of an occurrence policy in the short run, this type of policy is less common than claims-made policies for birth centers.

A third type of policy is a *slots* or *group policy*. The practice as a whole purchases a policy at the claims-made rates for experienced (usually Year 5) midwives. The policy covers a specified number of midwives. So long as the number of midwives remains constant, no tail needs to be purchased, even if the individual midwives change over time. Coverage for acts while a midwife is employed at the birth center is for the lifetime of each midwife. If the number of slots decreases, a tail is due for each one.

If there is a choice of reputable plans where the birth center is located, determining which plan is most advantageous financially depends on the expected turnover rate and the cost of the tail. It is likely that the prior acts coverage would cost a similar amount for all types of policies. For both claims-made and occurrence policies, new hires start at Year 1 rates for the premium, regardless of their prior experience, and the annual cost of coverage increases each year until about Year 5, when it levels out. This is because the insurance company is assuming responsibility for more and more potential cases. Although it is easy to compare the annual premium costs of the two types of policies, it can be difficult to get an estimate of the cost of tail coverage in advance. Once an estimate is obtained, then the longer a midwife is covered under a claims-made policy, the more years there are to amortize the cost of the tail.

One factor to consider in choosing a malpractice carrier is its A.M. Best rating. In the insurance industry, the A.M. Best Co. is the organization that assigns a rating to liability insurers on the basis of their ability to pay claims. These ratings are available to the public following a free registration on the A.M. Best website (www.ambest.com). In addition, it is important to determine how much experience the carrier has in covering and defending midwives and birth centers. Carriers without much experience are drawn to this market by the lower incidence of lawsuits than is true with obstetricians and hospitals. However, when there is an adverse outcome that requires a payout, that payout tends to be the same without respect to the provider or place of service. For the first 3 years, it is unlikely that the carrier will have any payouts, since it takes time to file and settle lawsuits. But once the normal, often unavoidable birth-related lawsuits start requiring payouts, many carriers leave the market, as they have not underwritten the premiums for the policy correctly. Policies often do not specify in advance what the "tail" will cost, as it is determined at the end of the policy period based on the experience of the carrier in making payouts. Companies that enter the midwife/birth center market and then exit in 3 to 4 years often charge very high premiums for tail coverage. Although it may seem like a good deal to get the cheaper rates from a new carrier, it is also important that the company be there to provide coverage when needed.

For more tips on choosing malpractice coverage, visit the American College of Nurse-Midwives (ACNM, n.d.) website (www.midwife.org).

Credentialing With the Birth Center

All providers who care for women in the birth center need to be credentialed, whether they are employees or not. Orientation for new midwives should be checked off by an experienced midwife in their personnel records to ensure that all steps are completed. The tasks that need to be completed prior to the first day that clients are seen include a signed and dated new hire letter, a resume, midwifery (and RN, if applicable) license for the state where the birth center is located, American Midwifery Certification Board (AMCB) certificate for certified nurse-midwives (CNMs), North American Registry of Midwives (NARM) certificate for certified professional midwives (CPMs), a National Provider Identifier (NPI) number, a DEA number if narcotics will be prescribed, signed collaborative agreement with a physician only in states where that is required for practice, current Neonatal Resuscitation Program and Cardio-Pulmonary Resuscitation cards, a background check that includes information about child abuse, evidence of immunizations that are required in the state (or documentation of refusal), and a negative tuberculosis skin test. Finally, midwives should be credentialed with all of the birth center's payers and have a signed W-9 form that assigns the revenue they generate to the birth center.

Credentialing With Hospitals

Midwives who practice in birth centers may choose to apply for hospital privileges, so women who transfer from birth center care may still be attended by birth center staff in the hospital setting. Each hospital has different requirements for gaining privileges, but essentially a detailed application is required that is usually reviewed by the administrative staff and the obstetrical (and pediatric, if well-baby privileges are sought) staff. The process may take many weeks. Some hospitals may grant provisional privileges and many do not. Hospitals usually require an orientation, training on their electronic health record, and orientation to the unit that often involves proctored admissions and births.

Credentialing With Payers

In order to receive payment from third parties for the services of midwives and the birth center, each provider must be credentialed by each payer. The application process is designed so that the insurer can be assured that the provider base will provide good care for the enrollees. The Council for Affordable Quality Healthcare (CAQH) website is a useful place to start the application process, because many insurance companies are able to access the same uniform credentialing application. License updates and other credentialing necessities can be efficiently managed on the CAQH site so that the information does not have to be sent to each one of the participating payers separately. Many of the larger health insurers, including Anthem BCBS, Cigna, Kaiser Permanente, and United Health Group, use the CAQH platform to credential providers. Then, because nearly half of all births are paid for by Medicaid, providers will need to apply to be credentialed both with "straight/open/state" Medicaid and with each of the Medicaid-managed care organizations (MMCOs) that operate in the service area. Finally, providers should be credentialed with any other payer that insures a significant number of potential clients in the service area.

The birth center itself must also be credentialed with each insurer. Insurance companies may not have a category on the facility credentialing application that accurately describes the birth center facility. Most births occur in hospitals, which are in-patient facilities, and a birth center is considered an outpatient facility. Network management staff may need to be educated about the birth center facility and what is considered routine and nonroutine care in a birth center facility. Routine facility items are included in the maternity facility service fee billing code. Items that are not considered routine in a birth center (e.g., IVs and medications) can be negotiated as separately reimbursed. Facility applications will require copies of the state license and proof of malpractice insurance, as well as accreditation for an increasing number of insurers. It can be challenging to complete all the tasks required for credentialing each provider and the

BOX 13.2
Helpful Credentialing Sites

National Provider Identifier (NPI): https://nppes.cms.hhs.gov/NPPES/Welcome.do

Drug Enforcement Administration (DEA): www.deadiversion.usdoj.gov/drugreg

Council for Affordable Quality Healthcare (CAQH): www.caqh.org

American Midwifery Certification Board (AMCB): www.amcbmidwife.org

North American Registry of Midwives (NARM): www.narm.org

Commission for the Accreditation of Birth Centers (CABC): www.birthcenteraccreditation.org

facility far enough in advance of opening to be fully credentialed with insurance carriers on opening day. Helpful credentialing websites are listed in Box 13.2.

Policies and Procedures

Midwives need to be on staff well before opening day so that they can be credentialed with the various entities, be accepted for coverage by the malpractice carrier, and be oriented to begin work. There are likely to be downtimes with these processes; these can be used to develop policies and procedures (P&P) that are evidence-based and a quality improvement plan to maximize the likelihood that safe care is always provided. Work can also begin on gathering the materials necessary for accreditation. However, the priority is to have all clinicians legally ready to provide care on opening day, and get reimbursed for it.

It is recommended that the clinical P&P be a separate document from administrative or personnel policies. A dated copy of each edit of the P&P, signed by a representative of the birth center's governing body, should be kept in a secure location. Even if there are no edits, the P&P should have a signed and dated affirmation that it was reviewed no less than annually. In the event of a lawsuit, the P&P for the appropriate date may be subpoenaed. Documentation of a recent review to ensure that the P&P manual included current evidence at the time, along with proof that the midwife adhered to the P&P, will be helpful to the defense attorney. Examples of P&P manuals are included in the "How to Start a Birth Center" workshop. Members of AABC can request additional examples from successful birth centers via the Members Only listserv. CABC also provides guidance on what must be included in the P&P (CABC, 2015).

Continuous Quality Improvement

In order to provide the best care to clients, promote sustainability, and enhance the reputation of the birth center, each center should have a formal continuous quality improvement (CQI) program. The list of subjects reviewed by the CABC to indicate compliance with the CQI Standards for Birth Centers is extensive (see Chapter 8). The purpose of a CQI program is to ensure that there are policies that address each subject, the policies are regularly reviewed and updated as necessary, and the policies are followed. When a review shows an opportunity for improvement, it is important that there be evidence of correction, either via updating a policy or counseling a staff member.

Other Clinical Staff

Some birth centers have two midwives attend each birth, one who is the primary provider, and the other who serves as a birth assistant. Birth assistants may be registered nurses, medical assistants, or specially trained staff who are not licensed by the state. They can be contracted hourly or on a per birth basis, or they can be employees of the birth center if the volume is sufficient.

Other Staff and Contractors

Some states still require that birth centers have a medical director (MD), and all birth centers need consulting obstetricians and pediatricians. In some cases, contracts with the physician(s) do not involve direct compensation; the MDs expect that all necessary referrals will be made to them, and they will bill for the services they provide to referred clients. In other cases, the MDs require a monthly retainer fee paid directly to them by the birth center. In either case, it is good practice to keep a file with a current license, hospital-privileging evidence, and a malpractice policy for the primary physician consultants.

Because there are still so few birth centers in the United States, very few medical billers are experts in billing birth center services. Although the global professional fee, prenatal care, and postpartum outpatient care are relatively straightforward, many other professional services provided in birth centers are not. It is even more challenging to correctly bill for the facility service fees, as there is no standardized way to do that billing; every insurance company requires a different process. Hospitals that own birth centers and have in-house billing departments are advised to seek training from billers experienced in birth center billing. For entrepreneurs, it may be tempting to save money by keeping the billing function in-house, but it is no more expensive to contract for the billing function with experienced companies and they may bring in more revenue.

Marketing

All the elements of the marketing plan influence each other to create a brand for the birth center. If they are well coordinated, they can give the business great success. Prior to launch, the marketing plan requires a careful analysis, market research, and consultation with several people, including users and other birth centers. Marketing activities include advertising, word of mouth, press reports, and incentives. Direct marketing, contests, and prizes may also be included.

Goals with measurable results should be part of the start-up plan so that the plan can be modified as needed. For example, the number of potential clients that come to each open house/information session is one key indicator of the success of the marketing plan. Another is how many calls are made to the center requesting information about the center and whether callers are appropriate clients. Asking each new client how he or she heard about the birth center can provide feedback about which marketing activities are most effective.

Examples of techniques current birth centers use to attract clients include:

- Purchasing Facebook ads and "boosting" the brand on search engines and pregnancy sites (e.g., pregnancy.org, stork.net, WebMD)
- National Public Radio and local AM station ads, including Spanish language stations
- Blog distributed via e-mail
- Being a site to obtain breast pumps, which are now free to consumers and paid for by insurers
- Holding a baby fair at the center
- Holding a sports physical day for young female athletes
- Annual picnics, often on "Labor" Day, which may include a parade of babies born at the center and live news coverage (Labor Day is usually a slow news day)

- Free movie and pizza nights, where films of interest to women of childbearing age are shown
- Participation in local parades, fun runs, county fairs, and similar community activities
- Distributing cards for free pregnancy tests in laundromats, on Facebook pages, and on community services boards
- Media coverage of visits by government officials who support the center
- Presentations at service clubs (Rotary, Kiwanis, chamber of commerce)
- "Meet the Midwife" open house and tours of the birth center
- Prominent listings on payers' websites, which list "in-network" providers

Utilization

A utilization worksheet such as that shown in Table 13.3 can help predict whether the marketing plan is providing sufficient clients to sustain the birth center. In the following example, the number of women that attend birth center orientation is the driver for all other numbers. Impressing participants enough to register for care and then having a low to average hospital transfer rate has a significant impact on total utilization and income.

Attrition is a big factor to consider when determining utilization, and includes those women who register for care at the birth center, but who are no longer eligible to give birth at the center prior to admission in labor, or who have chosen not to (Table 13.3). The Perinatal Data Registry (PDR) outcomes data collected by the AABC reports an average prenatal attrition rate for nonmedical reasons or for a first-trimester loss of 19% (Stapleton, Osborne, & Illuzzi, 2013; see Figure 13.1).

In our utilization examples, we use this attrition rate for a newly opened birth center. An additional 18% of the remainder transfer out of birth center care for medical reasons, either in the antepartum period or in labor prior to being admitted to the birth center. The first example shows utilization stabilizes by Year 2 if there is no growth in orientation attendance. The second example shows utilization with very rapid growth of 50% per year, reflecting the increase in orientations and registrants.

In the high-growth scenario, by Year 3 there have to be 45 potential clients attending the orientation session each and every month, and fewer than half of them will deliver in the birth center. However, the number of required registrants from the orientation session can be reduced by the number of "repeat customers" that register for care each month. It is much easier to retain a current client than to attract a new one.

TABLE 13.3
Utilization

SAMPLE UTILIZATION WORKSHEET—No Growth

Utilization	**Year 1**	**Year 2**	**Year 3**
Orientation attendance	240	240	240
Registrants (90%)	216	216	216
Attrition: SAB, nonmedical (19% of registrants)	(41)	(41)	(41)
Caseload	175	175	175
Caseload due this year (50%)	87	87	87
Carried from previous year, due this year (50%)		88	88
Total caseload due this year	87	175	175
Transfers: AP and Pre-Admit IP (18%)	(16)	(32)	(32)
Admitted to BC in labor	71	143	143
Transfers: IP after admission (12%)	(9)	(17)	(17)
Births at Birth Center	**62**	**126**	**126**

Example Utilization Worksheet—50% Growth per Year

Utilization	**Year 1**	**Year 2**	**Year 3**
Orientation attendance	240	360	540
Registrants (90%)	216	324	486
Attrition: SAB, nonmedical (19% of registrants)	(41)	(62)	(92)
Caseload	175	262	394
Caseload due this year (50%)	87	131	197
Carried from previous year, due this year (50%)		87	131
Total caseload due this year	87	218	328
Transfers: AP and Pre-Admit IP (18%)	(16)	(39)	(59)
Admitted to BC in labor	71	179	269
Transfers: IP after admission (12%)	(9)	(21)	(32)
Births at Birth Center	**62**	**158**	**237**

AP, antepartum; BC, birth center; IP, intrapartum; SAB, spontaneous abortion.

Reprinted with permission from American Association of Birth Centers (AABC).

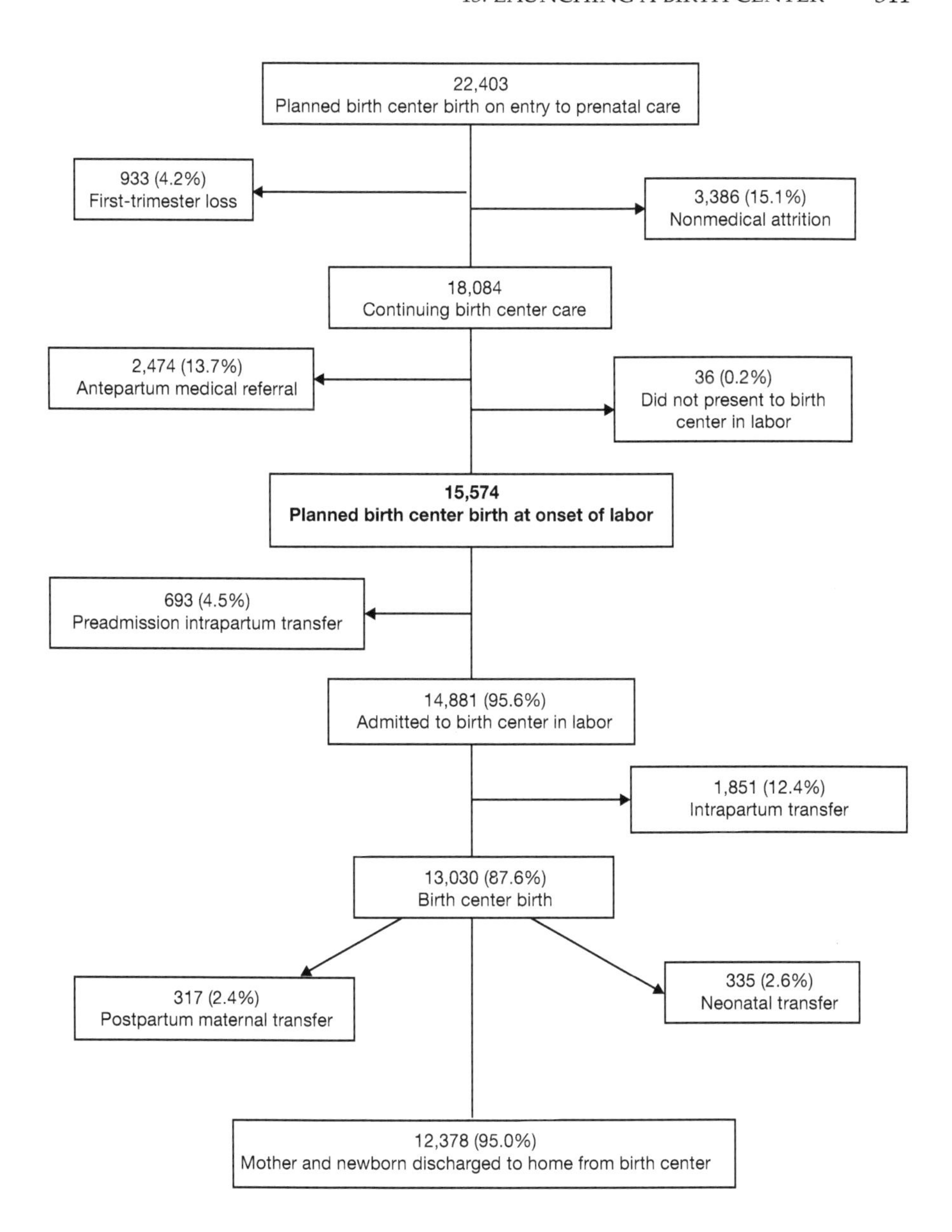

FIGURE 13.1 Attrition in number of actual birth center deliveries from planned deliveries.

Source: Stapleton, Osborne, & Illuzi (2013). Outcomes of care in birth centers: Demonstration of a durable model. Journal of Midwifery and Women's Health, 58(1), 3–14.

Start-Up Budget Categories

To summarize, during the period before the birth center opens, many tasks need to be accomplished. Some tasks can be accomplished by the founder or investor, and others must be done by newly hired employees and contractors. A worksheet containing a checklist of items that require time and/or cash budgets is shown in Table 13.4.

TABLE 13.4
Start-Up Time and Cash Expenditures Worksheet

Start-Up Time	Cash Expenditures
Building	
Rent or mortgage	
Regulatory fees: Incorporation, license, accreditation	
Taxes (state and federal)	
General liability, D&O, property insurance	
Preparation and securing of Certificate of Need	
AABC developing birth center dues	
Utilities	
Capital expenses	
Furniture and furnishings	
Office equipment	
Medical equipment	
Medical supplies	
Office supplies	
IT (EHR fees and staff training)	
Recruiting and contracting with staff	
Start-up salaries & benefits	
First year malpractice pre-pay	
Contracting with insurance payers (professional and facility)	

(continued)

TABLE 13.4
Start-Up Time and Cash Expenditures Worksheet *(continued)*

Start-Up Time	Cash Expenditures
Marketing	
Accounting, bookkeeping set-up	
TOTAL START-UP EXPENSES	

AABC, American Association of Birth Centers; D&O, Directors' and Officers' Liability Insurance; EHR, Electronic Health Record; IT, information technology

Reprinted with permission from American Association of Birth Centers.

Note: These expenses are incurred prior to opening the doors for business. Sufficient capital must be obtained to meet these expenses whether the birth center opens or not.

BUSINESS PLAN

Although the costs outlined for early planning and start-up efforts are not reimbursable, once the birth center opens, revenue is generated to defray some of the initial operating costs. Over time, if the birth center reaches full capacity and costs are managed well, there is a net profit in the current period. This profit can be used to repay the expenses incurred prior to opening, along with the deficits incurred prior to breaking even. This section describes factors to consider in creating the operating budget for the first 3 to 5 years, along with a description of how to put all the elements together to make the actual business plan.

Revenues

Financing

New birth centers are financed in a variety of ways. In some cases, an entrepreneur (or small group of entrepreneurs) pools his or her own resources to fund the project. Loans from banks or government agencies, such as the SBA, are potential sources. Founders who are women and/or minorities may have access to special funds from the SBA. Another potential source is "angel financing," which is usually in the $1 to $3 million range. "Angels" will expect that you form a C-corporation, that you have a board of directors, that they own a percentage of the business and have a seat on the board, that they earn a return on their investment, and that there is a plan for them to cash out. Another option is to assemble a pool of individuals who create self-directed individual retirement accounts (IRAs), that is, they use some or all of their IRA funds to invest in the birth center (instead of the stock market) for a share of the ownership. Finally, it may be possible to interest a large investor that is already starting birth centers to do so in your location. Not-for-profit birth centers can also seek tax-deductible donations from individuals and grants from foundations.

Contracting With Payers

The financial success of the business depends heavily upon how well the birth center is compensated for services rendered. It is critical to be clear about the actual cost of providing services in order to negotiate a reimbursement rate that can sustain the birth center over time. Calculating actual costs per birth should be an annual exercise once each year's books are closed, and every effort should be made to minimize those costs without sacrificing the quality of care.

Table 13.5 is an example of cost calculations from a birth center that has been in operation for some time.

TABLE 13.5
Cost Per Birth Calculation

Expense Item	Total Costs ($)	Professional Costs ($)	Facility Cost ($)
Administrative Expenses			
Accounting	62,000		62,000
Advertising	9,500		9,500
Internet/TV/computer	4,800		4,800
Copier	2,800		2,800
Drugs/medical/lab	21,000		21,000
Mortgage/rent	72,000		72,000
Office supplies & postage	16,700		16,700
Cleaning and supplies	1,700		1,700
Equipment/facility repairs and fees	1,700		1,700
Payroll processing fees	600		600
Fees/lic	3,700		3,700
Accreditation	3,000		3,000

(continued)

TABLE 13.5
Cost Per Birth Calculation *(continued)*

Expense Item	Total Costs ($)	Professional Costs ($)	Facility Cost ($)
Reserve fund	1,000		1,000
Other, misc	1,400		1,400
SUBTOTAL Administrative	**201,900**		**201,900**
Insurance			
Business liability	4,600		4,600
Birth center malpractice	35,000		35,000
Directors' and officers'	1,000		1,000
Midwife and nurse practitioner malpractice	27,000	27,000	
SUBTOTAL Insurance	**67,600**	**27,000**	**40,600**
Personnel			
Nurses (all)	37,500		37,500
Administrative	111,500	25,000	86,500
Med director/consult	30,000		30,000
Midwives and nurse practitioners	218,000	218,000	
Clinical/birth assistant	57,100		57,100
Travel	2,000	2,000	
Health and life insurance	18,200	15,200	3,000
Conference and prof dues	9,600	9,600	
Payroll taxes	34,300	19,300	15,000
Workers comp	1,800	1,100	700
SUBTOTAL Personnel	**520,000**	**290,200**	**229,800**
Utilities			
Gas & electric	8,800		8,800
Phone	9,600		9,600

(continued)

TABLE 13.5
Cost Per Birth Calculation *(continued)*

Expense Item	Total Costs ($)	Professional Costs ($)	Facility Cost ($)
Lawn maint	1,800		1,800
Water & sewage/garbage pick-up	2,200		2,200
SUBTOTAL Utilities	**22,400**		**22,400**
TOTAL Expenses	**811,900**	**317,200**	**494,700**

Reprinted with permission from American Association of Birth Centers (AABC).

Once the total expenses to run the birth center have been calculated, the next step is to calculate the revenue per birth that must be collected in order to break even. In the example in Table 3.5, $811,900 would need to be divided by the number of births projected for a given year in the birth center to calculate the break-even revenue that must be collected per birth. The revenue per birth required must then be collected in a combination of professional and facility fees, which will vary widely from state to state and between payers.

It may be easier to negotiate better reimbursement for the facility fee than the professional fee. Professional fees tend to be similar for all providers billing the same code in the same geographical area to the same payer. However, the real benefit to payers of contracting with birth centers comes from the codes *not* billed. Even if the payer reimburses the birth center facility service fee at the same rate he or she reimburses hospitals for the "room charge," birth centers do not bill for epidurals, anesthesiologists, routine IVs, extended stays due to medical inductions, and a host of other add-ons that are billed when healthy women choose to birth in the hospital. Most importantly, for the 70+% of pregnant women in the United States who qualify to give birth in a birth center, most choose to give birth in the hospital, and the cesarean rate for these women is about 26%; for similar women who choose a birth center, the cesarean rate is 6% (Stapleton et al., 2013). Since the cost (and reimbursement) of a cesarean is significantly higher than for a vaginal birth, each avoided cesarean represents savings for the payer. These savings can be shared with the birth center to ensure adequate reimbursement.

When negotiating for adequate reimbursement, it is best not to refer to midwifery or birth center services as "cheaper." Refer to the birth center and midwifery care as safe, high-quality care in a lower cost, outpatient (or community) setting. Demonstrate that compared with hospitals, birth centers meet the triple aim of better outcomes at lower cost with higher patient satisfaction. Birth centers should be compensated for the effort it takes to achieve these results at a rate that is sustainable for the centers, while ensuring that payers continue to average more profit from birth center deliveries than hospital deliveries for healthy women. Contracts are usually made for a 2- to 3-year period, and should include annual escalator clauses to account for the increased cost of providing services.

Contracts with each payer specify what will be paid for birth center services, but they do not specify what the birth center will charge. Birth centers are required to have a single fee schedule that specifies what they charge to all payers and those who self-pay. Most insurance carriers "allow" only a portion of invoiced charges to be paid, and the allowed amount is what is described in the contract. If any payer is reimbursing at the full amount charged, it is likely that the birth center is not charging enough.

Legally, health care providers may not give away their services to one without doing so for all, and must charge the amounts on their fee schedule to everyone. However, a birth center can have a uniformly applied policy stating that self-pay clients who pay in advance (unlike insurance companies) will receive a discount, so that self-pay clients actually pay an amount similar to what is received for insured clients.

Payer Mix

One reimbursement challenge is that, in most cases, Medicaid payment directly from the state (also known as "straight" Medicaid) does not pay the full cost of care. The amount paid is determined by the legislature as part of the overall state budgeting process. Reimbursement rates for each state are available to the public and cannot be negotiated by individual providers. If Medicaid pays less than the cost of providing care, other payers need to make up the difference to ensure sustainability. The vital statistics division of your state department of health will be able to provide information on the number of births in the county(s) near your service area and the numbers of women insured under Medicaid for their pregnancy. The figures listed typically include women insured both by "straight" Medicaid and by MMCOs. MMCOs typically negotiate with the state for a fixed payment per pregnancy that is a multiple of the "straight" Medicaid rate for pregnancy. Like private insurers, they can then negotiate with individual service providers regarding reimbursement rates.

In the example shown in Table 13.6, the fast-growing birth center has a payer mix that includes Managed Care Organization #1 (MCO #1), Managed Care Organization #2 (MCO #2), Medicaid, and Self-Pay.

The birth center's contracted rates determine its estimated revenue. Commercial (private) insurance is not shown in this example. The next example shows only revenue generated from birth center care, although some practices will have other sources of income. By Year 3, the combined reimbursement for professional and facility fees is $5,618 per birth, which should be more than the costs per birth of providing the service.

Note that MCO #2 pays more than other payers, especially Medicaid, for both total OB care (the professional fee for the mother) and the mother's facility service fee. In the example, this good payer constitutes 30% of the total number of clients, and Medicaid is 40% of the total. Simply by taking the time to assist a quarter of the Medicaid clients to enroll in MCO #2, so that there are more clients in MCO #2 than in Medicaid, revenues for the birth center would increase noticeably with no change in the number of clients or even the specific clients that are enrolled.

Collection Timing

The birth center begins earning income the day the birth center begins providing services to clients. However, the only way the center can require payment at the time of service is not to accept insurance, which severely restricts access to the birth center. If the birth center provides well-woman gynecological care, insurers pay claims for the service on a time schedule similar to most other health care services, that is, it takes at least a week for the claim to go from the provider to the biller to the clearinghouse to the insurer, and then the insurer reviews the claim for accuracy and eventually pays the claim, usually within 90 days if there are no disagreements between the provider and the payer that the payment is owed, and no other problems with the claim (it is "clean").

However, in the case of maternity care, typically the insurer requires that prenatal, birth, and postpartum care be "bundled" into a global charge that is not submitted until after the birth. The claim then goes through the process specified for gynecological claims. What this means, in effect, is that if the woman seeks care early in her pregnancy, it will be nearly a year before payment for the first visit will be received, even though the expenses associated with providing the service have to be paid much sooner.

TABLE 13.6
SAMPLE REVENUE WORKSHEET: Birth Center Only

INCOME BUDGET			Year 1		Year 2		Year 3	
Patient Revenue	**% Clients**	**Amt. Pd**	**Volume**	**Revenue**	**Volume**	**Revenue**	**Volume**	**Revenue**
Total OB Care			62		158		237	
MCO #1	0.20	$1,600	12	$19,200	32	$51,200	47	$75,200
MCO #2	0.30	$3,000	19	$57,000	47	$141,000	71	$213,000
Medicaid	0.40	$1,500	25	$37,500	63	$94,500	95	$142,500
Self-Pay	0.10	$1,900	6	$11,400	16	$30,400	24	$45,600
Facility Services Fee			62		158		237	
MCO #1	0.20	$3,000	12	$36,000	32	$96,000	47	$141,000
MCO #2	0.30	$3,500	19	$66,500	47	$164,500	71	$248,500
Medicaid	0.40	$1,900	25	$47,500	63	$119,700	95	$180,500
Self-Pay	0.10	$2,500	6	$15,000	16	$40,000	24	$60,000
Initial Newborn Care			62		158		237	
MCO #1	0.20	$400	12	$4,800	32	$12,800	47	$18,800
MCO #2	0.30	$300	4	$1,200	47	$14,100	71	$21,300
Medicaid	0.40	$300	8	$2,400	63	$18,900	95	$28,500

(continued)

TABLE 13.6
SAMPLE REVENUE WORKSHEET: Birth Center Only *(continued)*

INCOME BUDGET			Year 1		Year 2		Year 3	
Patient Revenue	**% Clients**	**Amt. Pd**	**Volume**	**Revenue**	**Volume**	**Revenue**	**Volume**	**Revenue**
Self-Pay	0.10	$400	3	$1,200	16	$6,400	24	$9,600
Newborn Facility Services Fee			62		158		237	
MCO #1	0.20	$700	12	$8,400	32	$22,400	47	$32,900
MCO #2	0.30	$500	19	$9,500	47	$23,500	71	$35,500
Medicaid	0.40	$–	25	$–	63	$–	95	$–
Self-Pay	0.10	$600	6	$3,600	16	$9,600	24	$14,400
Transfers & Attrition								
AP attrition: initial OB visit		$75	41	$3,075	62	$4,650	92	$6,900
AP transfers: prenatal care		$700	16	$11,200	39	$27,300	59	$41,300
IP transfers: facility services fee		$500	9	$4,500	21	$10,500	32	$16,000
Office procedures								
Education								
Other								
Total Patient Revenue				**$339,975**		**$887,450**		**$1,331,500**

AP, antepartum; IP, intrapartum; MCO, Managed Care Organization

Reprinted with permission from American Association of Birth Centers (AABC).

Some states, such as Washington, have recognized that the usual system of health care payment places an undue burden on small businesses that provide health care. In effect, the birth center is "loaning" money to the insurance company at no interest for the period after the service is rendered and before it is paid. Each day that the insurance company delays payment is a day when it can earn interest on the money that is owed to the provider. Washington's legislature passed a bill requiring insurance companies to pay "clean" claims within 30 days. Insurance companies are required to report their payment history to the state and there are fines associated with late payments.

Cash Flow

For budgeting purposes, assume that half of the clients who register for care in Year 1 will deliver in Year 1 and the other half will deliver the following year. Assume payment 90 days after the birth. Since services cannot be billed until after the birth, the income for the first year is limited by when it is possible to bill, skill in collecting claims payment quickly, and how soon the client base grows. Good planning will make it possible to have an orientation session or two prior to opening day, with the possibility of attracting women who are already pregnant to transfer in for birth center deliveries. This will ease some of the cash flow problems for the first year.

Expenses

Fixed Versus Variable Expenses

Once the space for the birth center is purchased or leased, the mortgage or lease payment must be paid every month, whether the birth center has one delivery or 30. This is an example of a *fixed* cost of doing business that does not vary with the volume of services delivered. *Variable* costs depend on how much business is done. For instance, the cost of disposable supplies for birth, such as underpads and gloves, varies by the number of births. Birthing tubs are fixed costs, but the water to fill them for each birth is a variable cost. Some costs resemble a combination, as they vary via a step function. An example is hiring a midwife. When she starts, her volume may be low, but she is a "fixed cost" until such time as her volume is high enough to support a second midwife. Unless the practice has ready access to per diem midwives who are willing to flex the time they work up and then down (when a new midwife is hired), the total for salaries paid to midwives is not a simple function of the number of births, but rather a step function.

All of the start-up costs and many of the operating costs are fixed. The birth center is most profitable when all fixed cost items are used to maximum capacity, but not beyond, in which case a "step" expenditure needs to be made. When a "step" expenditure is made, the profit will decrease for a time; once the additional expenditure is used to maximum capacity, the profit should be larger than before the step was taken. If there is not good evidence that taking the step can lead to full utilization of the resource in the future, the step should not be taken.

Capital Fund

Things wear out. Even with leased space, carpets will need to be replaced periodically, computers become outdated, and new furniture and equipment needs to be purchased. Space that is owned has an even longer list of items that will eventually need replacement, such as roofs, landscaping, and mechanical systems. Each birth center should have a list of major expenditures that will need to be made in the future to ensure the smooth running of the birth center, with an expected date of replacement and estimated cost. It is better to replace an item before the end of its useful life so that birth center operations are not disrupted. Without a specific fund for this purpose that has been built up month by month, unexpected expenses can even bankrupt the center.

Reserves

Some businesses combine their capital fund with their reserves, but this is not recommended for a birth center. Reserves should be used for specific purposes that are described in advance, to the extent possible. Examples are:

- Business interruptions, such as natural disasters or fires. Although insurance is available for this purpose, it may not be sufficient to keep the birth center running smoothly.
- Significant unanticipated collections problems. For instance, if a major payer changes computer systems and does not program the new system to pay birth centers properly, it may take months for payments everyone agrees are owed to actually be paid.
- Unexpected death or disability of the founder, in which case staff will need to be engaged quickly to perform his or her duties. Having outside contractors do his or her work may be more expensive.
- Addition of a new service or location. When profits have repaid start-up expenses and early deficits, and reserves have grown beyond the

amount needed to cover 3 to 6 months of operation without concomitant income, reserves may be used to expand the business.

Note that there may be limitations on how much reserve a not-for-profit can carry; an accountant experienced in working with not-for-profits can advise the birth center as to any limitations.

Expense Allocation

Although many aspects of not-for-profit and for-profit business accounting are similar, such as the tracking and reporting of income and expenses and payroll taxes, there are significant differences. These arise out of the not-for-profit organization's duty to drive its resources toward accomplishing its mission. For example, not-for-profit organizations are required to itemize expenses across management (general and administrative), fund raising, and program areas. Not-for-profits are required to allocate these "functional expenses" across the various functional areas and to specific programs. For example, let's say that those involved in administrative functions take up 20% of the office space. Then, 20% of an expense like paper would be allocated to the administrative functional area. The not-for-profit tax return form 990 requires documentation of the amount of money allocated to direct programs related to the charitable mission; the amount allocated to administration and top paid employees, such as the executive director; and the amount allocated to fund raising.

Direct Versus Indirect Costs

Businesses classify costs as direct or indirect based on whether or not they are used to produce specific goods or services. Direct costs related to birth center services can be tracked directly to the specific client being served or the specific program being offered. Direct labor is the largest cost in a birth center (i.e., salaries for midwives and nurses who provide patient care). Indirect costs are not traceable to a specific program or patient. Examples of indirect costs include utilities, overall birth center maintenance, marketing, and all other expenses involved in running the birth center that cannot be related to a specific client. In a not-for-profit birth center, cost tracking is imperative if the birth center receives grants or other types of restricted funding.

Operating Budget

The sample operating budget shown in Table 13.7 uses the revenue shown in the sample revenue worksheet for a very fast-growing birth center (50% increase in registrants/year) and extends the revenue until this birth center with three birth rooms reaches maximum capacity at 300 births/year with the stated payer mix constant and the present value of the reimbursement also remaining constant.

For expenses, it is assumed that the present value of the costs remains constant, and that any actual rate of increase in expenses is not greater than the actual rate of increase in revenues. The assumptions have been simplified for educational purposes and, where possible, the way the cells were calculated is indicated in the first column. The assumptions made for some cells require further explanation:

- In this example, the birth center is founded by a midwife, who is the chief administrator for the center. In the first year of operation, the center averages just over one birth per week. Although the volume is not sufficient to justify hiring a second midwife, a new graduate is hired by opening day at a salary of $80,000, and the founder mentors her as she orients. As the new graduate midwife assumes more responsibility and the volume grows, the founder decreases her call time and concentrates on management of the new enterprise. She remains available for consultation, vacation coverage, and support on busy days.
- By the middle of the second year, another new graduate is hired and oriented. Similarly, midwives are hired mid-year to accommodate the increasing volume of clients until the full complement of four full-time midwives is reached in Year 4.
- In this example, birth assistants (BAs) are either trained as such or as midwives' assistants who wish to work flex time. Three BAs share the call evenly and decide among themselves who is on call when. The birth center is informed a month in advance of the schedule. The BAs are paid $50/day when they are on call plus $250 for every birth they attend. Ideally, they are expected to complete any birth they begin.
- Once there is sufficient volume, an RN is hired to help the midwife with office visits and lab draws. As the volume increases, the nursing staff can assist more with educating clients, callbacks, normal lab reviews, and so forth.

TABLE 13.7
OPERATING EXPENSE BUDGET: Utilization Assumption 50% Growth

Births	**62**	**158**	**237**	**300**	**300**
OPERATING EXPENSES	Year 1	Year 2	Year 3	Year 4	Year 5
Personnel					
Executive director/lead midwife	$90,000	$90,000	$90,000	$90,000	$90,000
Midwives @ $80,000	$80,000	$120,000	$200,000	$240,000	$240,000
Birth assistants/MAs @250/birth + $50/day	$33,750	$57,750	$77,500	$93,250	$93,250
Nurses @$50,000		$50,000	$50,000	$100,000	$100,000
Receptionist/administration support	$24,000	$60,000	$90,000	$90,000	$90,000
Maintenance/housekeeping @$90/birth	$5,580	$14,220	$21,330	$21,330	$21,330
Subtotal	**$233,330**	**$391,970**	**$528,830**	**$634,580**	**$634,580**
Payroll taxes—10%	$23,333	$39,197	$52,883	$63,458	$63,458
Worker's comp—5%	$11,667	$19,599	$26,442	$31,729	$31,729
Benefits—20%	$46,666	$78,394	$105,766	$126,916	$126,916
Total Personnel	**$314,996**	**$529,160**	**$713,921**	**$856,683**	**$856,683**

(continued)

TABLE 13.7
OPERATING EXPENSE BUDGET: Utilization Assumption 50% Growth *(continued)*

Births	**62**	**158**	**237**	**300**	**300**
OPERATING EXPENSES	Year 1	Year 2	Year 3	Year 4	Year 5
Insurance					
Malpractice insurance @$15,000/midwife	$30,000	$45,000	$60,000	$60,000	$60,000
Comprehensive business insurance	$2,500	$2,500	$2,500	$2,500	$2,500
Directors & officers insurance	$10,000	$10,000	$10,000	$10,000	$10,000
Total Insurance Premiums	**$42,500**	**$57,500**	**$72,500**	**$72,500**	**$72,500**
Contracted Services					
Consulting physicians	$30,000	$30,000	$30,000	$30,000	$30,000
Legal	$2,500	$2,500	$2,500	$2,500	$2,500
Billing @7% of total revenue	$22,601	$59,161	$88,732	$112,319	$112,319
IT support @$20/birth	$1,240	$3,160	$4,740	$4,740	$4,740
Accounting/bookkeeping @3% of total revenues	$8,928	$22,752	$34,128	$34,128	$34,128
Total Contracted Services	**$65,269**	**$117,573**	**$160,100**	**$183,687**	**$183,687**

Facility Expenses					
Rent/mortgage/property tax	$88,000	$88,000	$88,000	$88,000	$88,000
Utilities	$6,000	$6,000	$6,000	$6,000	$6,000
Telephone/information technology	$4,800	$4,800	$4,800	$4,800	$4,800
Electronic records	$1,200	$1,200	$1,200	$1,200	$1,200
Answering service/cell phones	$6,000	$6,000	$6,000	$6,000	$6,000
Office supplies	$6,300	$6,300	$6,300	$6,300	$6,300
Housekeeping supplies/linen svc @$20/birth	$1,240	$3,160	$4,740	$6,000	$6,000
Marketing/public relations	$10,000	$10,000	$10,000	$10,000	$10,000
Membership and dues	$2,300	$3,100	$4,400	$4,400	$4,400
Licenses	$1,800	$1,800	$1,800	$1,800	$1,800
Accreditation	$4,000	$6,300	$3,000	$3,000	$3,000
Copier/equipment rental/postage	$5,700	$5,700	$5,700	$5,700	$5,700
Garbage pick-up/snow removal @$10/birth	$620	$1,580	$2,370	$2,370	$2,370
Total Facility Expense	**$137,960**	**$143,940**	**$144,310**	**$145,570**	**$145,570**

(continued)

TABLE 13.7
OPERATING EXPENSE BUDGET: Utilization Assumption 50% Growth *(continued)*

Births	62	158	237	300	300
OPERATING EXPENSES	Year 1	Year 2	Year 3	Year 4	Year 5
Client Care Expenses					
Medical supplies and drugs @$150/birth	$9,300	$23,700	$35,550	$35,550	$35,550
Home visit mileage @$20/birth	$1,240	$3,160	$4,740	$6,000	$6,000
Total Client Care Expenses	**$10,540**	**$26,860**	**$40,290**	**$41,550**	**$41,550**
Total Operating Expenses	**$571,265**	**$875,032**	**$1,131,121**	**$1,299,990**	**$1,299,990**
Contingency 5% of Total Operating Expenses	**$28,563**	**$43,752**	**$56,556**	**$64,999**	**$64,999**
TOTAL EXPENSES	**$599,828**	**$918,784**	**$1,187,677**	**$1,364,989**	**$1,364,989**
Revenue (birth center only)	$322,875	$845,150	$1,267,600	$1,604,556	$1,604,556
NET PROFIT (LOSS)	**($276,953)**	**($73,634)**	**$79,923**	**$239,567**	**$239,567**

IT, information technology; PR, public relations

Reprinted with permission from American Association of Birth Centers (AABC)

- By Year 3, there are three people in the office averaging $30,000/year. These would likely include an office manager, a front office receptionist, and someone whose main responsibility is incoming calls.
- The rest of the assumptions in this spreadsheet need to be adjusted to be consistent with local conditions.

SWOT Analysis

Prior to writing the formal business plan, it is helpful to perform a strengths, weaknesses, opportunities, threats (SWOT) analysis. This is one way to summarize the information that has been gathered so far, and to identify any further information that is needed. SWOT is an acronym for *strengths, weaknesses, opportunities,* and *threats,* and is a structured method of analyzing data that allows evaluation of those four elements of a business venture. It involves specifying the objective of the business venture, as outlined in the section on mission statements, and identifying the internal and external factors that are favorable and unfavorable to achieving that objective. It is important to include elements that are specific to the birth center's service area, but also to include elements that might be specific to the state where the birth center is located and national trends that might affect the business.

In addition to the usual challenges faced by any start-up, birth centers face some challenges that are unique to the industry. One example of a challenge for birth centers that can be included in a SWOT analysis is that there is no established market for selling a birth center business. In most cases to date, if the founder retires, moves away, or dies, the birth center closes and its assets are sold. Particularly in the case where the founder "does it all," other staff members are too often unwilling to be trained to take on the tasks the founder has done once she or he is no longer there. Many other challenges and opportunities that can be included in the SWOT analysis have already been described. When used as part of the planning process, SWOTs are used as inputs to the creative generation of possible strategies, by asking and answering the following four questions numerous times:

- How can we use each strength?
- How can we stop each weakness?
- How can we maximize each opportunity?
- How can we defend against each threat?

Constructing a Business Plan

Once all the pertinent data have been gathered and analyzed, the SBA has a simple tool for constructing a business plan, and for printing it out in a finished form (SBA, n.d.-b). They suggest that the plan consist of:

- **Cover page:** Contains the name of the company, its logo, its principals, and its contact information
- **Executive summary:** Written after the rest of the business plan is finished, it is a one-page summary of the company, its services, its customers, and its future
- **Company description:** Includes brief bios of key employees, a mission statement, a detailed description of the services provided, and reasons why the business will be successful
- **Market research:** This is essentially what was included in the community assessment plus the SWOT analysis
- **Services of the birth center:** How the services of the birth center meet the stated needs of its customers, and the competitive advantages of the birth center compared with other options for pregnant women
- **Marketing plan:** Description of how to attract sufficient clients to support start-up, growth, and sustainability, including communication and advertising plans
- **Financial projections:** Profit and loss, cash flow, balance sheet, and breakeven projections for the first 5 years. In the early years, the projections will be monthly or quarterly; then the projections can be annual.

When seeking a loan or equity financing, include an appendix containing the credit history of key employees, résumés of key employees, and letters of reference. This is also a good place to include any relevant information or documents that support the request for funds and demonstrate good planning. The SBA site includes a tool that can be used to help locate nearby SBA offices and resources when additional help with constructing the business plan is needed.

Sustainability

In most cases, the birth center will be a small business, and the failure rate for such start-ups is estimated at more than 40% in the first 4 years. The reasons include lack of knowledge of pricing, living too high for the net income of the business, lack of planning, lack of knowledge of financing and record-keeping, nonpayment of taxes, expansion that is too rapid, and a wasted advertising budget. Common management mistakes include taking advice from family and friends, being in the wrong place at the wrong time, not understanding the time requirements for a start-up, family pressures on time and money commitments, lack of market awareness, lack of financial responsibility and awareness, and lack of a clear focus (Statistic Brain, n.d.).

In 2016, the AABC sent a survey to every known birth center in the country. The survey included questions about the financial health of the birth centers, which were answered by 124 birth centers. Although the majority of the centers were meeting or exceeding their financial goals, 16% rated their finances as "Poor, we are struggling to keep our doors open due to financial concerns" or "Below average, we are not meeting our financial goals." The main problems the struggling centers mentioned were billing issues, collection issues, poor reimbursement from Medicaid, the costs of installing an electronic health record, insufficient volume of clients, overspending, and decreases in commercial insurance payments (AABC, 2016).

Birth centers are sustainable when they are managed well, are located in an area with sufficient demand for their services, and are able to negotiate adequate reimbursement to cover their costs. AABC, CABC, and the SBA all have resources available to help birth centers that are struggling with sustainability issues.

Soul Searching

Most birth centers to date have been founded either by an entrepreneur (or small group of entrepreneurs) or by large institutions, such as hospitals or investment funds. Each group has particular challenges that need to be thought through in advance.

In the case of entrepreneurs, consider:

➤ **Are you willing and able to bear substantial financial risk?**

Close to half of all start-ups close within 5 years, so it is important to be realistic about the financial risks. Be sure that if you lose your invested capital, it won't destroy your personal finances. Some people thrive on the financial risk; others are devastated by the thought of losing even a small sum. Don't assume you'll be able to lower your risk substantially by finding investors. Regardless of the economy, less than 10% of start-up financing comes from venture capitalists, angel investors, and loans from friends and family combined. Banks want to see that the start-up founder has a proven track record and they generally require personal financial collateral.

- **Are you willing to sacrifice your lifestyle, potentially for many years?**

In order to get a birth center off the ground, you may have to live on reduced income for several years. A successful start-up often entails putting in work weeks of 60 hours or more and any income is put back into the business, rather than paying yourself a livable salary. Having reduced or little income requires serious consideration during the planning process.

- **Is your significant other on board?**

Running a business may also affect your loved ones. Launching a business with the prospect of more working hours and reduced income can be stressful. Talking at length with your partner and family about the changes in schedules, daily chores, and time commitment and how it will affect your lives can help avoid disappointments down the road.

- **Do you like all the aspects of running a business?**

In the early stages of business, founders are often expected to handle everything from hiring employees and writing marketing materials to cleaning. Some new entrepreneurs become annoyed that they spend so much of their time doing administrative tasks rather than the aspects of the job that bring them more joy. If you don't have all the traits you need to run the business, find a business partner who has enthusiasm for the birth center concept and who complements your skill set. If you're not that exuberant about how you'll be spending your time—or the birth center concept itself—then opening a birth center will be a huge challenge.

- **How well have you sold and executed your ideas in the past?**

Your ability to execute your ideas is a big factor in determining success. Entrepreneurs possess a special mix of drive, persuasiveness, leadership skills, and keen intuition. As an entrepreneur, you sell your ideas to lenders, sell your mission and vision to your employees, and ultimately sell yourself as the service provider of the birth center. Strong communication and interpersonal skills are needed in order to get people to believe in your vision as much as you do.

➤ **Are you a self-starter?**

Entrepreneurs face lots of discouragement. Willpower and an unwavering optimism are needed to overcome the constant obstacles of opening a birth center. People who have practiced in large organizations where they primarily operate in "re-act" mode often find it a challenge to switch to "pro-act" mode, where no one directs them to take the next step.

In the case of a hospital planning to add a birth center, consider:

➤ **Does the birth center have the support of administration?**

Have funds and space been allocated? Has a project manager been identified and given sufficient time, support staff, and funds to make the project successful? Are all members of senior management in agreement and supportive?

➤ **Does the birth center have the support of staff obstetricians and midwives?**

Although it is common that the chief of obstetrics is on board, other obstetricians and midwives may not be. There may be differences of opinion among clinicians. It is important that the obstetricians who will serve as consultants to the birth center be especially supportive, but without the support of the full OB department, problems are likely to develop in the future. It may be helpful for a midwife to present a Grand Rounds on the Midwifery Pearls or to make copies of the Birth Center Study II available (Stapleton et al., 2013).

➤ **Does the birth center have the support of staff pediatricians and neonatologists?**

In many cases, it is more difficult to earn the support of the pediatric staff than the obstetric staff. Birth centers are perceived as possibly beneficial for the mother, but less so for the baby. It can help to invite them to emergency drills when the subject is neonatal resuscitation. This group may be especially resistant to water birth, as they are less familiar with the published evidence of its safety (American College of Nurse-Midwives, 2017).

- **Are you willing to continue to support the birth center even when a bad outcome occurs?**

Even with the best of care, eventually there may be a lawsuit, whether it was the fault of the birth center or not. Birth centers are often held to a much higher standard than hospitals for the care of low-risk women on the one hand; on the other hand, hospitals are excused for poor outcomes, such as complications of cesareans, when cesareans are more likely to occur if low-risk women choose hospital care for their delivery.

- **Are all the parties prepared for the birth center to be able to operate as a *birth center, rather than as a low-risk extension of a labor and delivery unit?***

A birth center is not just a "mini-hospital." It has a program of care that ideally requires a separate staff that fully subscribes to the midwifery model of care. It has a childbirth education class separate from the usual hospital classes, designed to prepare women for the birth center experience. It has its own management team that is responsible for its budget, for developing evidence-based P&P that promote safety, and for quality improvement. It ideally meets criteria for accreditation by CABC.

CONCLUSION

America is fortunate to have a "small but mighty" complement of birth centers, whose numbers have increased substantially in recent years. By far, the majority are doing well financially and providing a much-needed service to their communities. Increasingly, birth centers and midwives are recognized as an important part of the maternity care delivery system.

To date, most birth centers have been founded by entrepreneurial midwives who have each reinvented the wheels described in this chapter. Birth center owners are learning from each other, and becoming more skilled at the business aspects of sustaining a birth center. Still, most pregnant women in the United States do not have access to a birth center in their neighborhood. With only 0.5% of women using birth centers for giving birth at this time, and increasing recognition that some 70% of women are eligible for birth center care, the birth center industry is poised to expand dramatically. Disruptive innovators, who will use the information found in this volume and the available support provided by AABC, will place a birth center on every main street, so that all women and families have access to high-value, high-satisfaction care for the beginning of life.

Individuals or institutions considering launching a birth center are encouraged to attend the "How to Start a Birth Center" workshop, offered by the AABC several times each year (https://aabc.site-ym.com/?page=hsbc_workshops). The workshop is a full 2-day conference that addresses the many issues that should be considered when exploring the development of a birth center, including birth center operations, financial management, budgeting, community assessment, marketing, and next steps. It includes a tour of an accredited birth center and gives participants a chance to learn first-hand from birth center personnel. Participants receive a comprehensive digital manual with tools and resources to help throughout the development process. There are opportunities to engage with the experienced experts who present the workshop. This chapter is meant to provide a basic framework for understanding the scope of business concepts required in starting a birth center. Additional education about these concepts is recommended to avoid the pitfalls experienced by those who have come before you.

REFERENCES

American Association of Birth Centers. (2016). Birth center profile survey. (Unpublished data.)

American College of Nurse-Midwives. (n.d.). Ten questions midwives should ask when looking for professional liability insurance. Retrieved from http://www.midwife.org/Ten-Questions-Midwives-Should-Ask-Professional-Liability-Insurance

American College of Nurse-Midwives. (2017). A model practice template for hydrotherapy in labor and birth. *Journal of Midwifery & Women's Health, 62,* 120–126. doi:10.1111/jmwh.12587

American Institute of Architects Academy of Architecture for Health & Facility Guidelines Institute. (2011). Guidelines for design and construction of hospital and healthcare facilities. Retrieved from https://www.fgiguidelines.org/wp-content/uploads/2015/08/2001guidelines.pdf

B Corp. (n.d.). What are B Corps? Retrieved from http://www.bcorporation.net/what-are-b-corps

Boushey, H., & Glynn, S. J. (2012). There are significant business costs to replacing employees. Retrieved from https://cdn.americanprogress.org/wp-content/uploads/2012/11/16084443/CostofTurnover0815.pdf

CABC indicators for compliance with standards for birth centers. (2016, June 15). Retrieved from https://www.birthcenteraccreditation.org/go/get-cabc-indicators

Commission for the Accreditation of Birth Centers. (2015). Indicators of compliance with the standards for birth centers. Retrieved from https://www.birthcenteraccreditation.org/go/get-cabc-indicators

Chen, J. (2013). Should your business be nonprofit or for-profit? *Harvard Business Review.* Retrieved from https://hbr.org/2013/02/should-your-business-be-nonpro/#

Martin, J. A., Hamilton, B. E., Osterman, M. J. K., Curtin, S. C., & Mathews, T. J. (2015). Births: Final data for 2013. *National Vital Statistics Reports, 64*(1). Retrieved from http://www.cdc.gov/nchs/data/nvsr/nvsr64/nvsr64_01.pdf

McMurry University. (n.d.). Components of an effective mission statement. Retrieved from http://www.mcm.edu/~lapointp/missionstatementcomponents.html

National Conference of State Legislatures. (2016). CON-certificate of need state laws. Retrieved from http://www.ncsl.org/research/health/con-certificate-of-need-state-laws.aspx

National Fire Protection Association. (2015). NFPA 101 life safety codes. Retrieved from http://www.nfpa.org/codes-and-standards/all-codes-and-standards/list-of-codes-and-standards?mode=code&code=101&order_src=C900&gclid=CLHm2OfjwNICFUe5wAodSNMESQ

Stapleton, S. R., Osborne, C., & Illuzzi, J. (2013). Outcomes of care in birth centers: Demonstration of a durable model. *Journal of Midwifery and Women's Health, 58*(1), 3–14. doi:10.1111/jmwh.12003

Statistic Brain. (n.d.). Startup business failure rate by industry. Retrieved from http://www.statisticbrain.com/startup-failure-by-industry

U.S. Small Business Administration. (n.d.-a). Starting and managing. Retrieved from https://www.sba.gov/starting-business/choose-your-business-structure

U.S. Small Business Administration. (n.d.-b). Build your business plan. Retrieved from https://www.sba.gov/tools/business-plan/1

APPENDIX

Birth Centers in the Global Arena

KATHRYN M. SCHRAG

NOMENCLATURE AND DEFINITIONS

Any discussion of birth centers in the global context must begin with nomenclature. As noted in Chapter 1, use of the term *birth center* in the United States evolved over time. Although still often confused with some medical-model hospital labor and delivery units that adopted this name, the term is commonly accepted in the United States to refer to freestanding birth centers. Internationally, there is no standard term for these centers. A cursory review of English language medical and consumer materials reveals myriad terms: *alongside midwifery-led units, basic OB units, birth home, birth and family center, birth cottage, birthing house, community birthing home, home-from-home units, midwife-led unit, maternity home, maternity out-patient center, maternity waiting homes, midwifery-led birthing suites, normal birth unit, primary maternity units, stand-alone units,* and *out-of-hospital maternity unit.*

The European Midwives Association (EMA, 2016) has adopted the term *midwifery unit* to refer to "birth centers." The United Kingdom has created national standardized names and definitions for facility births. Its National Perinatal Epidemiology Unit (NPEU) designates three categories (Birthplace in England Collaborative Group, 2012):

1. Obstetric units (hospital labor and delivery units with either midwife or physician attendant)
2. Midwifery-led alongside units (within the hospital facility with midwife attendant)
3. Midwifery-led freestanding units (separate from the hospital with midwife attendant, called "freestanding birth centers" in the United States)

The challenge in reaching consensus on the label is not surprising: What is being referred to is more than a place for birth. A birth center is a place for the practice of midwifery and its philosophy of care, but midwifery is often misunderstood. A birth center is more than a facility for giving birth; it often includes prenatal care and education, as well as family services. Additionally, the model of care that is a birth center can be freestanding conceptually but within a hospital facility. As in the use of all languages, the terminology used will vary depending on the audience being addressed. Bridget Lynch, recent past president of the International Confederation of Midwives (ICM), suggested using the term *midwifery-led out-of-hospital facility-based unit* on a global policy level (Bridget Lynch, personal communication, June 13, 2016).

HISTORY OF INTERNATIONAL APPLICATION OF THE MODEL

An unanticipated benefit of the origination of the birth center concept in the United States, a country without a national health care system, was the independent creation of standards, policies, and systems of care for birth centers. The model that was rapidly developed by the birth center movement in the United States during the dynamic 1970s and 1980s provided guidance for other countries to adapt this approach as part of or parallel to their national health care systems.

In 1990, after consultation with the American Association of Birth Centers (AABC), the European Birth Center Network was formed under the leadership of midwife Hannah Beittel. AABC staff met with the midwives in Germany, and the AABC Standards were translated into German (Kate E. Bauer, personal communication, March 16, 2016). Per Mervi Jokinen, president of the EMA (personal communication, June 14, 2016), the original organization is no longer functioning.

Judith Rooks, in her 1997 classic textbook on midwifery, *Midwifery and Childbirth in America* (pp. 408–412), provided a snapshot of what was happening in global midwifery and birth centers during the early 1990s.

- Austria: 2% home births; 35 freestanding birth centers, some led by midwives and others by physicians
- Denmark: 2% home birth with a rising rate; four in-hospital birth centers in Copenhagen
- Germany: very few home births; 15 freestanding birth centers

- Sweden: very few home births; one hospital-based birth center
- Denmark: home birth 31%; "short stay normal-birth unit" in hospitals (no data provided on percentage of birth-unit births)

International randomized clinical trial (RCT) research on midwifery-led birth centers began emerging in the medical literature with the 1986 publication of a study from England (Chapman, Jones, Spring, De Swiet, & Chamberlain, 1986), followed by a trial from Scotland in 1994 (Hundley et al., 1994) and another from Sweden in 1997 (Waldenström, Nilsson, & Winbladh, 1997). The Cochrane Pregnancy and Childbirth Group (Hodnett, Downe, & Walsh, 2012) published a review of 10 RCTs on institutional birth settings from 1984 to 2011, including trials from Australia, Canada, Denmark, England, Ireland, Norway, Scotland, and Sweden. These trials included 11,795 women and all were in birth centers within a hospital. Primary results demonstrated fewer medical interventions, positive views of care from patients, and no apparent adverse outcomes.

International review articles on birth centers have been published by Walsh and Downe (2004) and Alliman and Phillippi (2016). Global research is challenging due to inconsistencies in definitions of the model of care and transfers, clinical eligibility guidelines, and the wide variation of how birth centers are integrated into a country's health care system. Not surprisingly, there have been no RCTs that have included a freestanding birth center outside the hospital setting.

LEADERSHIP FROM THE UNITED KINGDOM

For decades, the United Kingdom has provided leadership in guiding policy and examining the influence of the type of provider and place of birth to optimize choices and outcomes for healthy childbearing women. The number of birth centers in the United Kingdom has grown to 215 (116 alongside units and 99 freestanding units) compared with 198 obstetric units (Midwifery Unit Network [MUN], 2016a).

The medicalization of childbirth in the 1960s led to discontent among many UK midwives and consumers, resulting in the establishment of a few independently run birth centers, and culminating in a powerful national advocacy organization, the National Childbirth Trust, which is still active after nearly 60 years. Efforts by the trust resulted in formation of an Expert Maternity Group and the 1993 publication of *Changing Childbirth* (Expert Maternity Group, 1993). The report recommended that maternity services be community based, that every woman should have a midwife and the choice of birth site, and that a process for emergency transfers to the hospital should be in place. A year later, the recommendations were adopted as policy by Parliament, and endorsed by the Royal College of Midwives and the Royal College of Obstetricians (Rooks, 1997, pp. 416–418).

The National Health Service (NHS) published a consumer report, *Maternity Matters* (NHS, 2005), addressing the government's commitment to consumer choice, with a national goal that by the end of 2009 women would be able to choose among three different options: (a) a home birth, (b) birth in a local facility including a hospital under the care of a midwife, and (c) birth in a hospital with a team including midwives, anesthetists, and consultant obstetricians.

The Royal College of Midwives published *Birth Center Standards in England: A Standards Document* (Ackerman et al., 2009), and the following year published a second document, *Birth Centre Resource: A Practical Guide* (Walker & Jokinen, 2010) to provide operational assistance and guidance on the process of developing a birth center.

The Birthplace in England Collaborative, a project of the NPEU, undertook a large research project to evaluate the effect of birth settings on perinatal outcomes and cost. It studied 54,538 "low-risk" women and measured outcomes based on four birth sites: home, freestanding midwifery units (birth centers), alongside midwifery units (hospital-based birth centers), and obstetrical units. The results support a choice of birth setting (Birthplace in England Collaborative Group, 2011). Ongoing data analysis and publications can be found on the Birthplace website (www.npeu.ox.ac.uk/birthplace).

The National Institute for Health and Care Excellence (NICE, 2014) updated its maternity guideline "Intrapartum Care for Healthy Women and Babies" in 2014. The guidelines state that women at low risk of complications should be advised of the safety of midwifery-led units (either freestanding or hospital based); in fact, these units are "particularly suitable" because of lower rates of intervention and improved outcomes when compared to the hospital. This publication received wide coverage in the United States, including an editorial from *The New York Times* (2014), titled "Are Midwives Safer Than Doctors?"

INTERNATIONAL BIRTH CENTERS TODAY

No central repository of listings of international birth centers has been developed, although the newly organized GoodBirth Network (www

.goodbirth.net) is working to address this need. The GoodBirth Network proposes the following international categorization of the birth center model (S. Shaffer, MD, personal communication, July 19, 2016):

- High- and moderate-income countries where birth centers developed outside the country's health care system. These centers were often a consumer- and midwife-driven alternative to the physician-hospital model. Some examples in addition to the United States include Germany, France, and Italy.
- High- and moderate-income countries where birth centers were incorporated as integral to the national health care system. Examples include the United Kingdom, Canada, New Zealand, South Africa, Japan, and the Philippines.
- Low-income countries where the model had arisen to fill a need in the lack of available health services, and the gap between unsupervised home birth and hospital births. These centers are often funded by nongovernmental organizations (NGOs). Countries that are examples include Haiti and Uganda.
- Countries where birth centers have arisen in response to acute community crises. Such centers have opened in response to the tsunami in Indonesia, in response to Ebola in Sierra Leone, and to address internally displaced persons in Pakistan.
- Countries where midwives and/or birth centers are prohibited. Examples include Hungary and Cuba. The story of a Hungarian midwife, Agnes Gereb, is a well-known example. The successful *Ternovszky v. Hungary* legal case in the European Court of Human Rights in The Hague affirmed that childbirth is a human rights issue in which women are the ultimate decision makers (Harmon, 2017).

Birth Centers in Moderate- and High-Income Countries

During the second half of the 20th century, hospital labor units became the birth setting for most childbearing women in high- and moderate-income countries. The associated medicalization of childbirth led to the questioning of the benefits and risks to the healthy pregnant woman. The critique of this "technological" approach initially resulted in "bedroom-like" obstetrical units in most hospitals in developed countries. Parallel to changes within the hospitals, health care systems in some countries began offering alternative institutional birth settings, as compared with the conventional hospital labor ward. A common feature of the alternative units was that they are midwife-led versus consultant (physician)-led (Hodnett et al., 2012). The publication of standards, policies, and research has come from many high-income countries.

Birth Centers in Low-Income and Emerging Countries

In 2000, the world's leaders gathered to commit their nations to partnering to address the many dimensions of extreme poverty. The result of their summit was the adoption of the Millennium Development Goals (MDGs; Millennium Project, 2010) with a target to be met by 2015. The MDG-4 goal was to reduce under-five child mortality, and MDG-5 was to reduce maternal mortality. The Partnership for Maternal, Newborn and Child Health (PMNCH), formed in 2005 to address MDG-4 and -5, reports that in spite of progress, newborn mortality remains high and 800 women die daily during pregnancy or during and after birth, largely from preventable causes (PMNCH, 2015). The most recent set of goals is part of the new sustainable development agenda adopted by the countries of the United Nations in 2015. Number 3 of the 17 Sustainable Development Goals is to ensure healthy lives and promote well-being for all at all ages. Infant and maternal mortality, prenatal care, and contraception are addressed in this goal (United Nations, 2016).

Solutions to the problems are complex, but there is general consensus that resources need to be spent to increase skilled birth attendants (professional midwives, physicians, or nurses) rather than supporting traditional birth attendants, and to strengthen health care systems and encourage facility-based birth (PMNCH, 2015; World Health Organization [WHO], 2008). Worldwide, 32% of women are not attended by a skilled birth attendant, and 37% give birth at home. In the least developed countries, 54% of women are giving birth without a skilled birth attendant and 57% are not in a health care facility (UNICEF, 2014).

The Maternal Survival Series: Executive Summary, published in 2006 by the *Lancet*, presents evidence for strategies to reduce the persistent unacceptably high rates of maternal death and injury. Their recommendations are summarized in a single statement: "making sure women throughout the world can give birth in a health facility, in the presence of a midwife, is the best strategy for substantially reducing maternal mortality worldwide, according to a landmark series of papers" (Maternal Survival Series Steering Group, 2006).

The second paper in the series (Campbell & Graham, 2006) calls for prioritizing the intrapartum period, and "that the best intrapartum-care strategy is likely to be one in which women routinely choose to deliver in a 'health center,' with midwives as the main providers, but with other attendants working with them in a team." The recommendation is that the centers would aim to "maintain the normality of the birthing process, with an emphasis on nonintervention and timely watchfulness, and on preservation of the psychosocial benefits of a positive birthing experience." The authors go on to contrast the health center intrapartum-care strategy with the physician/hospital strategy and conclude that although "few data are available for the relative merits of health-centre package versus hospital packages for normal birth, that the risks of unnecessary intervention for normal births are likely to be most extreme in hospitals, as are the costs of care" (Campbell & Graham, 2006).

The 2009 Monitoring Emergency Obstetric Care: A Handbook (EmONC; WHO, 2009) focuses on the critical role of emergency care in reducing maternal and child mortality, and recommends that maternity care be provided by skilled birth attendants, and in a facility categorized either as "health centers for basic care" (basic emergency obstetric and newborn care: BEmONC) or "hospitals for comprehensive care" (comprehensive emergency obstetric and newborn care: CEmONC), with criteria identified for both levels of care (United Nations Population Fund [UNFPA], 2014; WHO, 2009). Jhpiego at Johns Hopkins University has published guidelines for in-service training in the levels of care (Dao, 2012). Although a birth center meets the criteria to be called a BEmONC, and is often included in the international lexicon of BEmONC, the midwifery model of birth centers embraces a philosophy that is omitted in the official definitions: the woman, her desires, and her community are at the heart of the care the center provides (Jennifer Stevens, CNM, personal communication, July 13, 2016).

The *Lancet*'s Midwifery Series (Renfrew et al., 2014) of four papers on international midwifery called for scaling up midwifery globally to reduce the persistent global crisis of infant and maternal mortality. The program proposals are team based, with midwives as the essential link in the continuum of care, and bringing women into the health care system at the most effective and efficient time, and at the appropriate level of services. The authors state that the application of the evidence presented in the series could avert more than 80% of maternal and newborn deaths. "Midwifery therefore has a pivotal, yet widely neglected, part to play in accelerating progress to end preventable mortality of women and children" (Horton & Astudillo, 2014).

In the first paper in the *Lancet* series (Renfrew et al., 2014), more than 50 outcomes were identified that could be improved by care within the scope of midwifery. The authors' recommendations include a system of care that strengthens women's capabilities, is individualized and respectful, and includes effective interdisciplinary teamwork and facility integration. Their category on organization of care includes midwife-led care, community-based programs, and alternative institutional settings for birth.

In spite of consensus within the international public health community that giving birth in a high-quality obstetric facility reduces maternal and perinatal mortality, the move from a traditional birth attendant/home birth model has been disappointingly low. A recent review of studies from 17 moderate- and low-income countries on facilitators and barriers to facility-based delivery found the perception by women and their families is that the emphasis on facility birth has led to childbirth becoming medicalized and dehumanized (Bohren et al., 2014).

ORGANIZATIONAL STATEMENTS AND POLICIES

Where births should take place and who should attend them has been debated for hundreds of years not only in the United States, but also around the world, and continues today. There is a disappointing lack of international professional organization statements, data collection, and guidance on the midwifery-led model of birth center care.

- The WHO consistently endorses midwifery, but has yet to address midwife-led units. In an opinion piece, Stanton (2008) states that the WHO "sidesteps the issue of where births should take place."
- The 2014 State of the World's Midwifery (SoWMy, 2014) is the latest triennial report published by the ICM, WHO, and the UNFPA. It focuses primarily on workforce issues (birth attendant), not the site of births, although it addresses EmONC. SoWMy's 2030 policy and planning guidance chapter (pp. 37–40) promotes models of practice and systems of care that include "first-level and next-level midwifery care." First-level care is described as midwifery services as close as possible to women's homes and communities, and in midwife-led units for births. The report cites the strong evidence from upper-middle and high-income countries that midwife-led care provides significant benefits with no identified adverse risks, and advocates for the model to be explored globally.

- International Confederation of Midwives (ICM) is the trade organization representing professional midwifery associations in all countries, with a current total of 130 midwifery organizations representing 112 countries across every continent (ICM, 2016). Its core document Bill of Rights for Women and Midwives (ICM, 2014a) identifies basic human rights for women and midwives across the globe, including a woman's "right to choose the place where she gives birth." The ICM has position statements on Appropriate Maternity Services for Normal Pregnancy, Childbirth and the Postnatal Period (ICM, 2011a), a statement on Keeping Birth Normal (ICM, 2014b), and one on Home Birth (ICM, 2011b). It has not yet published a position statement on birth centers.
- European Midwives Association (EMA) is a regional organization that supports the choice of birth setting including home and birth center as safe and beneficial options in its 2011 position paper on intrapartum care (EMA, 2011). According to Mervi Jokinen, president (personal communication, June 14, 2016), it has not yet published a position statement on birth centers, although it is a "standard item on our agenda."
- The newly formed Midwifery Unit Network (MUN) is a collaboration between the EMA and Royal College of Midwives, whose purpose is to support and promote the development and growth of birth centers, which are managed and staffed by midwives. It has published policy briefings on Philosophy of Care and Policy on Midwifery Unit Care and Evidence of Clinical Effectiveness (MUN, 2016b).
- In the United States, the American Association of Birth Centers (AABC) is the trade organization dedicated to the birth center model of care. A consensus statement on physiologic childbirth by the American College of Nurse-Midwives (ACNM), the Midwives Alliance of North America (MANA), and the National Association of Certified Professional Midwives (NACPM) advocates for processes, providers, and settings supportive of normal physiologic birth (ACNM, MANA, & NACPM, 2013). ACNM recently (ACNM, 2016) updated its Clinical Bulletin on home birth, but does not have a published statement regarding birth centers.
- GoodBirth Network is a new U.S.-based organization with the goal to support and develop a global "birth home" community. Its first network is among birth centers in Haiti, with plans to develop similar networks in other countries.

TABLE A.1
Lifetime Risk of Maternal Death in Selected Countries

Country Name	Estimated Risk
Uganda	1 in 44
Haiti	1 in 80
Indonesia	1 in 220
South Africa	1 in 300
Philippines	1 in 250
United States	1 in 1,800
Canada	1 in 5,200
New Zealand	1 In 6,600
United Kingdom	1 in 6,900
Japan	1 in 12,100

Source: UNICEF (2015).

BIRTH CENTERS IN SELECT COUNTRIES AND REGIONS

Africa

South Africa

The introduction of birth centers, called "midwife obstetric units," began in South Africa in the late 1970s within the public health sector in an attempt to move low-risk maternity care closer to the people who needed care. The public health system serves 85% of the country's population. In 2009, seven primary-level midwife units managed more than 17,000 women with 9,000 births in the midwife-led units. In spite of challenges due to HIV and AIDS, the system produced enviable clinical outcomes (UNPFA, 2011). Although not yet a national system-wide model, today between 15 and 20 midwife-led freestanding birth centers are funded from the provincial health budget. Additional (but few) private birth centers tend to have obstetrician involvement (Sheila Clow, professor in midwifery, personal communication, July 26, 2016).

Uganda

The Uganda Private Midwives Association (UPMA), an association of more than 700 midwives, began organizing in 1948. Professional midwives in Uganda are self-employed, but regulated through the Ministry of Health. During the political unrest of the 1960s, they were given permission to build or rent maternity houses to reduce the danger of traveling at night for births. These maternity units (birth centers) continue to operate providing prenatal care, births, family planning, HIV prevention and services, and general health services for women and children at the community level. Most of the birth centers are independently operated by midwives within their home or family compound. UPMA is currently working to educate more skilled birth attendants, and to increase the number of birth centers throughout the country (Mary Gorret Kigongo Musoke, president UPMA, personal communication, July 18, 2016). Shanti Uganda is an example of an NGO that began in 2008 to unite traditional birth practices with modern best practices to address poverty and AIDS in Uganda. It employs six registered Ugandan midwives who attend 15 to 20 births per month in their birth house, the only health facility in the village (Shanti Uganda, 2016).

Canada

Bridget Lynch, past president of the ICM and professor of midwifery in Ontario, reports on the growth of birth centers in Canada (Bridget Lynch, personal communication, July 12, 2016). There are currently 18 birth centers in four provinces in Canada, with British Columbia poised to become the fifth. All of these centers are midwife led with no physicians on staff, are publicly funded, and are fully integrated into the health care system with efficient and respectful transfers. In Quebec, the province with the largest number of birth centers, 80% of the births attended by midwives occur in these centers. In Ontario, there is a birth center on a First Nations reserve, and in Quebec there are three centers serving remote Inuit communities in the Arctic. A national professional association of birth centers is being discussed.

Europe

Mervi Jokinen, president of the EMA (personal communication, June 14, 2016), reports that there are few birth centers/birth houses in Europe, and many that exist are struggling to remain open due to health care governance issues, constant scrutiny, and economic sustainability. The EMA conducted an intrapartum survey of its members in 2010, in which it asked the question: "Which of the following choices are offered to women as a place to give birth?" Thirteen of 24 countries responded that birth center was an option; however, the question did not separate "alongside" (hospital based) from "freestanding" centers.

Haiti[1]

Haiti has the highest rate of maternal and newborn mortality of any country in the Western Hemisphere, and the risks for mothers and their newborns are greatest in rural areas. It is a useful country to spotlight because it illustrates the expression of the midwife philosophy of care in birth centers that have independently emerged to meet specific community needs.

The first birth center in Haiti, Maison de Naissance, was opened in 2004 by an NGO to determine if a midwife-led center could address maternal and newborn mortality in rural Haiti. Following its success (Shaffer, Fryzelka, Obenhaus, & Wickstrom, 2007), centers have recently been opened by other NGOs: Olive Tree Projects and Heartland Ministries. Another center, MamaBaby Haiti, was created in the aftermath of the massive 2010 earthquake. Midwives for Haiti, a training program for skilled birth attendants, has recently opened the Carrie Wortham Birth Center to provide services and educational opportunities. The UNFPA, in conjunction with Haiti's Ministry of Health, is planning to include midwifery birth services at some community health clinics, called Smile Clinics. In addition to labor and birth services in these various birth centers in Haiti, some provide community gardens, a women's small business loan program, matron (traditional midwives) training, men's business training, women's literacy, and a children's summer camp.

Because birth centers remain a new concept in Haiti, there are challenges for future development, and the organizations have had to work individually to forge political pathways and to discover their place in Haiti's fragmented health care system. In 2016, all Haiti's birth centers met together for the first time and established a country-wide network, GoodBirth Network (Réseau de Bonne Naissance).

Japan

Japan has more than 37,000 midwives and 441 "midwifery birth centers," with 0.8% of births occurring in the birth centers, and 0.2% home births. By

---

[1]This section is submitted by Stan Shaffer, MD, GoodBirth Network.

definition, a midwifery birth center is not in a hospital or a clinic, is midwifery led, and may not accommodate more than 10 women (Yaeko Kataoka, professor in midwifery, personal communication, July 21, 2016). According to a U.S. birth activist who toured Tokyo's dozens of "birth houses" in 2012, they are the "perfect union of modern and traditional" with family prenatal visits including a traditional meal, principles of Asian medicine throughout care, and a place supportive of physiologic birth (Lindberg, 2012).

New Zealand

New Zealand has a government-funded maternity service that provides care to all pregnant women with a single point of contact called a Lead Maternity Carer (LMC). Ninety-two percent of women have a midwife as their LMC. Women with a physician LMC also have a hospital-employed midwife involved in their care. The New Zealand College of Midwives is the professional association for midwives and their practice; there is not a trade organization specific to birth centers.

Healthy women are able to choose their site of birth, with all options supported by the government. Approximately 15% of women give birth outside the hospital: 10% in birth centers and 3% to 5% at home. All of the country's 56 birth centers (called "primary units") are freestanding and midwifery led. There are six tertiary-level maternity facilities and 18 secondary facilities in the towns and cities throughout New Zealand (Jacqui Anderson, midwifery advisor-quality, New Zealand College of Midwives, personal communication, July 19, 2016).

Philippines[2]

The Philippines provides an example of creative public and private partnerships to address high rates of maternal and infant mortality. In many low- to middle-income countries, much of the health care is influenced, and oftentimes provided, by the private sector, including NGOs and faith-based organizations. These organizations are often able to provide innovation and rapid actions, but being separate from the country's health care delivery system, they are usually not part of a long-term solution to problems.

The Philippine commitment to birth centers was built on government policy coupled with involvement with NGO organizations, such as

[2]This section is submitted by Jennifer Stevens, CNM, GoodBirth Network.

Mercy in Action (which runs free birth centers in the Philippines) and Progress Through Business/Called2Serve (which offers business classes to Filipinos on how to run a birth center). In 2010, the Aquino Health Agenda's "Achieving Universal Health Care for All Filipinos" was adopted. This national health care plan has a goal to entice women to give birth in health care facilities instead of home, and includes accredited nonhospital facilities: "health centers, lying-in clinics, birthing homes, and midwife-managed clinics" (PhilHealth, 2013). Additional support has been provided by the private sector franchise organization, Well-Family Midwife Clinic Partnerships Foundation, which, jointly with the Filipino government, receives U.S. Agency for International Development (USAID) funding to assist in the development and management of birth centers. UNICEF also contributes to the effort by providing standardized clinical training for the midwives in BEmONC. These public sector birth centers are owned, run, and licensed by Filipino midwives.

This example of multiorganizational partnerships has resulted in the rapid upscaling of birth centers, especially in rural areas. Data on the exact number of birth centers that are now operating is difficult to access. According to a private e-mail from Dr. Willibald Zeck of the UN Children's Fund, there are 1,639 birth centers in two of the three reported regions per the 2015 accomplishment report of the Department of Health's Safe Motherhood Program (see Table A.1).

CONCLUSION

Clearly, the birth center is emerging as the midwife's place of business focused on a woman-centered model of care. The international conversation about place of birth has been polarized between home (the mother's place) and hospital (the doctor's place) for birth. Within high-income countries, the controversy about home birth led to strong organizational statements about the importance of the option of home birth within a functional health system, but silence regarding the now well-established option of "birth center/midwife-led-unit." The recommendation for birth in low-income countries to be facility based has not moved beyond the distinction between the medical-model hospital and the medical-model health center. It is time that the international organizations issue position statements and begin the work of standardized nomenclature and definition, issues of birth center eligibility, and reliable data collection and research to further explore the midwifery-led unit model of care. The concept is a high-quality, cost-effective part of the solution to global maternity problems:

the overuse of medical interventions in developed countries, and the underuse of midwifery care to address maternal and newborn mortality in low-income countries.

REFERENCES

Ackerman, B., Cooke, P., Hutcherson, A., Jokinen, M., Shallow, H., & Walker, J. (2009). *Birth center standards in England: A standards document.* Royal College of Midwives. Retrieved from https://www.rcm.org.uk/clinical-practice-and-guidelines

Alliman, J., & Phillippi, J. (2016). Maternal outcomes in birth centers: An integrative review of the literature. *Journal of Midwifery and Women's Health, 61*(1), 21–51.

American College of Nurse-Midwives. (2016). Midwifery provision of home birth services. *Journal of Midwifery and Women's Health, 61*(1), 127–133.

American College of Nurse-Midwives, Midwives Alliance North America, & National Association of Certified Professional Midwives. (2013). Supporting healthy and normal physiologic childbirth: A consensus statement by ACNM, MANA, and NACPM. *Journal of Perinatal Education, 22*(1), 14–18.

Birthplace in England Collaborative Group. (2011). Perinatal and maternal outcomes by planned place of birth for healthy women with low risk pregnancies: The Birthplace in England national prospective cohort study. *British Medical Journal, 343.* Retrieved from http://www.bmj.com/content/343/bmj.d7400

Birthplace in England Collaborative Group. (2012). Birthplace terms and definitions: Consensus process. Retrieved from http://www.nets.nihr.ac.uk/__data/assets/pdf_file/0004/84946/FR2-08-1604-140.pdf

Bohren, M. A., Hunter, E. C., Munthe-Kaas, H. M., Souza, J. P., Vogel, J. P., & Gülmezoglu, A. M. (2014). Facilitators and barriers to facility-based delivery in low-and middle-income countries: A qualitative evidence synthesis. *Reproductive Health, 11*(1), 71. Retrieved from http://apps.who.int/rhl/pregnancy_childbirth/complications/preterm_birth/101401/en

Campbell, M., & Graham, W. (2006). Strategies for reducing maternal mortality: Getting on with what works. *Lancet, 368,* 1284–1299.

Chapman, M., Jones, M., Spring, J., De Swiet, M., & Chamberlain, G. (1986). The use of a birthroom: A randomized controlled clinical trial comparing delivery with that in the labour ward. *British Journal of Obstetrics and Gynaecology, 93,* 182–187.

Dao, B. (2012). Guidelines for in-service training in basic and comprehensive emergency obstetric and newborn care. Retrieved from http://reprolineplus.org/system/files/resources/Guidelines_for_Basic_and_Comprehensive_InService_Final.pdf

European Midwives Association. (2011). Statement of the European Midwives Association on intrapartum care. Retrieved from http://www.europeanmidwives.com/upload/filemanager/content-galleries/position-papers/statement_of_the_european_mid wives_association_on_intrapartum_caredraft_1.pdf

Expert Maternity Group. (1993). Changing childbirth: The report of the Expert Maternity Group (part 1). London, UK: HMSO.

Harmon, T. (2017). Agnes Gereb and the case for human rights in childbirth. Retrieved from http://www.huffingtonpost.com/toni-harman/filming-agnes-gereb_b_1539595.html

Hodnett, E., Downe, S., & Walsh, D. (2012). Alternative versus conventional institutional settings for birth. Retrieved from http://www.cochrane.org/CD000012/PREG_alter native-versus-conventional-institutional-settings-for-birth

Horton, R., & Astudillo, O. (2014). The power of midwifery. *Lancet, 384*(9948), 1075–1076. Retrieved from http://www.thelancet.com/series/midwifery

Hundley, V., Cruickshank, F., Lang, G. D., Glazener, C., Milne, J., Turner, M., . . . Donaldson, C. (1994). Midwife-managed delivery unit: A randomized controlled comparison with consultant led care. *British Medical Journal, 309*, 1400–1404.

International Confederation of Midwives. (2011a). Appropriate maternity services for normal pregnancy, childbirth and the postnatal period. Retrieved from http://internationalmidwives.org/assets/uploads/documents/Position%20Statements%20-%20English/PS2011_001%20ENG%20Appropriate%20maternity%20services%20for%20normal%20pregnancy.pdf

International Confederation of Midwives. (2011b). Home birth. Retrieved from http://www.internationalmidwives.org/assets/uploads/documents/Position%20Statements%20-%20English/PS2011_010%20ENG%20Home%20Birth.pdf

International Confederation of Midwives. (2014a). Bill of rights for women and midwives. Retrieved from http://www.internationalmidwives.org/who-we-are/policy-and-practice/bill-of-rights-what-does-a-midwife-do

International Confederation of Midwives. (2014b). Keeping birth normal. Retrieved from http://internationalmidwives.org/assets/uploads/documents/Position%20Statements%20-%20English/Review

International Confederation of Midwives. (2017). Retrieved from http://www.internationalmidwives.org/who-we-are

International Confederation of Midwives. (2017). Governance. Retrieved from http://internationalmidwives.org/who-we-are/governance/

Lindberg, J. (2012, June 26). Neglected art of midwifery is national asset. *The Japan Times Community*. Retrieved from http://www.japantimes.co.jp/community/2012/06/26/voices/neglected-art-of-midwifery-is-national-asset/#.V5rUTJMrJTY

Maternal Survival Series Steering Group. (2006). *Lancet*. Retrieved from http://www.thelancet.com/series/maternal-survival

Midwifery Unit Network. (2016a). What is a midwifery unit? Retrieved from http://www.midwiferyunitnetwork.com/what-is-a-midwifery-unit

Midwifery Unit Network. (2016b). Policy research briefing 2: Evidence of clinical effectiveness. Retrieved from http://static1.squarespace.com/static/553ca2bee4b00f34b152cc73/t/55884483e4b0751e884ab081/1434993795804/Midwifery+Unit+Network+-+policy+research+briefing+2+Evidence+of+clincial+effectiveness+FINAL.pdf

Millennium Project. (2010). Millennium development goals. Retrieved from http://www.unmillenniumproject.org/goals

National Association of Certified Professional Midwives. (2012). Physiologic birth. Retrieved from http://mana.org/pdfs/Physiologic-Birth-Consensus-Statement.pdf

National Health Service. (2005). *Maternity matters: Choice, access and continuity of care in a safe service*. Retrieved from http://webarchive.nationalarchives.gov.uk/20130107105354/http:/www.dh.gov.uk/prod_consum_dh/groups/dh_digitalassets/@dh/@en/documents/digitalasset/dh_074199.pdf

National Institute for Health and Care Excellence. (2014). Intrapartum care for healthy women and babies. Retrieved from http://www.nice.org.uk/guidance/cg190/chapter/1-recommendations#place-of-birth

Newburn, M., Byrom, S., Rocca-Ihenacho, L., & Cardona, F. C. (2016). Policy research briefing 1: Philosophy of care and policy on midwifery unit care. Retrieved from https://static1.squarespace.com/static/553ca2bee4b00f34b152cc73/t/559ac055e4b0050728db9bd0/1436205141945/Midwifery+Unit+Network+-+policy+research+briefing+1+Philosophy+and+policy+FINAL.pdf

Partnership for Maternal, Newborn and Child Health. (2015). Retrieved from http://www.who.int/pmnch/knowledge/publications/pmnch_2015_report/en

PhilHealth. (2013). PhilHealth benefit for mother and child. Retrieved from http://www.philhealth.gov.ph/news/2013/mother_child.html

PMNCH: The Partnership for Maternal Newborn and Child Health. Retrieved from http://www.who.int/pmnch/about/en/

Renfrew, M. J., McFadden, A., Bastos, M. H, Campbell, J., Channon, A. A., Cheung, N. G., . . . Declercq, E. (2014). Midwifery and quality care: Findings from a new evidence-informed framework for maternal and newborn care, *The Lancet, 384*(9948), 1129–1145. http://www.thelancet.com/journals/lancet/article/PIIS0140-6736(14)60789-3/abstract

Rooks, J. (1997). *Midwifery and childbirth in America*. Philadelphia, PA: Temple University Press.

Shaffer, S., Fryzelka, D., Obenhaus, C., & Wickstrom, E. (2007). Improving maternal health-care access and neonatal survival through a birthing home model in Rural Haiti. *Social Medicine Journal, 2*, 177–185.

Shanti Uganda. (2016). Maternal health. Retrieved from http:/shantiuganda.org/programs/maternal-health

Stanton, C. (2008). Bulletin of the World Health Organization: Steps toward achieving skilled attendance at birth. *Birth, 86*(4). Retrieved from http://www.who.int/bulletin/volumes/86/4/08-052928/en

The Midwifery Series. (2014). *Lancet*. Retrieved from http://www.thelancet.com/series/midwifery

The New York Times. (2014, December 14). Are midwives safer than doctors? (editorial). Retrieved from http://www.nytimes.com/2014/12/15/opinion/are-midwives-safer-than-doctors.html

The State of the World's Midwifery. (2014). A universal pathway: A woman's right to health. Retrieved from http://www.unfpa.org/sowmy

UNICEF. (2015). State of the world's children 2015: Executive summary. Retrieved from http://www.unicef.org/publications/files/SOWC_2015_Summary_and_Tables.pdf

United Nations. (2016). Sustainable Development Goal 3: Ensure healthy lives and promote well-being for all at all ages. Retrieved from http://www.un.org/sustainabledevelopment/health/inabledevelopment/health

UNICEF. (2014). State of the world's children 2014 in numbers. Retrieved from http://www.unicef.org/publications/files/SOWC2014_In_Numbers_28_Jan.pdf

United Nations Population Fund. (2014). Setting standards for emergency obstetric and newborn care. Retrieved from http://www.unfpa.org/resources/setting-standards-emergency-obstetric-and-newborn-care

UNPFA. (2011). The state of the world's midwifery: *Delivering health, saving lives*. Retrieved from http://www.unfpa.org/sowmy/resources/docs/main_report/en_SOWMR_Full.pdf

Waldenström, U., Nilsson, C.-A., & Winbladh, B. (1997). The Stockholm birth center trial: Maternal and infant outcome. *British Journal of Obstetrics and Gynaecology, 104*, 410–418.

Walker, J., & Jokinen, M. (2010). *Birth centre resource: A practical guide.* London, United Kingdom: The Royal College of Midwives.

Walsh, D., & Downe, S. (2004). Outcomes of free-standing, midwife-led birth centers: A structured review. *Birth, 31*(3), 222–229.

World Health Organization. (2008). Fact sheet on skilled birth attendant. Retrieved from http://www.who.int/maternal_child_adolescent/events/2008/mdg5/factsheet_sba.pdf

World Health Organization. (2009). Monitoring emergency obstetric care: A handbook. Retrieved from http://apps.who.int/iris/bitstream/10665/44121/1/9789241547734_eng.pdf

Index